W9-AAY-524

Teen Health Series

Asthma
SOURCEBOOK

Third Edition

Health Reference Series

Third Edition

Asthma

SOURCEBOOK

Basic Consumer Health Information about Allergic, Exercise-Induced, Occupational, and Other Types of Asthma, Including Facts about Causes, Risk Factors, Symptoms, and Diagnostic Tests and Featuring Details about Treating Asthma with Medication and Other Therapies, Minimizing Indoor and Outdoor Asthma Triggers, Recognizing and Handling Asthma Attacks, Monitoring Symptoms and Developing an Action Plan, and Dealing with Co-Existing Conditions

Along with a Detailed Look at Childhood Asthma Concerns and Asthma in Older Adults, Pregnant Women, Athletes, and Other Special Populations, a Glossary of Related Terms, and a List of Resources for Additional Help and Information

Edited by
Sandra J. Judd

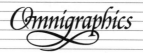

155 W. Congress, Suite 200, Detroit, MI 48226

Bibliographic Note
Because this page cannot legibly accommodate all the copyright notices, the Bibliographic Note portion of the Preface constitutes an extension of the copyright notice.

Edited by Sandra J. Judd

Health Reference Series

Karen Bellenir, *Managing Editor*
David A. Cooke, MD, FACP, *Medical Consultant*
Elizabeth Collins, *Research and Permissions Coordinator*
Cherry Edwards, *Permissions Assistant*
EdIndex, Services for Publishers, *Indexers*

* * *

Omnigraphics, Inc.
Matthew P. Barbour, *Senior Vice President*
Kevin M. Hayes, *Operations Manager*

* * *

Peter E. Ruffner, *Publisher*

Copyright © 2012 Omnigraphics, Inc.

ISBN 978-0-7808-1224-6

Library of Congress Cataloging-in-Publication Data

Asthma sourcebook : basic consumer health information about allergic, exercise-induced, occupational, and other types of asthma, including facts about causes, risk factors, symptoms, and diagnostic tests and featuring details about treating asthma with medication and other therapies ... / edited by Sandra J. Judd. -- 3rd ed.
   p. cm.
   Summary: "Provides basic consumer health information about diagnosis, treatment, and management of asthma, including facts about coping with the disease and minimizing triggers, along with a special section on asthma in children. Includes index, glossary of related terms, and other resources"-- Provided by publisher.
   Includes bibliographical references and index.
   ISBN 978-0-7808-1224-6 (hardcover : alk. paper) 1. Asthma--Popular works. I. Judd, Sandra J.
   RC591.A84 2011
   616.2'38--dc23
                                                        2011039923

Table of Contents

Visit www.healthreferenceseries.com to view *A Contents Guide to the Health Reference Series*, a listing of more than 16,000 topics and the volumes in which they are covered.

1507521

Part II: Recognizing and Diagnosing Asthma

Part III: Medications and Asthma Management

Part VI: Asthma in Other Special Populations

Part VII: Additional Help and Information

Preface

About This Book

Asthma is a chronic disorder characterized by inflammation of the air passages, resulting in the temporary narrowing of the passageways that transport air to the lungs. Although asthma can be managed with proper prevention and treatment, poorly controlled asthma can lead to reduced productivity, missed days at work or school, and acute medical emergencies, or even death.

The number of people with asthma in the United States is large and growing. According to the American Academy of Allergy Asthma and Immunology, approximately 23 million Americans, including almost 7 million children—an average of one out of every ten school-aged children—have asthma. From 2001 to 2009 the prevalence of asthma in the United States grew by more than 18 percent (an increase of more than 4 million cases), and that trend is expected to continue.

Despite asthma's prevalence, many Americans are unaware of the basic facts about the disorder and the progress being made in preventing and controlling it. New forms of treatment are being developed that make asthma easier to control, and with increased understanding of the causes and triggers of the disease, it is easier to prevent a flare-up.

Asthma Sourcebook, Third Edition provides basic consumer information about the different types of asthma and how they are diagnosed and treated. It includes information about the most common asthma triggers and suggests strategies for minimizing or avoiding them. It provides tips for managing asthma at school and in daily life and discusses common asthma concerns among older adults, pregnant women, and athletes. The book concludes with a glossary of related terms and a list of resources for further help and information.

How to Use This Book

This book is divided into parts and chapters. Parts focus on broad areas of interest. Chapters are devoted to single topics within a part.

Part I: Asthma Basics explains how the lungs work and describes what happens when asthma occurs. It discusses what is known about the causes of asthma and describes the most common asthma triggers. Finally, it provides statistics on the prevalence of asthma, both in the United States and worldwide.

Part II: Recognizing and Diagnosing Asthma describes what asthma attacks are and explains what to do when one occurs. It provides details about the different types of asthma and describes the tests and procedures most often used to diagnose the disorder.

Part III: Medications and Management discusses the different types of medications used to treat asthma. It explains the differences between reliever and controller medications and discusses when each should be used. It discusses the adverse effects related to the use of asthma medications and describes how the different medication delivery mechanisms should be used and maintained. It concludes with a description of the latest developments in asthma treatment.

Part IV: Living with Asthma provides tips on overcoming the challenges that are part of living with asthma. It describes asthma triggers and explains how to minimize or avoid them. It discusses the conditions that most commonly co-occur with asthma and offers suggestions for keeping asthma under control through lifestyle management. Finally, it outlines strategies for safely traveling with asthma and discusses the laws protecting the rights of those with the disorder.

Part V: Pediatric Asthma deals with common concerns about asthma in children. It explains how asthma is diagnosed in babies and young children and discusses the safety and effectiveness of the different treatments for children. It provides tips for handling asthma flare-ups in children and discusses how to deal with asthma at school and when children are participating in sports and other physical activity.

Part VI: Asthma in Other Special Populations discusses the particular challenges of managing asthma in pregnant women, older adults, and athletes. It describes the differing incidence rates of asthma among minority populations and discusses the disorder's disproportionate affect on low-income populations.

Part VII: Additional Help and Information includes a glossary of terms related to asthma and a directory of resources for further help and support.

Bibliographic Note

This volume contains documents and excerpts from the following U.S. government agencies: Centers for Disease Control and Prevention; National Center for Complementary and Alternative Medicine; National Heart Lung and Blood Institute; National Institute of Arthritis and Musculoskeletal and Skin Diseases; National Institute of Environmental Health Sciences; National Institutes of Health; *NIH News*; U.S. Department of Health and Human Services; U.S. Environmental Protection Agency; and the U.S. Food and Drug Administration.

In addition, this volume contains copyrighted documents from the following organizations: About.com; A.D.A,M., Inc.; Allergy and Asthma Network Mothers of Asthmatics; American Association for Respiratory Care; American College of Allergy, Asthma and Immunology; American College of Sports Medicine; American Lung Association; American Society of Health System Pharmacists; Asthma and Allergy Foundation of America; Asthma Foundation NSW; Asthma Initiative of Michigan; Asthma Society of Canada; Breathe Easy Play Hard Foundation; British Heart Foundation National Centre for Physical Activity and Health; California Environmental Protection Agency-Air Resources Board; CBC/Radio-Canada; Children's Asthma Education Centre; Cleveland Clinic; Colorado Allergy and Asthma Centers; Dietitians Association of Australia; European Federation of Allergy and Airways Diseases Patients Associations; Family Allergy and Asthma; Firestone Institute for Respiratory Health; Haz-Map.com; Imperial College London; Johns Hopkins Children's Center; McGill University; MyDR.com.au; National Asthma Council of Australia; National Jewish Health; National Lung Health Education Program; Nemours Foundation; Partners Asthma Center; *Respiratory Research*; University of California–Los Angeles Health System; University of California–San Francisco News Office; University of Chicago Asthma and COPD Center; University of Chicago Medical Center; University of Georgia News Service; University of Houston Today; University of Iowa Hospital and Clinics; University of Sunderland News; Utah Department of Health Asthma Program; Vanderbilt Kennedy Center; Virtual Medical Centre; West Virginia Asthma Education and Prevention Program; West Virginia University Health News; Woolcock Institute of Medical Research; and the Yale Daily News.

Acknowledgements

Thanks go to the many organizations, agencies, and individuals who have contributed materials for this *Sourcebook* and to medical consultant Dr. David Cooke and prepress services provider WhimsyInk. Special thanks go to managing editor Karen Bellenir and permissions coordinator Liz Collins for their help and support.

About the Health Reference Series

The *Health Reference Series* is designed to provide basic medical information for patients, families, caregivers, and the general public. Each volume takes a particular topic and provides comprehensive coverage. This is especially important for people who may be dealing with a newly diagnosed disease or a chronic disorder in themselves or in a family member. People looking for preventive guidance, information about disease warning signs, medical statistics, and risk factors for health problems will also find answers to their questions in the *Health Reference Series*. The *Series*, however, is not intended to serve as a tool for diagnosing illness, in prescribing treatments, or as a substitute for the physician/patient relationship. All people concerned about medical symptoms or the possibility of disease are encouraged to seek professional care from an appropriate healthcare provider.

A Note about Spelling and Style

Health Reference Series editors use *Stedman's Medical Dictionary* as an authority for questions related to the spelling of medical terms and the *Chicago Manual of Style* for questions related to grammatical structures, punctuation, and other editorial concerns. Consistent adherence is not always possible, however, because the individual volumes within the *Series* include many documents from a wide variety of different producers and copyright holders, and the editor's primary goal is to present material from each source as accurately as is possible following the terms specified by each document's producer. This sometimes means that information in different chapters or sections may follow other guidelines and alternate spelling authorities. For example, occasionally a copyright holder may require that eponymous terms be shown in possessive forms (Crohn's disease *vs.* Crohn disease) or that British spelling norms be retained (leukaemia *vs.* leukemia).

Locating Information within the Health Reference Series

The *Health Reference Series* contains a wealth of information about a wide variety of medical topics. Ensuring easy access to all the fact sheets, research reports, in-depth discussions, and other material contained within the individual books of the series remains one of our highest priorities. As the *Series* continues to grow in size and scope, however, locating the precise information needed by a reader may become more challenging.

A Contents Guide to the Health Reference Series was developed to direct readers to the specific volumes that address their concerns. It presents an extensive list of diseases, treatments, and other topics of general interest compiled from the Tables of Contents and major index headings. To access *A Contents Guide to the Health Reference Series*, visit www.healthreferenceseries.com.

Medical Consultant

Medical consultation services are provided to the *Health Reference Series* editors by David A. Cooke, MD, FACP. Dr. Cooke is a graduate of Brandeis University, and he received his M.D. degree from the University of Michigan. He completed residency training at the University of Wisconsin Hospital and Clinics. He is board-certified in Internal Medicine. Dr. Cooke currently works as part of the University of Michigan Health System and practices in Ann Arbor, MI. In his free time, he enjoys writing, science fiction, and spending time with his family.

Our Advisory Board

We would like to thank the following board members for providing guidance to the development of this series:

Dr. Lynda Baker, Associate Professor of Library and Information Science, Wayne State University, Detroit, MI

Nancy Bulgarelli, William Beaumont Hospital Library, Royal Oak, MI

Karen Imarisio, Bloomfield Township Public Library,
Bloomfield Township, MI

Karen Morgan, Mardigian Library,
University of Michigan-Dearborn, Dearborn, MI

Rosemary Orlando, St. Clair Shores Public Library,
St. Clair Shores, MI

Health Reference Series *Update Policy*

The inaugural book in the *Health Reference Series* was the first edition of *Cancer Sourcebook* published in 1989. Since then, the *Series* has been enthusiastically received by librarians and in the medical community. In order to maintain the standard of providing high-quality health information for the layperson the editorial staff at Omnigraphics felt it was necessary to implement a policy of updating volumes when warranted.

Medical researchers have been making tremendous strides, and it is the purpose of the *Health Reference Series* to stay current with the most recent advances. Each decision to update a volume is made on an individual basis. Some of the considerations include how much new information is available and the feedback we receive from people who use the books. If there is a topic you would like to see added to the update list, or an area of medical concern you feel has not been adequately addressed, please write to:

Editor
Health Reference Series
Omnigraphics, Inc.
155 W. Congress, Suite 200
Detroit, MI 48226
E-mail: editorial@omnigraphics.com

Part One

Asthma Basics

Chapter 1

What Is Asthma?

Chapter Contents

Section 1.1

Asthma: An Overview

"What Is Asthma?" National Heart, Lung, and Blood Institute, National Institutes of Health, February 2011.

Asthma is a chronic (long-term) lung disease that inflames and narrows the airways. Asthma causes recurring periods of wheezing (a whistling sound when you breathe), chest tightness, shortness of breath, and coughing. The coughing often occurs at night or early in the morning.

Asthma affects people of all ages, but it most often starts during childhood. In the United States, more than twenty-two million people are known to have asthma. Nearly six million of these people are children.

Overview

The airways are tubes that carry air into and out of your lungs. People who have asthma have inflamed airways. This makes the airways swollen and very sensitive. They tend to react strongly to certain inhaled substances.

When the airways react, the muscles around them tighten. This narrows the airways, causing less air to flow into the lungs. The swelling also can worsen, making the airways even narrower. Cells in the airways may make more mucus than normal. Mucus is a sticky, thick liquid that can further narrow your airways.

This chain reaction can result in asthma symptoms. Symptoms can happen each time the airways are inflamed.

Sometimes, asthma symptoms are mild and go away on their own or after minimal treatment with an asthma medicine. Other times, symptoms continue to get worse.

When symptoms get more intense and/or more symptoms occur, you're having an asthma attack. Asthma attacks also are called flare-ups or exacerbations.

It's important to treat symptoms when you first notice them. This will help prevent the symptoms from worsening and causing a severe asthma attack. Severe asthma attacks may require emergency care, and they can be fatal.

Outlook

Asthma can't be cured. Even when you feel fine, you still have the disease and it can flare up at any time.

However, with today's knowledge and treatments, most people who have asthma are able to manage the disease. They have few, if any, symptoms. They can live normal, active lives and sleep through the night without interruption from asthma.

You can take an active role in managing your asthma. For successful, thorough, and ongoing treatment, build strong partnerships with your doctor and other healthcare providers.

Section 1.2

How the Lungs Work

Excerpted from "How the Lungs Work," National Heart, Lung, and Blood Institute, National Institutes of Health, June 2010.

What Are the Lungs?

Your lungs are organs in your chest that allow your body to take in oxygen from the air. They also help remove carbon dioxide (a waste gas that can be toxic) from your body.

The lungs' intake of oxygen and removal of carbon dioxide is called gas exchange. Gas exchange is part of breathing. Breathing is a vital function of life; it helps your body work properly.

Other organs and tissues also help make breathing possible.

The Respiratory System

The respiratory system is a group of organs and tissues that help you breathe. The main parts of this system are the airways, the lungs and linked blood vessels, and the muscles that enable breathing.

5

Airways

The airways are pipes that carry oxygen-rich air to your lungs and carbon dioxide, a waste gas, out of your lungs. The airways include the following:

- Your nose and linked air passages (called nasal cavities)
- Your mouth
- Your larynx, or voice box
- Your trachea, or windpipe
- Tubes called bronchial tubes or bronchi, and their branches

Air first enters your body through your nose or mouth, which wets and warms the air. (Cold, dry air can irritate your lungs.) The air then travels through your voice box and down your windpipe. The windpipe splits into two bronchial tubes that enter your lungs.

A thin flap of tissue called the epiglottis covers your windpipe when you swallow. This prevents food or drink from entering the air passages that lead to your lungs.

Except for the mouth and some parts of the nose, all of the airways have special hairs called cilia that are coated with sticky mucus. The cilia trap germs and other foreign particles that enter your airways when you breathe in air.

These fine hairs then sweep the particles up to the nose or mouth. From there, they're swallowed, coughed, or sneezed out of the body. Nose hairs and mouth saliva also trap particles and germs.

Lungs and Blood Vessels

Your lungs and linked blood vessels deliver oxygen to your body and remove carbon dioxide from your body. Your lungs lie on either side of your breastbone and fill the inside of your chest cavity. Your left lung is slightly smaller than your right lung to allow room for your heart.

Within the lungs, your bronchi branch into thousands of smaller, thinner tubes called bronchioles. These tubes end in bunches of tiny round air sacs called alveoli.

Each of these air sacs is covered in a mesh of tiny blood vessels called capillaries. The capillaries connect to a network of arteries and veins that move blood through your body.

The pulmonary artery and its branches deliver blood rich in carbon dioxide (and lacking in oxygen) to the capillaries that surround the air sacs. Inside the air sacs, carbon dioxide moves from the blood into the air. At the same time, oxygen moves from the air into the blood in the capillaries.

The oxygen-rich blood then travels to the heart through the pulmonary vein and its branches. The heart pumps the oxygen-rich blood out to the body.

The lungs are divided into five main sections called lobes. Some people need to have a diseased lung lobe removed. However, they can still breathe well using the rest of their lung lobes.

Muscles Used for Breathing

Muscles near the lungs help expand and contract (tighten) the lungs to allow breathing. These muscles include the following:

- Diaphragm

- Intercostal muscles

- Abdominal muscles

- Muscles in the neck and collarbone area

The diaphragm is a dome-shaped muscle located below your lungs. It separates the chest cavity from the abdominal cavity. The diaphragm is the main muscle used for breathing.

The intercostal muscles are located between your ribs. They also play a major role in helping you breathe.

Beneath your diaphragm are abdominal muscles. They help you breathe out when you're breathing fast (for example, during physical activity).

Muscles in your neck and collarbone area help you breathe in when other muscles involved in breathing don't work well, or when lung disease impairs your breathing.

What Happens When You Breathe?

Breathing In (Inhalation)

When you breathe in, or inhale, your diaphragm contracts (tightens) and moves downward. This increases the space in your chest cavity, into which your lungs expand. The intercostal muscles between your ribs also help enlarge the chest cavity. They contract to pull your rib cage both upward and outward when you inhale.

As your lungs expand, air is sucked in through your nose or mouth. The air travels down your windpipe and into your lungs. After passing through your bronchial tubes, the air finally reaches and enters the alveoli (air sacs).

Through the very thin walls of the alveoli, oxygen from the air passes to the surrounding capillaries (blood vessels). A red blood cell protein called hemoglobin helps move oxygen from the air sacs to the blood.

At the same time, carbon dioxide moves from the capillaries into the air sacs. The gas has traveled in the bloodstream from the right side of the heart through the pulmonary artery.

Oxygen-rich blood from the lungs is carried through a network of capillaries to the pulmonary vein. This vein delivers the oxygen-rich blood to the left side of the heart. The left side of the heart pumps the blood to the rest of the body. There, the oxygen in the blood moves from blood vessels into surrounding tissues.

Breathing Out (Exhalation)

When you breathe out, or exhale, your diaphragm relaxes and moves upward into the chest cavity. The intercostal muscles between the ribs also relax to reduce the space in the chest cavity.

As the space in the chest cavity gets smaller, air rich in carbon dioxide is forced out of your lungs and windpipe, and then out of your nose or mouth.

Breathing out requires no effort from your body unless you have a lung disease or are doing physical activity. When you're physically active, your abdominal muscles contract and push your diaphragm against your lungs even more than usual. This rapidly pushes out the air in your lungs.

What Controls Your Breathing?

A respiratory control center at the base of your brain controls your breathing. This center sends ongoing signals down your spine and to the nerves of the muscles involved in breathing.

These signals ensure your breathing muscles contract (tighten) and relax regularly. This allows your breathing to happen automatically, without you being aware of it.

To a limited degree, you can change your breathing rate, such as by breathing faster or holding your breath. Your emotions also can change your breathing. For example, being scared or angry can affect your breathing pattern.

Your breathing will change depending on how active you are and the condition of the air around you. For example, you need to breathe more often when you do physical activity. In contrast, your body needs to restrict how much air you breathe if the air contains irritants or toxins.

To adjust your breathing to changing needs, your body has many sensors in your brain, blood vessels, muscles, and lungs.

Sensors in the brain and in two major blood vessels (the carotid artery and the aorta) detect carbon dioxide or oxygen levels in your blood and change your breathing rate as needed.

Sensors in the airways detect lung irritants. The sensors can trigger sneezing or coughing. In people who have asthma, the sensors may cause the muscles around the airways in the lungs to contract. This makes the airways smaller.

Sensors in the alveoli (air sacs) detect a buildup of fluid in the lung tissues. These sensors are thought to trigger rapid, shallow breathing.

Sensors in your joints and muscles detect movement of your arms or legs. These sensors may play a role in increasing your breathing rate when you're physically active.

Lung Diseases and Conditions

Many steps are involved in breathing. If injury, disease, or other factors affect any of the steps, you may have trouble breathing.

For example, the fine hairs (cilia) that line your upper airways may not trap all of the germs you breathe in. These germs can cause an infection in your bronchial tubes (bronchitis) or deep in your lungs (pneumonia). These infections cause a buildup of mucus and/or fluid that narrows the airways and limits airflow in and out of your lungs.

If you have asthma, breathing in certain substances that you're sensitive to can trigger your airways to narrow. This makes it hard for air to flow in and out of your lungs.

Over a long period, breathing in cigarette smoke or air pollutants can damage the airways and the air sacs. This can lead to a condition called chronic obstructive pulmonary disease (COPD). COPD prevents proper airflow in and out of your lungs and can hinder gas exchange in the air sacs.

An important step to breathing is the movement of your diaphragm and other muscles in your chest, neck, and abdomen. This movement lets you inhale and exhale. Nerves that run from your brain to these muscles control their movement. Damage to these nerves in your upper spinal cord can cause breathing to stop, unless a machine is used to help you breathe. (This machine is called a ventilator or a respirator.)

A steady flow of blood in the small blood vessels that surround your air sacs is vital for gas exchange. Long periods of inactivity or surgery can cause a blood clot called a pulmonary embolism (PE) to block a lung artery. A PE can reduce or block the flow of blood in the small blood vessels and hinder gas exchange.

Section 1.3

How Asthma Works: A Physiological View

"How Asthma Works," © 2011 University of Chicago Asthma and COPD Center. Reprinted with permission. For additional information, visit http://asthma.bsd.uchicago.edu.

Inflammation

The most important thing to know about how asthma works is that it is a disease of inflammation. All of the other components of asthma stem from that central problem.

Inflammation is a common process throughout the body, and it is not all bad. For instance, picture scratching your arm accidentally on a nail. The area right around the scratch becomes dark pink, maybe somewhat hot and puffy. And it hurts. Warmth, redness, swelling, and pain are the hallmarks of inflammation. A small amount of fluid may also seep out—this is common in inflamed tissues (medically, the fluid is called "exudate").

In the case of a nasty scratch, inflammation is the process the body uses to reduce the likelihood of infection and to promote repair. The symptoms will probably last a couple of days and then go away once the wound has effectively healed. There are times, though, when the standard (and usually useful) bodily process of inflammation gets out of hand, resulting in an inflammatory disease. Asthma is not the only inflammatory disease. Some others include:

- rheumatoid arthritis (inflammation in the joints);
- inflammatory bowel disease (inflammation in the intestine);
- lupus (an inflammatory disease that can affect many different parts of the body, including the skin, kidneys, and lungs).

In asthma, of course, the inflammation is located in the airways. Even when a person with asthma is not having an asthma attack and seems to be breathing okay, the walls of his or her airways remain inflamed. They are swollen and produce too much mucus, dramatically shrinking the space available for air to get through. This is why medicines to reduce inflammation (especially inhaled corticosteroids) are at the center of most asthma treatment plans.

In addition to its direct effects, inflammation contributes (in ways we do not fully understand) to the other two major problems in asthma—airway hyperresponsiveness and excessive bronchoconstriction.

Airway Hyperresponsiveness

Physicians often refer to asthmatic airways as "twitchy" because they are terribly sensitive to things that would cause no noticeable effect on the airways of non-asthmatics. (The medical term for this "twitchiness" is hyperresponsiveness.) Just walking into cold air, or sitting near someone wearing perfume, for example, can trigger a big reaction in the airways of an asthmatic. The airway walls swell up even more, the airway muscles squeeze, and the person with asthma can find himself wheezing, coughing, and maybe even having trouble breathing at all.

Doctors have noted, however, that if the inflammation in an asthmatic person's airways is controlled by medicines, the airways become much less "twitchy."

Excessive Bronchoconstriction

Airways are hollow tubes through which air passes. The tubes themselves are made up of different layers of tissue, one of which is a layer of smooth muscle. In a person with asthma, the airway muscles tend to be particularly large and strong.

When a response of the airways is triggered, the muscles contract, squeezing the airway and narrowing the space that air can get through. The smooth muscle of the airway in a person with asthma contracts too easily, too hard, and too long. As discussed above, the airways of asthmatics are already swollen and partly filled with mucus, so the extra squeezing of the airway smooth muscle can make it difficult or even impossible for any air to get through at all.

Excessive contraction of airway muscle appears to be directly related to airway inflammation. Controlling the inflammation with anti-inflammatory medicines helps prevent the muscles squeezing so easily and so hard, and thus, helps prevent asthma episodes.

11

"Rescue" or "reliever" medicines (such as albuterol, Ventolin, and Proventil) work by making the airway smooth muscle relax, to temporarily stop them from squeezing the airway closed. They do nothing, though, for the inflammation that is at the root of the problem.

Section 1.4

Physical, Emotional, and Social Effects of Asthma

Reprinted from "Physical Effects" and "Emotional and Social Effects," © 2011 University of Chicago Asthma and COPD Center. Reprinted with permission. For additional information, visit http://asthma.bsd.uchicago.edu.

Physical Effects

Having asthma can affect a person in many ways. Physical effects can range from the somewhat annoying (an occasional cough) all the way to the life threatening (not being able to breathe). The frequency and seriousness of asthma symptoms are dependent on how well a person's asthma is controlled (with medicines and other measures) as well as how severe that individual's asthma was to begin with.

The psychological and social effects of asthma are less often acknowledged but can for some people be at least as troubling as the physical ones.

Physical Symptoms

Asthma symptoms and severity vary substantially from person to person. Most people with asthma do not have symptoms constantly. Bothersome asthma symptoms can mean that asthma is not controlled sufficiently, or that an acute asthma episode may be starting. Common asthma symptoms include:

- cough;
- wheeze;
- tight feeling in the chest;

- shortness of breath;
- awakening at night from cough or wheeze.

Children are not always able to express in words that their asthma symptoms are worsening. They may have noticeable coughing and wheezing, but these are not always the first indications of breathing distress. Different children show asthma trouble in different ways. Some possible indications of the beginning of an asthma episode include:

- unusual tiredness or restlessness;
- trouble sitting still;
- crankiness;
- looking worried or scared;
- pale, sweaty skin;
- fast breathing;
- slouching over.

If you do not have asthma, you can help yourself imagine what it feels like to have an asthma episode. (No need to try these if you do have asthma—you already know what it feels like, and you don't want to risk triggering a real episode.)

1. Run in place for a minute or two, until you can feel your heart start to beat fast. Take a plastic drinking straw and put it in your mouth. Hold your nose closed and continue to breathe through the straw. OR

2. Take a deep breath in and hold it a moment. Now let out about a tenth of the air in your lungs. Breathe back in. Breathe out that same small amount of air. Breathe back in. Repeat until you can't stand it anymore.

Asthma Severity

Just as we do not yet know exactly what causes asthma, we do not know why the disease is mild in some people and very severe in others. National guidelines, developed by an expert committee in 1997, classify asthma severity into four levels:

- Mild intermittent:
  - wheeze or cough two or fewer times per week;
  - symptoms at night two or fewer times per month.

- Mild persistent:
  - wheeze or cough three to six times per week;
  - symptoms at night three to four times per month;
  - increased symptoms with activity.
- Moderate persistent:
  - daily symptoms;
  - daily inhaled beta-2 agonist (bronchodilator) medication use;
  - symptoms at night five or more times per month;
  - decreased exercise capacity.
- Severe persistent:
  - continual symptoms limiting activity;
  - frequent exacerbations;
  - frequent symptoms at night.

A single individual's asthma does not necessarily remain in the same category permanently. With effective ongoing asthma control, a person can move into a less severe category. A person with seasonal asthma triggers may find that at a certain time of year (for instance, when ragweed pollen is in the air) she is in a higher severity group than she is the rest of the year. Asthma that starts during childhood may also become less severe as a person grows, and his airways become wider.

Emotional and Social Effects

The psychological impact that asthma has on any individual person is determined by many factors, such as:

- asthma severity;
- limitation of activities due to asthma;
- social and family support available;
- age at which asthma symptoms started;
- level of asthma-related skills and knowledge;
- overall personality and coping style.

Each person's asthma experience is unique, but there are some feelings that many people with asthma experience at one time or another.

Fear and anxiety: Difficulty breathing, leading to the sensation of "air hunger," can of course be terribly upsetting. It is common for people with asthma to experience fear that they are going to die during an asthma episode. The fear of dying then can become more general and continue when the person is not having active symptoms. Asthma episodes are for most people somewhat unpredictable, and unpredictable events are known to be more stressful than events that can be anticipated and prepared for. Feeling that another asthma episode could start at any time may cause a person to feel anxious constantly.

Hypervigilance: To be vigilant is to be watchful, so hypervigilance is being too watchful. A person with asthma can sometimes get so focused on when another asthma episode might occur as to be alarmed by even small and normal bodily changes (for example, heart rate increasing with activity).

Loss of control: Asthma (especially asthma that is not effectively controlled) can lead a person to feel out of control in life. If you feel as if your efforts don't do any good anyway, it may make you stop even trying to take care of yourself. People who feel out of control in one area may also try to make themselves feel more secure by exerting extra control in other areas (such as the workplace, or relationships with family and friends).

Denial: Having asthma can involve a lot of anxiety and fear. Denial is one natural mechanism that humans have to deal with an excess of anxiety and fear. We seem to "forget" the thing that is causing us to feel anxious so that we can keep functioning and not be paralyzed by our emotions. Unfortunately, denial can also prevent a person with asthma from doing the things he needs to do to stay healthy and prevent serious asthma episodes.

Anger: As with other diseases, the basic truth is that asthma isn't fair. It places demands on the people affected by it. It causes discomfort and worry. It can limit a person's activities. And nobody deserves it. Most people with asthma will feel angry at some point about having the disease. This may be a part of a person's reaction to the initial diagnosis of asthma, or may crop up much later. If you don't have a chance to acknowledge and talk about feeling angry, the unresolved emotion can sometimes make it difficult for you to take the best possible care of yourself.

Guilt: Even if you understand that asthma is not something you caused, and that you can't make it go away, you can still sometimes have irrational feelings of guilt. Children may be especially prone to blame themselves for the disruption their asthma causes on their families. Frequent reassurances that asthma is nobody's fault can help.

Embarrassment: It can, for most of us, be uncomfortable at times to feel different from those around us. Aspects of having asthma such as using an inhaler or avoiding triggers, as well as the asthma symptoms themselves, can make a person feel conspicuous and set apart from others. These feelings can be particularly difficult for children and adolescents. The desire to fit in with a peer group or not to appear different can sometimes lead people with asthma to neglect important parts of their own asthma care.

Confusion: Especially in the period following the initial asthma diagnosis, a person can feel overwhelmed by all of the information there is to take in. Asthma is a complex disease, with many aspects to understand and, often, many steps to take (such as taking medicines, watching for symptoms, taking peak-flow measurements, keeping a daily record, deciding when to seek urgent care, and so on). If the feelings of confusion are too severe, a person may give up on trying to understand asthma and the steps to take to stay well.

There is, of course, no one right way to go about dealing with the emotions that asthma can cause. There are some strategies, though, that many people find particularly useful.

Acknowledge and accept the feelings you're having. Pretending you don't feel a certain emotion doesn't make it go away. It just makes it more difficult for you to address the feeling and its underlying cause.

Take an active role in taking care of yourself. Learn about the disease and what you can do to stay as healthy as possible. Ask questions when you see your healthcare provider, and make it clear you want to participate in your own care. Make the changes you know you need to make. Not only will your asthma get better, but you will feel more in control of what happens to you.

Learn and practice relaxation exercises or meditation. These have been shown not only to reduce asthma-related stress and anxiety but also, in some cases, actually to reduce the physical symptoms of asthma.

Find yourself a healthcare provider you feel comfortable with. A healthcare provider who is patient and understanding, and who has the time to explain things and answer questions, can be of significant help. Talk with your healthcare provider about the emotions that asthma causes for you. They are an important part of how you experience the disease. Also, pay attention to your own preferences. Even if other people swear by Dr. X, you may find you actually communicate better with Dr. Y.

It is important, too, to note that psychological factors do not cause asthma. Half a century ago, psychoanalytic theories of the origin of asthma were popular, but these have fallen out of favor as we have learned more about the biology of asthma and its genetic and environmental elements. Emotions can, however, be asthma triggers. Some people find they are more susceptible to asthma episodes when they are under a lot of stress. Emotional responses like laughing and crying can also sometimes trigger an attack.

Chapter 2

Asthma Causes and Risk Factors

Chapter Contents

Section 2.1

What Do We Know about the Causes of Asthma?

"Asthma in Adults, " © 2011 A.D.A.M., Inc. Reprinted with permission.

Causes

The exact cause of asthma is unknown. Asthma is most likely caused by a combination of genetic (inherited) factors and environmental triggers (such as allergens and infections). Asthma tends to run in families, so children whose parents have asthma are more likely to develop it themselves.

The Allergic Response (Allergens)

Nearly half of adults with asthma have an allergy-related condition, which in most cases developed first in childhood. (In patients who first develop asthma during adulthood, the allergic response usually does not play a strong causal role.)

In people with allergies, the immune system overreacts to exposure to allergens. Allergic asthma is triggered by inhaling certain substances (allergens), such as:

- Dust mites, specifically mite feces, which are coated with enzymes that contain a powerful allergen. These are the primary allergens in the home.

- Animal dander. Cats harbor significant allergens, which can even be carried on clothing; dogs usually cause fewer problems. People with asthma who already have pets and are not allergic to them probably have a low risk for developing such allergies later on.

- Molds.

- Cockroaches. Cockroach dust is a major asthma trigger and may reduce lung function even in people without a history of asthma.

- Pollen, from plants.

Environmental Factors (Irritants)

An asthma attack can also be induced or aggravated by direct irritants to the lungs. Important irritants involved in asthma include cigarette smoke, indoor chemicals, and air pollution.

Infections

Respiratory viral and bacterial infections play a role in some cases of adult-onset asthma. In both children and adults with existing allergic asthma, an upper respiratory tract infection often worsens an attack.

Risk Factors

About twenty-two million Americans have asthma.

Gender

Before puberty, asthma occurs more often in males, but after adolescence, it is more common in females. In adults, women are more likely to report severe symptoms than men.

Hormonal fluctuations or changes in hormone levels may play a role in the severity of asthma in women. Between 30 and 40 percent of women with asthma experience fluctuations in severity that are associated with their menstrual cycle. Some women first develop asthma during or shortly after pregnancy, while others first develop it around the time of menopause (perimenopause).

Race and Ethnicity

African Americans have higher rates of asthma than Caucasians or other ethnic groups. They are also more likely to die of the disease. Ethnicity and genetics, however, are less likely to play a role in these differences than socioeconomic differences, such as having less access to optimal healthcare, and greater likelihood of living in an urban area (another asthma risk factor).

Obesity

Studies report a strong association between obesity and asthma. Evidence also suggests that people who are overweight (body mass index greater than 25) have more difficulty getting their asthma under control. Weight loss in anyone who is obese and has asthma or shortness of breath helps reduce airway obstruction and improve lung function.

Other Risk Factors

Gastroesophageal reflux disease (GERD): At least half of patients with asthma have GERD, the cause of heartburn. It is not entirely clear which condition causes the other or whether they are both due to common factors. Treating GERD does not appear to improve asthma control.

Aspirin-induced asthma: Aspirin-induced asthma (AIA) is a condition in which asthma gets worse after taking aspirin or other nonsteroidal anti-inflammatory drugs (NSAIDs). AIA often develops after a viral infection. It is a particularly severe asthmatic condition, associated with many asthma-related hospitalizations. In about 5 percent of cases, aspirin is responsible for a syndrome that involves multiple attacks of asthma, sinusitis, and nasal congestion. Such patients also often have polyps (small benign growths) in the nasal passages. Patients with aspirin-induced asthma (AIA) should avoid aspirin and other NSAIDs, including ibuprofen (Advil) and naproxen (Aleve).

Section 2.2

Study Shows Genetic Ties to Asthma

Excerpted from "Largest Genetic Study of Asthma Points Towards
Better Treatments," September 23, 2010. © Imperial College London
(www3.imperial.ac.uk). Reprinted with permission.

An international study looking at deoxyribonucleic acid (DNA)
from over twenty-six thousand people has identified several genetic
variants that substantially increase susceptibility to asthma in the
population. The findings, published in the *New England Journal of
Medicine*, will help scientists to focus their efforts to develop better
therapies for the illness.

The study, which was coordinated by researchers from Imperial
College London, was performed by the GABRIEL consortium, a collaboration of 164 scientists from nineteen countries in Europe, along
with other groups in the United Kingdom, Canada, and Australia. It
analyzed DNA samples from ten thousand children and adults with
asthma and sixteen thousand nonasthmatics.

The researchers performed more than half a million genetic tests on
each subject, covering all the genes in the human genome. The study
pinpointed seven locations on the genome where differences in the
genetic code were associated with asthma.

When the airway is irritated in a person with asthma, the airway
narrows and the lining becomes inflamed, causing difficulty breathing. The causes of the disease are poorly understood, but genetic and
environmental factors are thought to play roughly equal roles.

Today's research has a number of potential implications, according
to the study team. It suggests that allergies are probably a consequence of asthma, rather than a cause of the disease. It also suggests
that genetic testing would not help predict who is likely to develop
the disease.

The new variants linked to asthma were found in more than a third
of children with asthma in the study. The gene with the strongest effect
on children did not affect adults, and adult-onset asthma was more
weakly linked to other genetic differences, suggesting that it may differ biologically from childhood-onset asthma.

Childhood asthma, which affects boys more than girls and can persist throughout life, is often linked to allergies, and it has been assumed that these can trigger the condition. However, the study found that genes controlling the levels of antibodies that cause allergies had little effect on the presence of asthma, suggesting that allergies are more likely to be a consequence of asthma than a cause.

Professor Miriam Moffatt, professor of human genetics at Imperial College London and one of the study's leaders, said: "As a result of genetic studies we now know that allergies may develop as a result of defects of the lining of the airways in asthma. This does not mean that allergies are not important, but it does mean that concentrating therapies only on allergy will not effectively treat the whole disease."

Some of the genes identified are involved in signaling pathways that tell the immune system when the lining of the airways has been damaged. Other genes appear to control how quickly the airways heal after they have been injured. Identifying these genes should help direct research into new treatments for asthma, the researchers suggest.

"Asthma is a complex disease in which many different parts of the immune system can become activated," said Professor William Cookson, director of respiratory sciences at Imperial College London, who coordinated the study. "One of the problems with asthma research has been choosing where to intervene in the disease pathways. Our study now highlights targets for effective asthma therapies, and suggests that therapies against these targets will be of use to large numbers of asthmatics in the population."

Professor David Strachan, professor of epidemiology at St Georges, University of London, who also co-authored the study, said: "Asthma has often been considered a single disease, but our genetic findings suggest that childhood-onset asthma may differ biologically from asthma that is acquired in adult life. The GABRIEL consortium is now investigating whether the causes of asthma differ between people with and without these newly discovered genetic variants."

The study also found that the genes associated with asthma did not have strong enough effects to be useful for predicting early in life which children might eventually develop the disease. This indicates that environmental factors are also very important in causing asthma to develop. The GABRIEL consortium is working to identify environmental exposures that could protect against the illness.

The study was primarily funded by the European Commission, the French Ministry for Higher Education and Research, the charity Asthma UK, and the Wellcome Trust.

Although large multinational collaborations are becoming the norm with the study of many complex genetic diseases, the GABRIEL study is unique in that nearly all of the fifteen billion genetic tests were performed in a single institution, the Centre National de Genotypage (CEA-CNG) near Paris.

Professor Mark Lathrop, the director of the CEA-CNG and the scientific director of the Fondation Jean Dausset–Centre d'Etude du Polymorphisme Humain (CEPH), pointed out the crucial role of an integrated large-scale infrastructure like CEA-CNG, which has the capacity to perform all the steps from receiving the biological samples, to high throughput genotyping, quality control, and data analysis. The Fondation Jean Dausset–CEPH was also a major player in this study.

Professor Miriam Moffatt said: "It has been enormously gratifying to work with such a group of dedicated scientists from so many countries. This genetic study has taken five years from planning until completion, but it builds on many earlier years of work in which all the twenty-six thousand volunteers were recruited and studied in great detail. The study would not have been possible without the contribution of all of the GABRIEL members."

Professor Ivo Gut, former deputy director of the CEA-CNG and now director of the Centro Nacional de Análisis Genómico in Barcelona, said: "These results constitute a huge leap forward in the understanding of asthma that will lead to major advances in the treatment and quality of life of people suffering from the disease. It has been an immense effort to get this far but is well worth it. The generous support from the funding agencies, the kind donation of DNA by the research subjects, and the huge personal dedication of the collaborators of the Gabriel consortium have made this study possible."

Professor Florence Demenais, director of the Genetic Variation and Human Diseases Laboratory in Paris (UMR-946 Inserm-Université Paris Diderot, Fondation Jean Dausset), who led the statistical analysis that combined all of the data, said: "Large-scale genetic studies, such as this one, provide a powerful tool to decipher the genetic mechanisms underlying asthma and to unravel different types of disease that make up the asthma syndrome."

Professor Erika von Mutius at the University of Munich and co-coordinator of GABRIEL said: "The puzzle now is to work out what is causing the damage to the airway lining in asthma. The GABRIEL study has also been busy looking for clues as to the environmental causes of asthma, particularly by dissecting the strong protective effects of living on a farm. In the next year we will be combining the results from the genetic and environmental wings of the GABRIEL study, and we are greatly looking forward to what we may find."

Section 2.3

Researchers Identify New Asthma Genes

New research from Yale scientists has shown that asthma may be more complex than previously thought.

A few years ago, scientists focused on only two or three genes for asthma. Now about 250 genes are implicated.

At the Yale Center for Perinatal, Pediatric and Environmental Epidemiology, School of Public Health professor Michael Bracken designed several genetic studies to look for genes associated with increased susceptibility to asthma. Since there are already a few hundred genes linked to asthma, Bracken said he hopes the three newly identified genes may help doctors increase their understanding of how this common disease develops.

In the first study, School of Public Health professor Andrew DeWan analyzed the genetic makeup of 108 children in Connecticut and Massachusetts for 500,000 genetic markers. After sifting through the data, DeWan said he found one gene—associated with the muscle cells that line the lungs—that was different in asthmatic children.

In another study, researchers sifted through PubMed, a digital database run by the United States National Library of Medicine, for articles that cited genes associated with asthma. From a sample of five hundred papers related to 250 genes linked to asthma, they culled the 50 most-researched genes and searched for them in the 108 children. While they found mutations on two of these genes in the children, only one gene involved in repairing double-stranded DNA had a particularly strong relationship with asthma.

The final study examined the average number of copies asthmatic children have of the TCR (gamma) gene, which codes for markers on the surface of immune system cells. Immune cells use these markers to recruit additional cells to kill foreign invaders such as pollen and dust, which asthmatic children are especially sensitive to. The researchers found that compared to nonasthmatic children, asthma sufferers had on average fewer copies of the TCR (gamma) gene, but they are not sure what this means yet, researcher Kyle Walsh said.

Walsh said the difference in the number of copies is likely caused by mutations acquired after birth.

"If these are mutations you're not born with, then you may be able to prevent people from getting them," he said.

Bracken said these studies point to a new direction in asthma research. Only a few years ago, scientists were looking for just two or three genetic mutations that caused asthma. But as new studies have come out, Bracken said about 250 genes have been reported to be associated with asthma, with more to be discovered. In different combinations, these genetic mutations may interact together or with the environment to increase the risk of asthma, Bracken said. What was once believed to be a simple, chronic inflammatory lung disease, Bracken said, may instead have a whole spectrum of variants ranging from exercised-induced asthma to pollen-induced asthma.

Bracken said the next step is to determine how the pathways for asthma develop, which can lead to more effective treatments.

"The ultimate goal [is to] identify the child early," he said.

Asthma affects more than 6.5 million children in the United States.

Section 2.4

Mother's Depression a
Risk Factor in Childhood Asthma

"Mother's Depression a Risk Factor in Childhood Asthma Symptoms, Study Says," November 19, 2009. © Johns Hopkins Children's Center (www.hopkinschildrens.org). Reprinted with permission.

Asthma symptoms can worsen in children with depressed mothers, according to research from Johns Hopkins Children's Center published online in the *Journal of Pediatric Psychology*.

Analyzing data from interviews with 262 mothers of African American children with asthma—a population disproportionately affected by this inflammatory airway disorder—the Hopkins investigators found that children whose mothers had more depressive symptoms had more frequent asthma symptoms during the six months of the study. Conversely, children whose mothers reported fewer depressive symptoms had less frequent asthma symptoms.

Researchers tracked ups and downs in maternal depression as related to the frequency of symptoms among children.

"Even though our research was not set up to measure just how much a mom's depression increased the frequency of her child's symptoms, a clear pattern emerged in which the latter followed the earlier," says senior investigator Kristin Riekert, Ph.D., a pediatric psychologist and co-director of the Johns Hopkins Adherence Research Center.

But while maternal depression appeared to aggravate a child's asthma, the opposite was not true: How often a child had symptoms did not seem to affect the mother's depressive symptoms, an important finding that suggests maternal depression is an independent risk factor that can portend a child's symptoms, researchers say.

Past studies have shown that children with chronic health conditions fare worse if their primary caregiver is depressed, but none have teased out the exact interplay between the two.

"Intuitively, it may seem that we're dealing with a chicken-egg situation, but our study suggests otherwise," Riekert says. "The fact that mom's depression was not affected by how often her child had

28

symptoms really caught us off guard, but it also suggested which factor comes first."

Researchers did not study why and how a mother's depression affects a child's asthma status, but because depression often involves fatigue, memory lapses, and difficulty concentrating, it can affect a parent's ability to manage the child's chronic condition, which can involve daily, and sometimes complex, drug regimens and frequent visits to the doctor.

"Mom is the one who must implement the doctor's recommendations for treatment and follow-up, and if she is depressed she can't do it well, so the child will suffer," says lead investigator Michiko Otsuki, Ph.D., a behavioral medicine fellow at Johns Hopkins at the time of the study, now at the University of South Florida St. Petersburg.

Investigators say their findings should prompt pediatricians who treat children with asthma to pay close attention to the child's primary caregiver—whether or not it is the mother—and screen and refer them for treatment if needed.

"We ask these parents if they are smokers all the time, so maybe it's time to start asking them if they are coping well emotionally," said co-investigator Arlene Butz, Sc.D., a pediatric asthma specialist at Johns Hopkins Children's Center. "Doctors are trained to pick up on subtle clues, so if they see a red flag in mom, they should follow up with a depression screener and referral if needed."

Treating depressed mothers whose children are at high risk for asthma complications will likely benefit both mother and child, researchers say, while providing a clear treatment target to help reduce the burden of asthma in the United States. Asthma is the country's leading pediatric chronic illness, affecting 6.5 million children under the age of eighteen, according to the Centers for Disease Control and Prevention (CDC).

The Hopkins study included only mothers but investigators believe a similar pattern would emerge regardless of who the primary caregiver is.

Researchers caution that the mothers in their study were screened for depression with a standard questionnaire, which is a reliable detector of symptoms but not a firm diagnosis.

The Hopkins findings came from a high-risk, inner-city population and thus cannot be statistically extended to other ethnic and socioeconomic groups, but researchers say the effect of caregiver depression on a child's asthma likely transcends demographics.

The research was funded by the National Heart, Lung, and Blood Institute.

Other Hopkins researchers involved in the study included Michelle Eakin, Ph.D., Lisa Arceneaux, Psy.D., and Cynthia Rand, Ph.D.

Section 2.5

Respiratory Syncytial Virus Can Increase Risk of Asthma

What sounds like a cold, looks like a cold, and acts like a cold—but sends more babies to the hospital than any other condition?

Respiratory syncytial virus, or RSV: the common disease with the uncommon name.

RSV tends to pop up in the winter and early spring. It starts as an upper respiratory infection, with familiar cold symptoms—runny nose, mild cough, low fever. And for most people, that's where it ends.

By the time children are two or three years old, most have likely been infected by RSV at least once, with few problems. However, for premature babies and infants; children with asthma; and patients of all ages with underlying lung, heart, or immune system problems, the virus can be life-threatening.

What makes RSV so dangerous is its ability to quickly spread down from the nose and throat into the lower respiratory tract, where it infects and causes inflammation in the tissues of the lungs (causing pneumonia) and the tiny bronchial air tubes (causing bronchiolitis). Inflammation is the body's natural process for fighting infection, but in tiny infant airways or those already inflamed by asthma, it can cause increased airway obstruction and difficulty in breathing.

Another danger of RSV is that a serious RSV infection in young children often leads to later development of asthma and allergies. Researchers do not know exactly why this happens. It may be a cause-and-effect reaction, where the RSV infection damages the lung, which leads to asthma; or it may just be an association, where a child who is at risk for asthma may also be at risk for a more serious RSV infection.

Over the past ten years, researchers have realized that RSV is also quite common among adults, especially senior citizens living in group settings. People most at risk of exposure to RSV are those in close contact with large numbers of people. The highly contagious virus spreads quickly through human contact, often before the infected person shows any obvious signs of the disease. To make things worse, the RSV virus can live on surfaces such as doorknobs and tabletops for days.

Prevention

The key to controlling RSV is preventing infection and identifying early symptoms. Prevention centers on strict hygiene:

- Wash hands frequently, especially before eating or before handling babies.

- Wash toys, tabletops, and other shared surfaces.

- Avoid sharing cups, eating utensils, or food.

- Stay away from people with obvious cold symptoms.

- Stay away from cigarette smoke, which can increase the risk of infection and severity of symptoms.

Identification

Identifying RSV depends on recognizing the danger signs. Call your physician if cold symptoms last longer than a week, or if they evolve into any of these complications:

- high fever (above 100.4° in babies under three months old; above 101° in babies three to six months; above 103° in babies older than six months);

- fast breathing or other breathing problems;

- wheezing;

- worsening cough;

- blueness around the mouth (indicating lack of oxygen).

Treatment

There is no medical cure for RSV. Physicians focus instead on treatments that reduce congestion and open the airways so the patient can breathe. Serious cases require hospital care, intravenous fluids, nebulizer medications, and oxygen treatments. Some high-risk babies may qualify to receive a preventive medicine called palivizumab, given by injection every month during RSV season (fall and winter).

Parents and caregivers of children with asthma, premature babies and infants—as well as elderly people—need to take extra precautions during the RSV season, learn to recognize the warning signs, and seek medical treatment as soon as possible.

Section 2.6

Early Antibiotic Use May Increase Childhood Asthma Risk

"Early Antibiotic Use May Increase Childhood Asthma Risk: Study," CBC News, June 11, 2007. Copyright © 2007. CBC/Radio-Canada. All rights reserved. Reprinted with permission.

Children who are given antibiotics before they turn one seem to be significantly more likely to develop asthma by age seven, Canadian researchers say.

A team from the University of Manitoba and McGill University in Montreal looked at the medical records of more than thirteen thousand children up to seven years old.

"Antibiotics are prescribed mostly for respiratory tract infections, yet respiratory symptoms can be a sign of future asthma. This may make it difficult to attribute antibiotic use to asthma development," said lead author Anita Kozyrskyj of the University of Manitoba.

"Our study reported on antibiotic use in children being treated for nonrespiratory tract infections, which distinguishes the effect of the antibiotic," she added in a release.

Previous research has also suggested early antibiotic use may be linked to an increased risk of asthma, but some studies relied on parents recalling what antibiotics their children were given after the youngsters had grown up.

In the June 2007 issue of the journal *Chest*, the researchers found 6 percent of children had asthma at age seven. Reasons for antibiotic during the first year of life included:

- otitis media or middle-ear infection—40 percent;

- other upper respiratory tract infections such as bronchitis or pneumonia—28 percent;

- lower respiratory tract infections—19 percent;

- non–respiratory tract infections such as urinary infections—7 percent.

The risk for asthma rose as the number of antibiotic prescriptions went up, with children who had more than four courses showing 1.5 times the risk of the lung condition compared with those who did not receive any antibiotics.

Children who received multiple courses of antibiotics and were born to women without a history of asthma were twice as likely to develop the condition than those who never received the drugs.

"Understanding the relationship between antibiotic use and asthma can help clinicians make more informed decisions about treatment options for children," said Dr. Mark Rosen, president of the American College of Chest Physicians, which publishes the journal.

Fido Favored

Asthma risk also appeared to be doubled among children who did not have a family dog during their first year of life.

"Dogs bring germs into the home, and it is thought that this exposure is required for the infant's immune system to develop normally," Kozyrskyj said. "Exposure to germs is lower in the absence of a dog. The administration of an antibiotic may further reduce this exposure and increase the likelihood of asthma development."

A ten-year study published in 2002 also suggested that infants who live in homes with two or more cats or dogs appeared to be at lower risk for developing allergic reactions that may lead to asthma.

The researchers also accounted for asthma risk factors such as gender, urban or rural location, neighborhood income, and number of siblings.

Chapter 3

Do Dietary Factors Contribute to the Development of Asthma?

Chapter Contents

Section 3.1

Imbalanced Diet and Inadequate Exercise May Underlie Asthma

"Metabolic Link to Asthma Seen in Children," September 16, 2010, West Virginia University Health News, © 2010 West Virginia University Robert C. Byrd Health Sciences Center (www.hsc.wvu.edu). All rights reserved. Reprinted with permission.

Children of any weight who have an imbalanced metabolism due to poor diet or exercise may be at increased risk of asthma, according to new research at West Virginia University (WVU). The findings, derived from data on nearly eighteen thousand West Virginia children, challenge the widespread assumption that obesity itself is a risk factor for asthma.

"Our research showed that early abnormalities in lipid and/or glucose metabolism may be associated to the development of asthma in childhood," said Giovanni Piedimonte, M.D., chairman of pediatrics at WVU and physician-in-chief at WVU Children's Hospital, who led the study. "Our findings also imply a strong and direct influence of metabolic pathways on the immune mechanisms involved in the pathogenesis of asthma in children."

The research, which was published online September 16, 2010, ahead of the print edition of the American Thoracic Society's *American Journal of Respiratory and Critical Care Medicine*, implicates metabolic disorders directly in the development of asthma, and points to a new way of viewing diet and lifestyle as risk factors for asthma, even in children who are not obviously obese or overweight.

"The key takeaway message for parents is this: there's one more good reason to make sure your children eat healthy and exercise," said WVU pediatric researcher Lesley Cottrell, Ph.D. "Even healthy-looking children can be at higher risk for asthma if they are sedentary and have a poor diet."

The researchers gathered demographic data, estimates of body mass index, and asthma prevalence on thousands of children who were four to twelve years old and were participating in WVU's long-running Coronary Artery Risk Detection in Appalachian Communities Project. The large sample size is unusual in pediatric research.

The researchers found that while asthma prevalence generally increased with increasing body mass index (BMI), asthma prevalence in obese and morbidly obese children was significantly higher than in children with healthy BMI. Simple overweight status did not appear to be linked to increased asthma prevalence. However, after controlling for BMI and other confounding variables, asthma prevalence was significantly associated with triglyceride levels and the presence of a biomarker for diabetes, regardless of body weight.

"The association between asthma risk, triglyceride levels, and the diabetes marker, even among children who are a healthy weight or underweight, suggests that a subtle metabolic dysfunction may exist that is a central hub from which the asthma-obesity-diabetes triad originates, at least in a subpopulation of patients," said Dr. Piedimonte. "This opens a Pandora's box of questions concerning the role of pre- and early post-natal nutrition as a critical determinant of chronic diseases throughout life."

The article, "Metabolic Abnormalities in Children with Asthma," was authored by Drs. Cottrell and Piedimonte, along with William Neal, M.D., Christa Ice, Ph.D. and Miriam Perez, M.D., all of the WVU Department of Pediatrics and Pediatric Research Institute.

Section 3.2

Diet and Asthma: Some Research Results

"Diet and Asthma: Looking Back, Moving Forward," by June-Ho Kim, Philippa E. Ellwood, and M. Innes Asher. *Respiratory Research*, Volume 10, 2009. © 2009 Kim et al. All rights reserved.

Abstract

Asthma is an increasing global health burden, especially in the western world. Public health interventions are sought to lessen its prevalence or severity, and diet and nutrition have been identified as potential factors. With rapid changes in diet being one of the hallmarks of westernization, nutrition may play a key role in affecting the complex genetics and developmental pathophysiology of asthma. The present review investigates hypotheses about hygiene, antioxidants, lipids and other nutrients, food types and dietary patterns, breastfeeding, probiotics and intestinal microbiota, vitamin D, maternal diet, and genetics. Early hypotheses analyzed population level trends and focused on major dietary factors such as antioxidants and lipids. More recently, larger dietary patterns beyond individual nutrients have been investigated such as obesity, fast foods, and the Mediterranean diet. Despite some promising hypotheses and findings, there has been no conclusive evidence about the role of specific nutrients, food types, or dietary patterns past early childhood on asthma prevalence. However, diet has been linked to the development of the fetus and child. Breastfeeding provides immunological protection when the infant's immune system is immature and a modest protective effect against wheeze in early childhood. Moreover, maternal diet may be a significant factor in the development of the fetal airway and immune system. As asthma is a complex disease of gene-environment interactions, maternal diet may play an epigenetic role in sensitizing fetal airways to respond abnormally to environmental insults. Recent hypotheses show promise in a biological approach in which the effects of dietary factors on individual physiology and immunology are analyzed before expansion into larger population studies. Thus, collaboration is required by various groups in studying this enigma from epidemiologists to geneticists to immunologists. It is now apparent that this multidisciplinary approach is required to move forward and understand the complexity of the interaction of dietary factors and asthma.

Introduction

Asthma, particularly among children, has grown in prevalence and as a worldwide public health burden,[1] but has been an elusive target for public health interventions. Dietary factors have been a focus at both the cellular and population levels, and several theories have been proposed or abandoned, though no clear answer has emerged.[2-12] This review highlights the development of major promising hypotheses about diet and asthma and possible paths for future investigation.

Nature to Nurture

Asthma is an allergic disease of complex gene-environment interactions.[13-15] Twin studies show that over 70 percent of the variation in asthmatic tendency is explained by genetic factors, and several contributing genes have been identified.[16,17] However, individual genes have been ineffective in altering the expression of asthma, indicating the necessity of environmental factors.[14] Rapid increases in worldwide asthma prevalence in only the past couple decades, especially in westernized countries, signal an important role of the environment.[12]

It is known that environmental factors affect gene expression and manifestation of disease. Early fetal exposures to nutrition and other environmental factors may program organ development and future development of disease. For example, severe fetal malnutrition has been linked to increased risk for health problems in adulthood.[18] Thus, nutrition and diet may be important to the development of asthma through epigenetic effects. With rapid changes in diet as a hallmark of westernization, dietary factors may indeed play a key role in affecting the complex genetics and developmental pathophysiology of asthma.

Early Dietary Hypotheses

It is important to look back on the progression of dietary studies over the years to see how theories have evolved and adapted as new evidence has been brought forth and new ideas proposed.

Hygiene Hypothesis

Increased westernization and the correlated rise in asthma prevalence have prompted investigation of environmental factors related to westernization. One of the earliest theories became known as the "hygiene hypothesis," which suggested that increasing "cleanliness" and lack of exposure to infections at a critical point in the development of the immune system may lead to an increased risk of asthma and other atopic diseases.[19] This hypothesis has not been well supported by evidence, such as an increase of asthma in North and South American inner cities that are generally characterized by poor housing and a dirty environment.[12,20,21]

Antioxidant Hypothesis

Seaton et al. 1994 hypothesized that alteration in diet associated with westernization may be responsible for the increase in asthma prevalence.[22] Observations showed that consumption of foods rich in antioxidants had decreased in the United Kingdom diet while asthma prevalence rose. Thus the promising hypothesis was put forth that populations had become more susceptible to respiratory disease due to dietary antioxidant omission.

Antioxidant studies have focused on vitamin C, vitamin E, carotenoids, flavonoids, and antioxidant nutrients such as selenium and zinc. A wide range of cross-sectional studies has been done on the relationship of antioxidants with asthma. Vitamin C, beta-carotene, magnesium, and selenium were associated with reduction in asthma prevalence[23-27] and may prevent or limit an inflammatory response in the airways by reducing reactive oxygen species and inhibiting lipid peroxidation. Flavonoids may also be potential anti-allergic substances,[28] and a recent study on enzymatic and nonenzymatic antioxidant systems in childhood asthma suggested that antioxidant defenses such as glutathione peroxidase and superoxide dismutase were lowered in asthmatic children.[29]

However, not all studies on the role of antioxidants have been positive. A meta-analysis determined that dietary intake of antioxidants vitamins C and E and beta-carotene does not significantly influence the risk of asthma.[30] Furthermore, many studies have shown no association between selenium and asthma.[31] However, these results may still have significance in light of biological studies that show that selenium acts as an antioxidant but can also upregulate immune responses that characterize allergic asthma—a more complex effect that cannot be explained just by case-control studies.[32] The potential role of antioxidants as supplements has been explored,[33] but a number of studies have been inconclusive.[34] Overall, supplementation studies have suggested a minor role for individual antioxidants in asthma prevention,[4] perhaps working in larger food groups instead—the source of Seaton's original study.

Lipid Hypothesis

In 1997, Black and Sharpe cited evidence, which contradicted the antioxidant hypothesis, instead proposing that the rise of asthma prevalence may have stemmed from increased consumption of polyunsaturated fatty acids (PUFAs) and decreased consumption of saturated fat.[35] The omega-6 PUFAs may particularly have a role in regulating immune response and inflammation. These PUFAs are found largely as linoleic acid in foods such as margarine and vegetable oils, which have risen in consumption with westernization. Linoleic acid is a precursor of arachidonic acid that is converted into prostaglandin E2 (PGE2), which inhibits interferon-gamma and promotes an inflammatory environment that favors asthma development. Meanwhile, omega-3 PUFAs may have an anti-inflammatory role. Thus, the increase in omega-6 PUFA and decrease in omega-3 PUFA consumption may immunologically increase the susceptibility of the population. PUFAs may have other immunosuppressive mechanisms that require further study.[36]

Investigation of the lipid hypothesis found mixed results. A number of cross-sectional studies showed beneficial associations between foods containing omega-3 PUFAs and asthma, but studies on cord blood PUFA composition and development of atopic disease have been inconclusive.[5] There have been conflicting reports on the relationship between levels of PUFAs and wheeze.[37,38] Disappointingly, intervention studies have not found consistent results nor provided sufficient support for dietary supplementation with PUFAs.[36,37,39–41]

Other Nutrients

Other nutritional factors have recently been investigated using various methods ranging from cohort studies to ecological analyses with populations from schoolchildren to entire nations.

A sodium hypothesis was proposed in 1987 based on a correlation between table salt purchases and asthma mortality.[42] Sodium intake could potentially exacerbate asthma as hypersensitized bronchial smooth muscle could be leaky to sodium and thus lead to hyperpolarization of the muscle in response to increased sodium intake.[43] However, there is no clear relationship between airway responsiveness (a surrogate for asthma) and urinary sodium excretion (an indicator of sodium intake).[44] A more recent trial, in which participants adopted a variable sodium diet based on supplements or placebo, found no benefit for asthma either.[45]

Magnesium has been implicated through its possible effects on bronchial smooth muscle. Low magnesium intake has been correlated with decreased lung function in children,[46] and intravenous magnesium is recommended to control acute severe asthma in many emergency departments.[47] Nevertheless, due to a paucity of studies on magnesium and asthma prevalence, its importance remains to be seen.

Food Types and Dietary Patterns

Larger food groups have been studied as possible examples of synergy among multiple nutrients. Fruits and vegetables have been extensively studied as potent sources of antioxidants. A low dietary intake of fruit was associated with asthma in Norwich, United Kingdom.[25] Several other cross-sectional studies have indicated an inverse association between consumption of fruits and vegetables and symptoms of asthma, though the particular foods and symptoms varied.[8,48–52] Moving beyond individual country studies, Ellwood et al. conducted an ecological analysis on data from centers in fifty-three countries in the International Study of Asthma and Allergies in Childhood (ISAAC), which not only looked at single countries, but also compared diet and asthma globally using asthma prevalence data from ISAAC and dietary data from the Food and Agriculture Organization of the United Nations.[53] Together, these data suggested an inverse relationship between asthma prevalence rates and intake of vegetables and foods of plant origin such as starch and cereals. However, a smaller study of Dutch children found no clear association between fruit and vegetable intake and asthma symptoms.[54] Despite the plethora of cross-sectional data about fruits and vegetables, there is a lack of longitudinal studies and analyses to form a causal link between these foods and asthma prevalence.

The hypothesis of westernized diets affecting asthma prevalence has prompted studies of fast foods, Mediterranean diet, and obesity as potential factors. A cross-sectional study of children in Hastings, New Zealand, showed that hamburger consumption positively associated with asthma symptoms while takeaway consumption had a marginal effect on bronchial hyperresponsiveness.[55]

The Mediterranean diet, on the other hand, has been suggested as a healthy dietary pattern that may reduce the risk of asthma. In fact,

ISAAC data indicated lower asthma prevalence in Mediterranean countries with diet as a possible variable to explain this disparity.[1,56,57] There is a consistent relationship between a Mediterranean diet and asthma symptoms.[48,57,58] But additional studies are necessary to corroborate this association and define a possible mechanism.

Lastly, obesity is a major factor of diet that may have a role in asthma. Its role has been controversial as, yet again, different studies have found contrasting results.[58] Epidemiologic studies have suggested that asthma is more prevalent among obese than lean individuals. It is unclear, however, whether obesity merely exacerbates the asthmatic symptoms, creates susceptibility to onset of asthma, or develops concurrently with the respiratory disease. Obesity could have potential biological effects on lung function and systematic inflammation while also sharing certain co-morbidities and etiologies with asthma.[59] Nevertheless, the relationship between obesity and asthma remains an enigma despite evidence of a connection.

Overall, interesting hypotheses and some promising positive findings have made no definitive conclusions about the role of specific nutrients, food types, or dietary patterns on asthma prevalence.

Evolution of Dietary Hypotheses and Studies

Recent work has linked diet to the development of the fetus and child—an extrapolation from studies on other diseases indicating an effect of early diet on later onset of disease. This "thrifty phenotype hypothesis" argues that poor nutrition in early life is epidemiologically associated with poor fetal and infant growth and subsequent development of type 2 diabetes.[60] A large body of evidence shows that the intrauterine and early childhood environments are crucial for development of diabetes and coronary heart disease, and asthma has been increasingly included in a similar category of diseases "programmed" in utero,[61] hinting at a possible epigenetic component. This developmental model of the origins of disease possesses a variety of subcategories that have been recently explored for asthma from breastfeeding and intestinal microbiota to maternal nutrition.

Breastfeeding

Breastfeeding provides infants with nutrients for growth, development, and immunological protection during a critical period of the infant's life when its own immune system is immature.[62,63] There are many questions about exclusive breastfeeding over infant formula and the optimal length of breastfeeding in asthma development. A

2004 cohort study showed exclusive breastfeeding for more than four months reduced the risk of asthma at the child's age of four.[64] A separate 2008 cohort report on the Avon Longitudinal Study of Parents and Children (ALSPAC) agrees that breastfeeding has a modest protective effect against wheeze and asthma in early childhood.[65] However, the study found that this effect did not last beyond the sixth year of life. Despite some positive studies, others have seen an entirely converse effect,[66] leading to some heated controversy about breastfeeding recommendations.[67,68]

Breastfeeding is complex in its effects on the immunological health of the child. Regardless, not enough evidence exists to recommend guidelines for breastfeeding for asthma prevention.

Probiotics and Intestinal Microbiota

Breastfeeding is well known to modify the intestinal composition of commensal bacteria, which drives immune development in the infant. For example, exclusively formula-fed infants possessed more colonies of *E coli, C difficile, Bacteroides*, and lactobacilli compared to breastfed infants.[69] Instead, breastfed infants had the most potentially beneficial intestinal microbiota. The human gastrointestinal tract is sterile at birth, rapidly undergoing colonization of the gut with subsequent development of the immune system. Studies have shown that there are obvious differences in the composition of intestinal microbiota between healthy and allergic infants within the first week of life and before clinical symptoms for the latter group, suggesting that modifying microbiota composition may affect disease outcome.[70]

Probiotics are dietary supplements that contain beneficial bacteria such as *Lactobacillus GG* and may be effective in preventing early atopy in children through the modulation of intestinal microbiota.[71] Probiotics may enhance immunoglobulin A (IgA) responses in the gut as well as regulate inflammatory cytokines, both immunomodulatory effects that could prevent progression of atopy and potentially development of disease. Further study, possibly large-scale birth cohort analyses using molecular methods to test for microbiota,[72] is required before any recommendations can be given about probiotic administration for asthma prevention.

Vitamin D

Recently, Litonjua and Weiss hypothesized that vitamin D deficiency can increase the incidence of asthma in young children.[73,74] This idea stemmed from the discovery that the vitamin D receptor gene was associated with asthma.[75] (Albeit, more genetic work is necessary to clarify this since vitamin D receptor knockout mice do not develop the murine model for asthma.[76]) Vitamin D does not occur naturally in humans and is acquired through supplements and exposure to sunlight. The rise of asthma in westernized countries may be linked to the fact that people spend much more time indoors and away from sunlight. Furthermore, vitamin D has significant immunomodulatory functions through control of T regulatory cells, which modulate levels of CD4+ helper T cells. Vitamin D receptors have been identified in various immune cells from T cells to dendritic cells that have a potential role in asthma pathogenesis.

Observational studies in the United States and the United Kingdom have reported that maternal intake of vitamin D during pregnancy was associated with lung function, suggesting that increased vitamin D in maternal diet may reduce risk of wheeze and other symptoms of asthma.[77,78] As with other hypotheses, supplementation studies are necessary, especially in pregnancy.

Maternal Diet Hypothesis

Extending the "thrifty phenotype hypothesis" by Barker et al,[79,80] maternal nutrition has been recognized as a potential (and potent) factor in the development of the fetal airway and immune system. Nutrients during pregnancy may affect T helper cell differentiation toward a Th2 bias through cytokine regulation and promote normal airway formation in the fetus.[3]

With the prospect that diet during pregnancy may be more important than at any other point in life, many nutrients such as antioxidants and lipids have been tested. In 2002, Devereux et al found that increased maternal intake of vitamin E was associated with decreased proliferation of cord blood mononuclear cells in response to allergens, suggesting a beneficial effect of maternal nutrition against atopy.[81] Two separate maternal antioxidant studies showed an inverse relationship of antioxidants vitamin E, vitamin C, and zinc with wheeze.[82,83] The selenium status of a cohort of two thousand pregnant mothers was also inversely associated with wheezing in the child,[84] but this disappeared after the age of five years. While these results indicate a possible role of maternal intake of certain antioxidants, more studies are necessary to confirm this. Studying the effects of maternal PUFA intake has been sparser, largely tested through analysis of maternal fish consumption. One such study found that maternal oily fish consumption during pregnancy was protective for childhood asthma, particularly in children who have asthmatic mothers.[85] In keeping with many other diet studies, however, a longitudinal study of maternal consumption of various food types found no association between fish intake and asthma outcomes in children.[86] There was also no association between asthma and maternal consumption of foods such as vegetables, egg, and dairy. In contrast to the more specific antioxidant and vitamin D studies, the effect of broader food groups on asthma outcomes seems less significant.[87]

There is an obvious need for more intervention studies on dietary supplementation using nutrients and factors that have potential to impact the intrauterine environment and fetal immune and lung development.[88] Further understanding of dietary immunomodulation of the pregnant uterus is necessary.[41] With exciting developments elucidating the relationship between the in utero environment and subsequent onset of complex diseases, there is further motivation to explore the impact of diet on fetal development and risk of asthma.

Conclusion: The Road Ahead

Asthma is complex: comprised of a heterogeneous variety of diseases, initiated by disparate genetic and environmental factors, and unified by common symptoms such as airway constriction and wheeze.[89] Diet could modulate epigenetics, intestinal microbiota, physiological development, airway remodeling, and immune maturation—factors highly relevant to the etiology of asthma. Yet the literature on diet and asthma is "fragmentary and hard to summarize in a systematic way and difficulties with many small studies leave unexplained contradictions in the literature."[10]

Such complexity makes for a daunting task of identifying pathways for future intervention. Evidence for nutrient supplementation after early childhood to support any primary prevention is weak. A greater understanding of maternal diet is necessary, particularly for antioxidants and vitamin D, perhaps by supplementing pregnant mothers with vitamin D and following their children through childhood.[73] Additionally, mechanistic studies are needed through gene expression and association studies. Explaining the downstream effects of vitamin D on infant physiology and immunology is crucial to vetting vitamin D as a possible intervention. One novel approach may be through genetic epidemiology using DNA collected from cohorts to analyze the effect of a modifiable factor by measuring variations in relevant genes.[90] Lastly, more extensive animal studies are necessary. There have been many diet-related studies using murine models of asthma. Admittedly, such models are relatively weak. Nevertheless, discoveries in a controlled animal model environment have advantages over the epidemiological approach in pursuing specific modalities.[28,91,92]

Historically, studies have started from a population level formed from trends seen at the macro level with molecular mechanisms generally analyzed afterwards. With vitamin D[73] and maternal diet,[3,80] there is a subtle but important difference in approach: mechanistic hypotheses at the micro level are now being expanded into larger clinical and population-based studies. Though it is still too early to determine if such an approach is beneficial, early indications are promising.

On the road ahead, if hypotheses are to be derived from the micro level, there is need for more collaboration amongst various groups from epidemiologists to geneticists to immunologists. As we look back and move forwards, a multidisciplinary approach is increasingly necessary to understand the complexity of dietary factors and asthma.

References

1. Asher MI, Montefort S, Bjorksten B, Lai CK, Strachan DP, Weiland SK, Williams H. Worldwide time trends in the prevalence of symptoms of asthma, allergic rhinoconjunctivitis, and eczema in childhood: ISAAC Phases One and Three repeat multicountry cross-sectional surveys. *Lancet* 2006, 368(9537):733–43.

2. Baker JC, Ayres JG. Diet and asthma. *Respir Med* 2000, 94(10):925–34.

3. Devereux G. The increase in the prevalence of asthma and allergy: food for thought. *Nat Rev Immunol* 2006, 6(11):869–74.

4. Devereux G. Early life events in asthma—diet. *Pediatr Pulmonol* 2007, 42(8):663–73.

5. Devereux G, Seaton A. Diet as a risk factor for atopy and asthma. *J Allergy Clin Immunol* 2005, 115(6):1109–17.

6. Fogarty A, Britton J. The role of diet in the aetiology of asthma. *Clin Exp Allergy* 2000, 30(5):615–27.

7. Litonjua AA. Dietary factors and the development of asthma. *Immunol Allergy Clin North Am* 2008, 28(3):603–29.

8. McKeever TM, Britton J. Diet and asthma. *Am J Respir Crit Care Med* 2004, 170(7):725–29.

9. Romieu I, Trenga C. Diet and obstructive lung diseases. *Epidemiol Rev* 2001, 23(2):268–87.

10. S. Tricon et al. Nutrition and allergic disease. *Clinical & Experimental Allergy Reviews* 2006, 6(5):117–88.

11. Seaton A. From nurture to Nature—the story of the Aberdeen asthma dietary hypothesis. *QJM* 2008, 101(3):237–39.

12. Cooper PJ, Rodrigues LC, Cruz AA, Barreto ML. Asthma in Latin America: a public health challenge and research opportunity. *Allergy* 2009, 64(1):5–17.

13. Miller RL, Ho SM. Environmental epigenetics and asthma: current concepts and call for studies. *Am J Respir Crit Care Med* 2008, 177(6):567–73.

14. Castro-Giner F, Kauffmann F, de Cid R, Kogevinas M. Gene-environment interactions in asthma. *Occup Environ Med* 2006, 63(11):776–86.

15. Martinez FD. Gene-environment interactions in asthma: with apologies to William of Ockham. *Proc Am Thorac Soc* 2007, 4(1):26–31.

16. Sandford AJ, Pare PD. The genetics of asthma. The important questions. *Am J Respir Crit Care Med* 2000, 161(3 Pt 2):S202–6.

17. Skadhauge LR, Christensen K, Kyvik KO, Sigsgaard T. Genetic and environmental influence on asthma: a population-based study of 11,688 Danish twin pairs. *Eur Respir J* 1999, 13(1):8–14.

18. Hales CN, Barker DJ, Clark PM, Cox LJ, Fall C, Osmond C, Winter PD. Fetal and infant growth and impaired glucose tolerance at age 64. *BMJ* 1991, 303(6809):1019–22.

19. Cabana MD, McKean M, Wong AR, Chao C, Caughey AB. Examining the hygiene hypothesis: the Trial of Infant Probiotic Supplementation. *Paediatr Perinat Epidemiol* 2007, 21(Suppl 3):23–28.

20. Platts-Mills TA, Erwin E, Heymann P, Woodfolk J. Is the hygiene hypothesis still a viable explanation for the increased prevalence of asthma? *Allergy* 2005, 60(Suppl 79):25–31.

21. Platts-Mills TA, Woodfolk JA, Sporik RB. Con: the increase in asthma cannot be ascribed to cleanliness. *Am J Respir Crit Care Med* 2001, 164(7):1107–8.

22. Seaton A, Godden DJ, Brown K. Increase in asthma: a more toxic environment or a more susceptible population? *Thorax* 1994, 49(2):171–74.

23. Burns JS, Dockery DW, Neas LM, Schwartz J, Coull BA, Raizenne M, Speizer FE. Low dietary nutrient intakes and respiratory health in adolescents. *Chest* 2007, 132(1):238–45.

24. Greer FR, Sicherer SH, Burks AW. Effects of early nutritional interventions on the development of atopic disease in infants and children: the role of maternal dietary restriction, breast-feeding, timing of introduction of complementary foods, and hydrolyzed formulas. *Pediatrics* 2008, 121(1):183–91.

25. Patel BD, Welch AA, Bingham SA, Luben RN, Day NE, Khaw KT, Lomas DA, Wareham NJ. Dietary antioxidants and asthma in adults. *Thorax* 2006, 61(5):388–93.

26. Rubin RN, Navon L, Cassano PA. Relationship of serum anti-oxidants to asthma prevalence in youth. *Am J Respir Crit Care Med* 2004, 169(3):393–98.

27. Kalayci O, Besler T, Kilinc K, Sekerel BE, Saraclar Y. Serum levels of antioxidant vitamins (alpha tocopherol, beta carotene, and ascorbic acid) in children with bronchial asthma. *Turk J Pediatr* 2000, 42(1):17–21.

28. Kawai M, Hirano T, Higa S, Arimitsu J, Maruta M, Kuwahara Y, Ohkawara T, Hagihara K, Yamadori T, Shima Y, et al. Flavonoids and related compounds as anti-allergic substances. *Allergol Int* 2007, 56(2):113–23.

29. Sackesen C, Ercan H, Dizdar E, Soyer O, Gumus P, Tosun BN, Buyuktuncer Z, Karabulut E, Besler T, Kalayci O. A comprehensive evaluation of the enzymatic and nonenzymatic antioxidant systems in childhood asthma. *J Allergy Clin Immunol* 2008, 122(1):78–85.

30. Gao J, Gao X, Li W, Zhu Y, Thompson PJ. Observational studies on the effect of dietary antioxidants on asthma: a meta-analysis. *Respirology* 2008, 13(4):528–36.

31. Feary J, Britton J. Dietary supplements and asthma: another one bites the dust. *Thorax* 2007, 62(6):466–68.

32. Hoffmann PR. Selenium and asthma: a complex relationship. *Allergy* 2008, 63(7):854–56.

33. Trenga CA, Koenig JQ, Williams PV. Dietary antioxidants and ozone-induced bronchial hyperresponsiveness in adults with asthma. *Arch Environ Health* 2001, 56(3):242–49.

34. Kaur B, Rowe BH, Ram FS. Vitamin C supplementation for asthma. *Cochrane Database Syst Rev* 2001, (4):CD000993.

35. Black PN, Sharpe S. Dietary fat and asthma: is there a connection? *Eur Respir J* 1997, 10(1):6–12.

36. Shaikh SR, Edidin M. Polyunsaturated fatty acids and membrane organization: elucidating mechanisms to balance immunotherapy and susceptibility to infection. *Chem Phys Lipids* 2008, 153(1):24–33.

37. Almqvist C, Garden F, Xuan W, Mihrshahi S, Leeder SR, Oddy W, Webb K, Marks GB. Omega-3 and omega-6 fatty acid exposure from early life does not affect atopy and asthma at age 5 years. *J Allergy Clin Immunol* 2007, 119(6):1438–44.

38. Mihrshahi S, Peat JK, Marks GB, Mellis CM, Tovey ER, Webb K, Britton WJ, Leeder SR. Eighteen-month outcomes of house dust mite avoidance and dietary fatty acid modification in the Childhood Asthma Prevention Study (CAPS). *J Allergy Clin Immunol* 2003, 111(1):162–68.

39. Blumer N, Renz H. Consumption of omega3-fatty acids during perinatal life: role in immuno-modulation and allergy prevention. *J Perinat Med* 2007, 35(Suppl 1):S12–18.

40. Miyake Y, Sasaki S, Tanaka K, Ohya Y, Miyamoto S, Matsunaga I, Yoshida T, Hirota Y, Oda H. Fish and fat intake and prevalence of allergic rhinitis in Japanese females: the Osaka Maternal and Child Health Study. *J Am Coll Nutr* 2007, 26(3):279–87.

41. de Vries A, Howie SE. Diet and asthma—Can you change what you or your children are by changing what you eat? *Pharmacol Ther* 2009, 122(1):78–82.

42. Burney P. A diet rich in sodium may potentiate asthma. Epidemiologic evidence for a new hypothesis. *Chest* 1987, 91(6 Suppl):143S–48S.

43. Burney PG. The causes of asthma—does salt potentiate bronchial activity? Discussion paper. *J R Soc Med* 1987, 80(6):364–67.

44. Devereux G, Beach JR, Bromly C, Avery AJ, Ayatollahi SM, Williams SM, Stenton SC, Bourke SJ, Hendrick DJ. Effect of dietary sodium on airways responsiveness and its importance in the epidemiology of asthma: an evaluation in three areas of northern England. *Thorax* 1995, 50(9):941–47.

45. Pogson ZE, Antoniak MD, Pacey SJ, Lewis SA, Britton JR, Fogarty AW. Does a low sodium diet improve asthma control? A randomized controlled trial. *Am J Respir Crit Care Med* 2008, 178(2):132–38.

46. Gilliland FD, Berhane KT, Li YF, Kim DH, Margolis HG. Dietary magnesium, potassium, sodium, and children's lung function. *Am J Epidemiol* 2002, 155(2):125–31.

47. Beasley R, Aldington S. Magnesium in the treatment of asthma. *Curr Opin Allergy Clin Immunol* 2007, 7(1):107–10.

48. Chatzi L, Apostolaki G, Bibakis I, Skypala I, Bibaki-Liakou V, Tzanakis N, Kogevinas M, Cullinan P. Protective effect of fruits, vegetables and the Mediterranean diet on asthma and allergies among children in Crete. *Thorax* 2007, 62(8):677–83.

49. Chatzi L, Torrent M, Romieu I, Garcia-Esteban R, Ferrer C, Vioque J, Kogevinas M, Sunyer J. Diet, wheeze, and atopy in school children in Menorca, Spain. *Pediatr Allergy Immunol* 2007, 18(6):480–85.

50. Shaheen SO, Sterne JA, Thompson RL, Songhurst CE, Margetts BM, Burney PG. Dietary antioxidants and asthma in adults: population-based case-control study. *Am J Respir Crit Care Med* 2001, 164(10 Pt 1):1823–28.

51. Tsai HJ, Tsai AC. The association of diet with respiratory symptoms and asthma in schoolchildren in Taipei, Taiwan. *J Asthma* 2007, 44(8):599–603.

52. Okoko BJ, Burney PG, Newson RB, Potts JF, Shaheen SO. Childhood asthma and fruit consumption. *Eur Respir J* 2007, 29(6):1161–68.

53. Ellwood P, Asher MI, Bjorksten B, Burr M, Pearce N, Robertson CF. Diet and asthma, allergic rhinoconjunctivitis and atopic eczema symptom prevalence: an ecological analysis of the International Study of Asthma and Allergies in Childhood (ISAAC) data. ISAAC Phase One Study Group. *Eur Respir J* 2001, 17(3):436–43.

54. Tabak C, Wijga AH, de Meer G, Janssen NA, Brunekreef B, Smit HA. Diet and asthma in Dutch school children (ISAAC-2). *Thorax* 2006, 61(12):1048–53.

55. Wickens K, Barry D, Friezema A, Rhodius R, Bone N, Purdie G, Crane J. Fast foods—are they a risk factor for asthma? *Allergy* 2005, 60(12):1537–41.

56. Worldwide variations in the prevalence of asthma symptoms: the International Study of Asthma and Allergies in Childhood (ISAAC) *Eur Respir J* 1998, 12(2):315–35.

57. Castro-Rodriguez JA, Garcia-Marcos L, Alfonseda Rojas JD, Valverde-Molina J, Sanchez-Solis M. Mediterranean diet as a protective factor for wheezing in preschool children. *J Pediatr* 2008, 152(6):823–28.

58. Garcia-Marcos L, Canflanca IM, Garrido JB, Varela AL, Garcia-Hernandez G, Guillen Grima F, Gonzalez-Diaz C, Carvajal-Uruena I, Arnedo-Pena A, Busquets-Monge RM, et al. Relationship of asthma and rhinoconjunctivitis with obesity, exercise and Mediterranean diet in Spanish school-children. *Thorax* 2007, 62(6):503–8.

59. Shore SA. Obesity and asthma: possible mechanisms. *J Allergy Clin Immunol* 2008, 121(5):1087–93.

60. Hales CN, Barker DJ. The thrifty phenotype hypothesis. *Br Med Bull* 2001, 60:5–20.

61. Barker DJ. Fetal and infant origins of adult disease. *Monatsschr Kinderheilkd* 2001, 149:S2–S6.

62. Hoppu U, Kalliomaki M, Laiho K, Isolauri E. Breast milk—immunomodulatory signals against allergic diseases. *Allergy* 2001, 56(Suppl 67):23–26.

63. Rosetta L, Baldi A. On the role of breastfeeding in health promotion and the prevention of allergic diseases. *Adv Exp Med Biol* 2008, 606:467–83.

64. Kull I, Almqvist C, Lilja G, Pershagen G, Wickman M. Breast-feeding reduces the risk of asthma during the first 4 years of life. *J Allergy Clin Immunol* 2004, 114(4):755–60.

65. Elliott L, Henderson J, Northstone K, Chiu GY, Dunson D, London SJ. Prospective study of breast-feeding in relation to wheeze, atopy, and bronchial hyperresponsiveness in the Avon Longitudinal Study of Parents and Children (ALSPAC). *J Allergy Clin Immunol* 2008, 122(1):49–54.

66. Sears MR, Greene JM, Willan AR, Taylor DR, Flannery EM, Cowan JO, Herbison GP, Poulton R. Long-term relation between breastfeeding and development of atopy and asthma in children and young adults: a longitudinal study. *Lancet* 2002, 360(9337):901–7.

67. Peat JK, Allen J, Oddy W, Webb K. Breastfeeding and asthma: appraising the controversy. *Pediatr Pulmonol* 2003, 35(5):331–34.

68. Sears MR, Taylor DR, Poulton R. Breastfeeding and asthma: appraising the controversy—a rebuttal. *Pediatr Pulmonol* 2003, 36(5):366–68.

69. Penders J, Thijs C, Vink C, Stelma FF, Snijders B, Kummeling I, Brandt PA, Stobberingh EE. Factors influencing the composition of the intestinal microbiota in early infancy. *Pediatrics* 2006, 118(2):511–21.

70. Bjorksten B. Effects of intestinal microflora and the environment on the development of asthma and allergy. *Springer Semin Immunopathol* 2004, 25(3–4):257–70.

71. Kalliomaki M, Salminen S, Arvilommi H, Kero P, Koskinen P, Isolauri E. Probiotics in primary prevention of atopic disease: a randomised placebo-controlled trial. *Lancet* 2001, 357(9262):1076–79.

72. Penders J, Stobberingh EE, Brandt PA, Thijs C. The role of the intestinal microbiota in the development of atopic disorders. *Allergy* 2007, 62(11):1223–36.

73. Litonjua AA, Weiss ST. Is vitamin D deficiency to blame for the asthma epidemic? *J Allergy Clin Immunol* 2007, 120(5):1031–35.

74. Weiss ST, Litonjua AA. Maternal diet vs lack of exposure to sunlight as the cause of the epidemic of asthma, allergies and other autoimmune diseases. *Thorax* 2007, 62(9):746–48.

75. Raby BA, Lazarus R, Silverman EK, Lake S, Lange C, Wjst M, Weiss ST. Association of vitamin D receptor gene polymorphisms with childhood and adult asthma. *Am J Respir Crit Care Med* 2004, 170(10):1057–65.

76. Wittke A, Weaver V, Mahon BD, August A, Cantorna MT. Vitamin D receptor-deficient mice fail to develop experimental allergic asthma. *J Immunol* 2004, 173(5):3432–36.

77. Camargo CA Jr, Rifas-Shiman SL, Litonjua AA, Rich-Edwards JW, Weiss ST, Gold DR, Kleinman K, Gillman MW. Maternal intake of vitamin D during pregnancy and risk of recurrent wheeze in children at 3 y of age. *Am J Clin Nutr* 2007, 85(3):788–95.

78. Devereux G, Litonjua AA, Turner SW, Craig LC, McNeill G, Martindale S, Helms PJ, Seaton A, Weiss ST. Maternal vitamin

D intake during pregnancy and early childhood wheezing. *Am J Clin Nutr* 2007, 85(3):853–59.

79. Hales CN, Barker DJ. Type 2 (non-insulin-dependent) diabetes mellitus: the thrifty phenotype hypothesis. *Diabetologia* 1992, 35(7):595–601.

80. Barker DJ. Maternal nutrition, fetal nutrition, and disease in later life. *Nutrition* 1997, 13(9):807–13.

81. Devereux G, Barker RN, Seaton A. Antenatal determinants of neonatal immune responses to allergens. *Clin Exp Allergy* 2002, 32(1):43–50.

82. Litonjua AA, Rifas-Shiman SL, Ly NP, Tantisira KG, Rich-Edwards JW, Camargo CA Jr, Weiss ST, Gillman MW, Gold DR. Maternal antioxidant intake in pregnancy and wheezing illnesses in children at 2 y of age. *Am J Clin Nutr* 2006, 84(4):903–11.

83. Martindale S, McNeill G, Devereux G, Campbell D, Russell G, Seaton A. Antioxidant intake in pregnancy in relation to wheeze and eczema in the first two years of life. *Am J Respir Crit Care Med* 2005, 171(2):121–28.

84. Devereux G, McNeill G, Newman G, Turner S, Craig L, Martindale S, Helms P, Seaton A. Early childhood wheezing symptoms in relation to plasma selenium in pregnant mothers and neonates. *Clin Exp Allergy* 2007, 37(7):1000–1008.

85. Salam MT, Li YF, Langholz B, Gilliland FD. Maternal fish consumption during pregnancy and risk of early childhood asthma. *J Asthma* 2005, 42(6):513–18.

86. Willers SM, Wijga AH, Brunekreef B, Kerkhof M, Gerritsen J, Hoekstra MO, de Jongste JC, Smit HA. Maternal food consumption during pregnancy and the longitudinal development of childhood asthma. *Am J Respir Crit Care Med* 2008, 178(2):124–31.

87. Shaheen SO, Northstone K, Newson RB, Emmett P, Sherriff A, Henderson J. Dietary patterns in pregnancy and respiratory and atopic outcomes in childhood. *Thorax* 2009.

88. Moore DC, Elsas PX, Maximiano ES, Elsas MI. Impact of diet on the immunological microenvironment of the pregnant uterus and its relationship to allergic disease in the offspring—a review of the recent literature. *Sao Paulo Med J* 2006, 124(5):298–303.

89. Holgate ST. Pathogenesis of asthma. *Clin Exp Allergy* 2008, 38(6):872–97.

90. Shaheen SO. Prenatal nutrition and asthma: hope or hype? *Thorax* 2008, 63(6):483–85.

91. Eder W, Ege MJ, von Mutius E. The asthma epidemic. *N Engl J Med* 2006, 355(21):2226–35.

92. Haworth O, Cernadas M, Yang R, Serhan CN, Levy BD. Resolvin E1 regulates interleukin 23, interferon-gamma and lipoxin A4 to promote the resolution of allergic airway inflammation. *Nat Immunol* 2008, 9(8):873–79.

Chapter 4

Asthma Triggers

Chapter Contents

Section 4.1

Common Allergic and Non-Allergic Asthma Triggers

An asthma "trigger" is anything that brings on or aggravates asthma symptoms. Common asthma triggers can be divided into roughly two groups:

- substances called allergens that set off an allergic reaction in the body, a symptom of which may be asthma; and

- other substances and circumstances that aggravate asthma without involving an allergic reaction.

Knowing what your asthma triggers are, and then avoiding them, are important aspects in controlling your asthma.

Allergens

House dust mites: These are tiny creatures related to ticks and spiders that live by the tens of thousands in the dust of our houses, especially if the air is warm and humid. Inhaling dust mite droppings can trigger asthma symptoms.

Pollen (usually from grasses, trees or weeds): As well as causing hay fever in people with a pollen allergy, pollen can also trigger asthma attacks in susceptible people. Many of the pollens that trigger asthma are from introduced plant species such as ryegrass, the weeds Paterson's curse and pellitory ("asthma weed"), and street trees such as oaks, elms and birch. A phenomenon called "thunderstorm asthma" can happen in humid conditions, for example before a storm, when the high humidity causes pollen grains to break apart and release tiny starch granules, which can be breathed into the lungs more easily than larger, intact pollen grains, resulting in an increase in the number of people with asthma symptoms around the time of a storm.

Animal dander (skin scales or flakes from the hair or feathers of animals): Exposure to allergens from pets, especially cats, can trigger or worsen asthma symptoms. Animal allergens are present in household dust, so direct contact with an animal is not always needed for asthma symptoms to be triggered in those allergic to animal dander.

Molds or fungi: *Alternaria* is an outdoor fungus that is found on plants. It is known to trigger asthma, especially in agricultural regions when crops are harvested. *Cladosporium* is a plant mold that can also trigger asthma and can be a problem when grass is mown.

Molds that grow indoors—for example, on damp walls, especially in corners—can also trigger asthma.

Cockroach allergen: This allergen, which is found in cockroach droppings, can build up in the dust of houses that have cockroaches present, and can trigger asthma symptoms.

Food allergy: Being exposed to a food to which you are allergic can trigger asthma symptoms—often accompanied by other symptoms such as a rash. The foods that can trigger allergic asthma attacks include nuts, eggs, milk, shellfish, fish, or seeds (e.g., sesame seeds). Food allergy is not a common trigger of asthma, but in some cases—nut allergy, in particular—a severe and life-threatening allergic reaction (anaphylaxis), rather than asthma alone, can occur.

Occupational allergens: Some adults can develop an allergy to substances that are present in the air at their workplace and can trigger asthma symptoms, for example, flour, latex, and wood dusts. Some other workplace asthma triggers, such as isocyanates, which are used in the manufacture of pesticides, polyurethane foam, plastics, paints, and varnishes, may trigger asthma symptoms either via an allergy or because they irritate the airways directly.

Non-Allergic Triggers

Viral respiratory infections: Viral infection of the upper airways is a common trigger of asthma, especially in children, and often leads to a period of persistent coughing.

Medicines: Asthma can be triggered by certain medicines such as aspirin and other non-steroidal anti-inflammatory drugs (NSAIDs), as well as COX-2 inhibitors, which are often used for arthritis; heart and blood pressure medicines called beta blockers; certain eye drops; and complementary medicines, including echinacea and Royal Jelly, which has even resulted in death in some people with asthma.

Air pollution and other inhaled irritants: Exhaust fumes, in particular from diesel engines, are thought to contain particles that stick to common airborne allergens, for example broken-up pollen grains, and make them easily breathed into the lungs, where they can trigger asthma symptoms. Brushfire smoke is another trigger of asthma symptoms.

Cigarette smoke, some perfumes, and the fumes from paints and cleaning fluids can also provoke asthma symptoms.

Exercise: Exercise is a very common asthma trigger and may be the only trigger in some people with asthma. It is thought that breathing in cold, dry air while needing to breathe hard, as occurs with vigorous exercise, are the key elements of this trigger.

Emotions: Strong emotions such as stress, anxiety, and hearty laughing or crying can trigger asthma symptoms in some people.

Heartburn (reflux): A small amount of stomach acid refluxing or regurgitating into the lower esophagus, as occurs in heartburn, is a potential asthma trigger.

Cold air and ambient temperature changes: Breathing in cold air can trigger asthma symptoms, for example, outside air on a cold day or cold nighttime air in your bedroom.

Food additives: Some food additives can trigger asthma. These include sulfur dioxide and sulfites (food additive numbers 220 to 228)—found in sausages, dried apricots, wine, and many "fast foods." Sulfur dioxide (additive number 220) is the one thought most likely to trigger asthma symptoms. Tartrazine (a food dye, additive number 102) is another possible trigger of asthma, although research has not shown a firm link between tartrazine and asthma symptoms.

Glutamates are found in many foods naturally or are added as flavor enhancers (food additive numbers 620 to 625). One of these additives, monosodium glutamate (MSG; additive number 621), has been studied a great deal; however, research has not clearly shown that MSG can provoke asthma symptoms.

At the time of writing, there is not enough evidence to suggest that people with asthma should routinely avoid food additives without having first been referred by their doctor to an allergy specialist.

Section 4.2

Thunderstorms as an Asthma Trigger

"Link Shown Between Thunderstorms and Asthma Attacks in Metro At-
lanta Area by Team of Researchers from University of Georgia and Emory
University," by Philip Lee Williams, University of Georgia News Service,
June 7, 2010. Reprinted with permission.

In the first in-depth study of its kind ever done in the Southeastern
United States, researchers at the University of Georgia and Emory University have discovered a link between thunderstorms and asthma attacks in the
metro Atlanta area that could have a "significant public health impact."

While a relationship between thunderstorms and increased hospital
visits for asthma attacks has been known and studied worldwide for years,
this is the first time a team of climatologists and epidemiologists has ever
conducted a detailed study of the phenomenon in the American South.

The team, studying a database consisting of more than ten million
emergency room visits in some forty-one hospitals in a twenty-county
area in and around Atlanta for the period between 1993 and 2004, found
a 3 percent higher incidence of visits for asthma attacks on days following thunderstorms.

"While a 3 percent increase in risk may seem modest, asthma is quite
prevalent in Atlanta, and a modest relative increase could have a significant public health impact for a region with more than five million people,"
said Andrew Grundstein, a climatologist in the department of geography
at UGA and lead author on the research. Grundstein went on to say that
"3 percent is likely conservative because of limitations in this study."

The next step for the UGA and Emory team will be, for the first
time, to apply Doppler radar, modeling, and observational data to the
"thunderstorm asthma" problem based on what Grundstein calls an
intriguing initial finding. He points out that "radar data coupled with
the metro Atlanta database will allow us to correlate thunderstorm-
asthma interactions that we are probably missing today."

Paige Tolbert, professor and chair of the department of environmental and occupational health in the Rollins School of Public Health at
Emory and a co-author of the just-published study, said the expertise of
the two universities came together strongly in studying the problem.

61

"The Emory team has experience with a comprehensive emergency department database, and the UGA team can provide a much more refined characterization of thunderstorms than was performed in the previous studies of this question," she said. "The study will thus provide new insight into the mechanisms under the phenomenon of thunderstorm-induced asthma."

The research was published in the online edition of the medical journal *Thorax*. Other authors of the paper include: Marshall Shepherd and Thomas Mote from the UGA department of geography; Luke Naeher from the UGA department of environmental health science; and Stefanie Ebelt Sarnat and Mitchell Klein, who along with Tolbert are from the department of environmental and occupational health in the Rollins School of Public Health at Emory.

About twenty million Americans have asthma, according to the American Academy of Allergy, Asthma and Immunology. There also has been a dramatic increase in reported cases of the disease, with its prevalence increasing 75 percent between 1980 and 1994. Some five thousand Americans die annually from asthma attacks.

Approximately 210,000 Georgia children under the age of seventeen have asthma, according to the Division of Public Health of the Georgia Department of Human Resources. Some 65 percent of that number had an attack within the last year.

While associations between thunderstorm activity and asthma deaths and emergency room visits have been reported around the world, virtually no studies have been done in the American South, where hundreds of thousands suffer from asthma and thunderstorms are prevalent.

Some people may find it odd that thunderstorms, which supposedly "clear the air" of pollen and pollutants, are implicated in asthma attacks. The most prominent hypothesis as to why it happens, the authors of the paper say, is that "pollen grains may rupture upon contact with rainwater, releasing respirable allergens, and that gusty winds from thunderstorm downdrafts spread particles . . . which may ultimately increase the risk of asthma attacks."

The team used thunderstorm occurrences from meteorological data gathered at Atlanta's Hartsfield-Jackson International Airport and compared that information with the vast database of emergency room visits to arrive at the figure of a 3 percent increase in asthma-related emergency room visits following thunderstorms for the study period.

In all, during the eleven-year period, there were 564 thunderstorm days, and in order to better understand the physical mechanisms that relate thunderstorms and asthma, the team also mined the information on total daily rainfall and maximum five-second wind gusts, which they used as "a surrogate for thunderstorm downdrafts and to indicate the maximum wind speed of the storm."

In all, there were 215,832 asthma emergency room visits during the period and 28,350 of these occurred on days following thunderstorms. While the new study is the first of its kind in the South and does clearly indicate a relationship between thunderstorms and asthma in the metro Atlanta area, much more work remains, Grundstein said.

"Obtaining a better understanding of the mechanistic basis of the phenomenon of thunderstorm-induced asthma will allow for better intervention strategies and improved emergencies services planning," said Stefanie Ebelt Sarnat of Emory. "This will be particularly important in the era of climate change."

Grundstein added that in the Atlanta area conditions favorable for an estimated doubling of severe thunderstorms are expected within this century.

Section 4.3

Occupational Asthma Triggers

"Occupational Asthma (OA)," reprinted with permission from www.haz-map .com, © 2011. All rights reserved. Table 4.1—Chemicals Associated with Occupational Asthma and Table 4.2—Biological Agents Associated with Occupational Asthma, reprinted with permission from www.haz-map.com, Table 1 and Table 2 based on: Malo J-L, Chan-Yeung M. Appendix: Agents Causing Occupational Asthma with Key References. In: Bernstein LI, Chan-Yeung M. Malo J-L, Bernstein DI (eds). *Asthma in the Workplace, 3rd Ed.* New York: Taylor and Francis, 2006, with permission from Moira Chan-Yeung. For the up-to-date version, see www.asthme.csst.qc.ca.

Two Types of Occupational Asthma

Immunologic asthma develops after a variable period of time during which "sensitization" to an agent present in the workplace takes place. Irritant-induced asthma occurs without a latency period after an intense exposure to an irritating dust, mist, vapor, or fume. The pathophysiologic mechanism underlying irritant-induced asthma is not well understood, and it is not known why the asthmatic response persists in certain individuals.[1]

Two Types of Immunologic Occupational Asthma (OA)

The Haz-Map database focuses on immunologic asthma and the predictable and preventable occupational settings in which exposures occur. Immunologic asthma can be classified into that caused by high-molecular or low-molecular weight compounds. The high-molecular-weight compounds are animal- and plant-derived proteins or polysaccharides such as wheat flour and animal dander that cause an immunoglobulin E (IgE)–dependent immune response. The low-molecular-weight compounds are chemicals that can also initiate an immune response after repeated inhalation. The nature of the immune response is more complex for the low-molecular-weight chemicals than it is for the high-molecular-weight agents. "An IgE- or immunoglobulin G (IgG)–dependent mechanism has not been consistently seen with low-molecular-weight agents (isocyanates, for example). These agents can cause sensitization through a hapten-mediated effect. The role of lymphocytes or other immunologic mechanisms remains unclear."[2]

The Haz-Map database contains over 180 biological agents and chemicals that can cause immunologic OA based on a previously published table. (Chan-Yeung & Malo and Appendix B in Harber) In the two tables that follow, the high-molecular-weight compounds and wood dusts are listed as "Biological Agents," while the low-molecular-weight compounds are listed in the "Chemicals" table. Wood dusts are biological agents or products, but sensitization may occur through a low-molecular-weight chemical, as has been proven for the case of Western red cedar.

Incidence and Prevalence of Occupational Asthma

In a study done in the West Midlands Region of the United Kingdom, the average annual incidence of occupational asthma was found to be 43 cases per million workers, with a range of 1,833 per million for spray painters to 8 per million for clerks.[3]

The prevalence of occupational asthma in adults with asthma is estimated to be between 3 percent and 20 percent.

Prevention of Occupational Asthma

The diagnosis of occupational asthma is a sentinel event—an alert that engineering controls or protective equipment could prevent asthma from developing in workers in the same workplace or industry.

64

Table 4.1. Chemicals Associated with Occupational Asthma

Chemical Name	Alternate Name	Occupation or Industry
Acrylates and Methacrylates		
Ethyl cyanoacrylate	Ethyl-2-cyanoacrylate	Building airplane models
Methyl 2-cyanoacrylate		Using adhesives
Ethyl methacrylate		Manicurist
Methyl methacrylate		Nurse
Ethoxylated bisphenol A diacrylate		Auto body shop worker
Metals		
Aluminum		Solderer
Chromium and compounds		Printer, plater, welder, tanner
Cobalt		Hard metal grinder, diamond polisher
Nickel and compounds		Metal plating; welder
Palladium		Assembly line worker
Platinum		Platinum refinery
Tungsten carbide		Grinder
Zinc chloride fume		Solderer
Aldehydes		
Formaldehyde		Hospital staff
Glutaraldehyde	Cidex	Hospital endoscopy unit
Amines		
Ethylenediamine	1,2-Diaminoethane	Shellac handler; photographer
Hexamethylene tetramine		Lacquer handler
N,N-Dimethyl-1,3-propanediamine	DMAPA	Ski manufacturer
Triethylenetetramine		Manufacturing aircraft filters
EPO 60		Mold maker
Trimethylhexanediamine + Isophoronediamine		Floor covering material salesman
4-Methylmorpholine		Manufacturing polyurethane foam
Piperazine dihydrochloride		Pharmaceutical and chemical manufacturing

Table continues on next page.

Table 4.1. *continued*

Chemical Name	Alternate Name	Occupation or Industry
p-Phenylenediamine		Fur dyeing
Ethanolamine	2-Aminoethanol	Beauty culture
N,N-Dimethyl-ethanolamine		Spray painter
N-(2-hydroxyethyl)-ethylenediamine	Aminoethyl-ethanolamine	Solderer; cable jointer
Triethanolamine		Metal worker
Acid Anhydrides		
Chlorendic anhydride		Mechanic
Hexahydrophthalic anhydride		Chemical worker
Himic anhydride		Manufacturing flame retardant
Maleic anhydride		Manufacturing polyester resin
Methyltetrahydrophthalic anhydride		Using curing agent
Phthalic anhydride		Producing resins
Pyromellitic dianhydride		Using epoxy adhesives
Tetrachlorophthalic anhydride		Using epoxy resins
Trimellitic anhydride		Using epoxy resins
Preservatives/ Disinfectants		
Benzalkonium chloride		Using cleaning product
1,2-Benzisothiazolin-3-one		Chemical manufacturing
Chloramine T		Chemical manufacturing; brewery; janitorial/cleaning
Chlorhexidine	Hibiclens	Nurse
Hexachlorophene		Hospital staff
Isononanoyl oxybenzene sulfonate		Laboratory technician
Lauryl dimethyl benzyl ammonium chloride		Using floor cleaner
Methylchloroiso-thiazolinone		Chemical manufacturing

Table continues on next page.

Table 4.1. *continued*

Chemical Name	Alternate Name	Occupation or Industry
Isocyanates		
Dicyclohexylmethane 4,4-diisocyanate	Hydrogenated MDI	Manufacturing polyurethane products
Hexamethylene diisocyanate	HDI	Spray painter
Isophorone diisocyanate	IPDI	Spray painter
Methylene bisphenyl iso-cyanate	MDI; Diphenyl-methane diisocyanate	Foundry
Naphthalene diisocyanate	NDI	Rubber manufacturing
Polymethylene polyphenyl isocyanate	PPI	Paint shop worker
Toluene diisocyanate	TDI	Producing polyurethanes; floor varnisher
Plastic and Rubber Dusts		
Azodicarbonamide	1,1'-Azobisformamide	Rubber and plastic manufacturing
Plexiglass (dust)	Lucite; Methyl meth-acrylate polymer	Factory worker
Polyvinyl chloride (heated)		Meat wrapper's asthma
Polyvinyl chloride (dust)		Manufacturing bottle caps
Polyethylene (heated)		Paper wrapper's asthma
Polypropylene (heated)		Manufacturing bags
Pyrolysis Products		
Rosin core solder	Rosin flux pyrolysis products	Electronics worker; manufacturing solder flux
Zinc chloride fume		Solderer; locksmith
Fungicides		
Bis(tri-n-butyltin)oxide	Tributyltin oxide	Exposure to carpet deodorizer
Captafol	Difolatan®	Chemical manufacturing
Chlorothalonil	Tetrachloroisophtha-lonitrile	Farmer

Table continues on next page.

Table 4.1. *continued*

Chemical Name	Alternate Name	Occupation or Industry
Other Chemicals		
Aluminum smelting	Yet to be identified substance or mixture (? aluminum, ? fluorides) that can cause "potroom asthma" in workers at electrolytic reduction facilities	Potroom worker
Ammonium persulphate		Hairdresser
Diazonium salt	e.g., diazonium tetrafluoroborate and p-diethylaminobenzenediazonium chloride	Manufacturing photocopy paper; manufacturing fluorine polymer precursor
Dioctyl-phthalate		Polyvinyl chloride (PVC) production worker
Drugs		Pharmacist; pharmaceutical worker
Ethylene oxide		Nurse
Furfuryl alcohol		Foundry mold making; wool dye house
Ninhydrin		Laboratory worker
Nitrogen chloride		Indoor pool lifeguards
Oil mist, mineral	Metalworking or machining fluids, cutting oils (may contain numerous additives and contaminants)	Toolsetter and automobile plant
Styrene		Plastics factory
Sulfites		Water plant; food processor
Tetramethrin		Exterminator
Tetrazine		Detonator manufacturing
Textile dyes		Textiles, dye manufacturing
Triglycidyl isocyanurate		Spray painter
Urea formaldehyde	Kaurit S	Resin and foam manufacturing

Table 4.2. Biological Agents Associated with Occupational Asthma

Agent Name	Other Name or Comments	Industry or Occupation
Animal-Derived Proteins		
Frog		Frog catcher
Egg protein		Egg producer
Milk protein	Casein	Dairy industry, Tanner
Farm animals	Animal dander	Agricultural worker, Poultry worker, Butcher
Laboratory animals		Laboratory worker
Bat guano	Bat droppings	Various
Bovine serum albumin		Laboratory worker
Deer dander		Farmer
Endocrine glands		Pharmacist
Ivory dust		Ivory worker
Mink urine		Farmer
Monkey dander		Laboratory worker
Anisakis simplex (nematode)		Chicken breeder, Fish monger
Aquatic Animal Allergens		
Hoya	Sea-squirt	Oyster farm worker
Crab	Snow crab	Snow crab processor
Prawn		Prawn processor
Lobster		Fish shop worker
Fish		Trout processor, deep-sea fisher
Shrimp meal		Technician
Red soft coral	*Dendronephthytia nipponica*	Fisherman
Daphnia	Water flea (a small freshwater crustacean)	Fish food storage worker
Nacre	Mother-of-pearl	Nacre (mother-of-pearl) button maker
Cuttlefish bone		Fisherman
Marine sponge		Laboratory grinder

Table continues on next page.

69

Table 4.2. *continued*

Biological Enzymes	
Esperase	Detergent industry
Fungal amylo-glucosidase and hemicellulase	Baker
Fungal amylase	Baker
Papain	Pharmaceutical
Egg lysozyme	Pharmaceutical
Flaviastase	Pharmaceutical
Subtilisins	Detergent industry
Pancreatin	Pharmaceutical
Pepsin	Pharmaceutical
Trypsin	Plastic and pharmaceutical
Bromelin	Pharmaceutical
Serratial peptidase	Pharmaceutical
Fungal pectinase and glucanase	Food Processing
Fungal lactase	Formulating and Packaging
Fungal xylanase	Laboratory workers
Phytase	Animal-feed mixers

Insect-Derived Allergens		
L. Caesar larvae		Angler
Grain mite		Farmer, Grain storage worker
Locust		Laboratory worker
Screw worm fly		Flight crew
Cricket		Laboratory worker
Moth		Entomologist
Butterfly		Entomologist
Echinidorus larva	*Echinodorus plamosus*	Aquarium keeper
Fruit fly		Laboratory worker
Silkworm		Silk worker

Table continues on next page.

Table 4.2. *continued*

Insect-Derived Allergens, *continued*		
Sericin	Silk gum; gelatinous protein on raw silk	Hairdresser
Fowl mite		Poultry worker
Barn mite		Farmer
Acarians (mites)	*Panonychus ulmi, P. citri*	Apple and citrus growers
Sheep blowfly		Technician
Larva of silkworm		Sericulture
Lesser mealworm		Grain and poultry worker
Mexican bean weevil		Seed house worker
Bee moth		Fish bait breeder
Honeybee		Honey processor
Beetles	Coleoptera	Museum curator, Wool worker, Mechanic in rye plant
Chironomid midges	Bloodworms	Fish-food factory workers
Ground bugs		Bottling worker
Mealworm larvae		Fish-bait handlers
Sewer fly		Sewage plant workers
Wheat weevil		Mill workers
Plant-Derived Allergens		
Flour (wheat, rye and soya)		Bakers and millers
Tobacco leaf		Tobacco manufacturer
Lycopodium	Moss spores; A fine yellow powder used as an absorbent and lubricant	Condom manufacturer
Henna		Hairdresser
Garlic		Food packager
Onion		Homemakers
Tea		Tea processor
Castor bean		Oil industry

Table continues on next page.

Table 4.2. *continued*

Plant-Derived Allergens, *continued*

Coffee bean (green)		Food processor
Grain dust		Grain elevator worker
Latex		Glove manufacturer
Allergens, flowers	Limonium tataricum	Floral worker
	Decorative flowers	floral worker
	Spathe flowers	Floral worker
	Baby's breath (*Gypsophila paniculata*)	Florist
	Cyclamen (flowering plants)	Florists
	Roses	Rose grower
	Bells of Ireland (*Molucella laevis*)	Grower
Allergens, garden and greenhouse	Bell peppers	Greenhouse workers
	Amaryllis (Belladonna lily)	Greenhouse worker
	Chrysanthemum	Greenhouse worker
	Solanum melongena (egg-plant)	Greenhouse worker
	Stepanotis floribunda	Greenhouse workers
	Umbrella tree (Schefflera)	Landscape gardener
	Grass juice	Gardener
	Phoenix canariensis (canary palm pollen)	Gardener
	Weeping fig	Plant keeper
	Lathyrus odoratus (sweet pea)	Greenhouse worker
	Freesia	Horticulturist
	Paprika	Horticulturist
	Tetranychus urticae (red spider mite)	Farmers, greenhouse workers
	Amblyseius cucumeris (predatory mite used to control thrips, a common pest of bell peppers)	Horticulturists

Table continues on next page.

Table 4.2. *continued*

Plant-Derived Allergens, *continued*

Allergens, baking industry	Flour (wheat, rye, and soya)	Bakers or millers
	Gluten	Baker
	Buckwheat	Baker
	Lathyrus sativus (grass pea)	Flour handlers
	Soybean lecithin	Bakers
	Saccharomyces cerevisiae (baker's yeast)	Baker
Allergens, processing plant extracts	Rose hips	Pharmaceutical worker
	Herb material	Herbal worker
	Licorice root	Herbalist
	Sarsaparilla root	Herbal tea worker
	Brazil ginseng	Medicinal plant processor
	Voacanga africana (small tropical African tree used to produce drugs)	Spouse of chemist working in pharmaceutical company
	Passiflora alata and *Rhamnus purshiana*	Pharmacy technician
	Chamomile	Cosmetician
Allergens, spice processing	Spices	Spice processing
	Saffron spice	Saffron processors
	Fenugreek	Food industry
	Aniseed	Food industry
Allergens, food processing	Chicory	Vegetable wholesaler
	Carob bean	Jam factory
	Pectin	Christmas candy maker
	Cacoon seed	Decorator
	Onion seed	Seed packing
	Fennel seed	Sausage processing
	Courgette (zucchini)	Fruit warehouse
	Aromatic herbs	Butcher

Table continues on next page.

Table 4.2. *continued*

Plant-Derived Allergens, *continued*

Allergens, food
processing, *continued*

	Olive oilcake	Oil industry
	Peach	Factory worker
	Green bean	Homemaker
	Asparagus	Food processor
	Potato	Housewives
	Swiss chard	Housewives
	Mushroom	Mushroom soup processor
	Sunflower pollen	
	Hops	Brewery chemist

Vegetable Gums

Guar		Carpet manufacturer
Karaya		Hairdresser
Acacia		Printer
Tragacanth		Gum importer

Wood Dusts

Abiruana	*Lucuma* spp. (*Pouteria* spp.)	
African maple	*Triplochiton scleroxylon*	
African zebra	*Microberlinia* spp.	
American mahogany	*Swietenia mahogani*	
Antiaris	*Antiaris Africana*	Door manufacturing
Ash	*Fraxinus americana*	
Australian blackwood	*Acacia melanoxylon*	Furniture manufacturing
Brazilian walnut	*Cordia goeldiana* HUBER	Furniture manufacturing
Cabreuva	*Myyrocarpus fastigiatus* Fr. All.	Parquet floor layer
California redwood	*Sequoia sempervirens*	Wood carver, carpenter
Cedar of Lebanon	*Cedrus libani*	
Central American Walnut	*Juglans olanchana*	
Cinnamon	*Cinnamomum zeylanicum*	

Table continues on next page.

Table 4.2. *continued*

Plant-Derived Allergens, *continued*

Cocobolo	*Dalbergia retusa*	
Colophony	Gum rosin; wood rosin; tall oil rosin; abietic acid	
Eastern white cedar	*Thuja occidentalis*	Sawmill worker
Ebony	*Diospyros crassiflora*	
Fernambouc	*Caesalpinia echinata*	Bow making
Iroko	*Chlorophora excelsa*	Carpenter
Kejaat	*Pterocarpus angolensis*	
Kotibe	*Nesorgordonia papverifera*	
Makore	*Tieghemella heckelii*	Carpenter
Mukali	*Aningeria robusta*	
Oak	*Quercus* spp.	
Pau Marfim	*Balfourodendron riedelianum*	Woodworker
Philippine mahogany	*Swietenia macrophylla*	
Quillaja bark		Factory to produce saponin
Ramin	*Gonystylus bancanus*	Woodworker
Tanganyika aningre		
Western red cedar	*Thuja plicata* (Plicatic acid has been identified as the low-molecular-weight chemical sensitizer)	Carpentry, furniture making, cabinetmaking, sawmill worker

Mold and Algae

Dictyostelium discoideum		Technicians
Aspergillus niger	Technicians	
Aspergillus	Beet sugar workers	
Aspergillus alternaria		Baker
Trichoderma koningii		Sawmill workers
Plasmopara viticola		Agricultural workers
Chlorella		Pharmacists
Neurospora		Plywood factory worker
Chrysonilia sitophila		Logging worker
Rhizopus nigricans		Coal miner

References

1. Balmes JR. *Occupational Lung Diseases*. p. 315 in LaDou.

2. Malo JL, Cartier A. *Occupational Asthma*, p. 424 in Harber.

3. Gannon PF, Burge PS. The SHIELD scheme in the West Midlands Region, United Kingdom. *Br J Ind Med* 1993 Sep;50(9):791–96. Read Shield reports at the website of the Oasys research group.

4. PubMed Abstracts.

5. See Table 2 from page 6 in *Asthma in the Workplace*.

6. Diagnosis and management of work-related asthma: American College Of Chest Physicians Consensus Statement.

Chapter 5

Asthma Prevalence, Health Care Use, and Mortality in the United States

Asthma is a chronic respiratory disease characterized by episodes or attacks of impaired breathing. Symptoms are caused by inflammation and narrowing of small airways and may include shortness of breath, coughing, wheezing, and chest pain. Disease severity ranges from mild with occasional symptoms to severe with persistent symptoms that impact quality of life. However, even people with mild disease may suffer severe attacks. Common attack triggers include airway irritants (e.g., tobacco smoke and air pollution), allergens, respiratory infections, stress, and exercise.[1]

Although little is understood about preventing asthma from developing, the means for controlling and preventing symptoms are well established. Treatment includes the use of medication for short-term relief; daily use of preventive medication to avert attacks; monitoring of early symptoms; avoiding factors that trigger attacks; and removing risks (e.g., tobacco smoke or mold) from the home, school, and work environments. Nevertheless, morbidity, direct healthcare costs, indirect costs such as lost productivity, and mortality due to asthma continue pose a high burden in the United States. This section presents estimates for asthma prevalence in the United States, as well as for asthma-related healthcare use and mortality. Differences between groups are presented where data are available.

Excerpted from "Asthma Prevalence, Health Care Use, and Mortality: United States, 2005–2009," National Center for Health Statistics, Centers for Disease Control and Prevention, January 12, 2011.

77

Table 5.1. Asthma Period Prevalence, Current Asthma Prevalence, and Asthma Attack Prevalence for All Ages, United States, 1980–2009

Year	Asthma Period Prevalence	Current Asthma Prevalence	Asthma Attack Prevalence
	Percentage (standard error)	Percentage (standard error)	Percentage (standard error)
1980	3.1 (0.2)	---	---
1981	3.2 (0.2)	---	---
1982	3.5 (0.2)	---	---
1983	3.8 (0.2)	---	---
1984	3.6 (0.2)	---	---
1985	3.7 (0.2)	---	---
1986	4.1 (0.3)	---	---
1987	4.0 (0.2)	---	---
1988	4.1 (0.2)	---	---
1989	4.8 (0.2)	---	---
1990	4.2 (0.2)	---	---
1991	4.7 (0.2)	---	---
1992	4.9 (0.2)	---	---
1993	5.1 (0.3)	---	---
1994	5.6 (0.3)	---	---

Table continues on next page.

Data Sources

Estimates for asthma prevalence, school and work absences, and asthma control measures are based on data from the National Health Interview Survey (NHIS). NHIS serves as a principal source of health information for the U.S. civilian noninstitutionalized population. Questions used to ascertain asthma prevalence are contained in the core questionnaire asked of one sample adult in each family included in NHIS, and, if children are present, one sample child in the family for whom a responsible adult responds. Periodically, supplements with special content for asthma are included in the survey. In 2008, an asthma supplement ascertained aspects of disease control and asthma-specific absences from school and work.

Ambulatory visit numbers and rates were estimated using data from the National Ambulatory Medical Care Survey (NAMCS) and the National Hospital Ambulatory Medical Care Survey (NHAMCS). Visits to private physician offices were estimated using NAMCS, which samples visits made in the United States to offices of non–federally

Table 5.1. *continued*

Year	Asthma Period Prevalence	Current Asthma Prevalence	Asthma Attack Prevalence
	Percentage (standard error)	Percentage (standard error)	Percentage (standard error)
1995	5.7 (0.3)	---	---
1996	5.5 (0.3)	---	---
1997	---	---	4.1 (0.1)
1998	---	---	3.9 (0.1)
1999	---	---	3.9 (0.1)
2000	---	---	4.0 (0.1)
2001	---	7.4 (0.1)	4.3 (0.1)
2002	---	7.2 (0.2)	4.3 (0.1)
2003	---	7.0 (0.2)	3.9 (0.1)
2004	---	7.1 (0.2)	4.1 (0.1)
2005	---	7.6 (0.2)	4.2 (0.1)
2006	---	7.8 (0.2)	4.2 (0.1)
2007	---	7.7 (0.2)	4.2 (0.1)
2008	---	7.8 (0.2)	4.3 (0.1)
2009	---	8.2 (0.2)	4.2 (0.1)

Source: CDC/NCHS, National Interview Survey.

employed physicians. Visits to private, nonhospital-based clinics, community health centers, and health maintenance organizations were included. Telephone contacts and visits made outside of physician's offices were excluded. Visits to outpatient departments (OPDs) and emergency departments (EDs) were estimated using NHAMCS, which samples visits made to these departments in nonfederal short-stay hospitals (average stay fewer than thirty days) and in general hospitals (medical or surgical) and children's general hospitals. EDs that operate fewer than twenty-four hours were included in the OPD component.

Data for asthma hospitalization numbers and rates were obtained from the National Hospital Discharge Survey (NHDS). NHDS is a national probability survey that collects data from a sample of inpatient records acquired from a national sample of nonfederal short-stay hospitals in the United States. Only hospitals with an average length of stay of fewer than thirty days for all patients, and general hospitals and children's general hospitals were included in the survey.

Asthma death data were obtained from the National Vital Statistics System (NVSS). NVSS includes data on births and deaths based on U.S. standard certificates. The mortality component was used to report asthma death rates.

Results

Asthma Prevalence Continues to Increase

In 2009, current asthma prevalence was 8.2 percent, affecting 24.6 million people in the United States (17.5 million adults and 7.1 million children aged birth to seventeen years) (See Table 5.1). Asthma attack prevalence—the proportion of the population with at least one attack in the previous year—was 4.2 percent. That is, 12.8 million people (8.7 million adults and 4.0 million children aged birth to seventeen), or 52 percent of those with current asthma, had attacks and were at risk for adverse outcomes such as ED visits or hospitalization. The most rapid growth in asthma prevalence occurred from 1980 to 1996, when asthma period prevalence grew from 3.5 percent to 5.5 percent, an annual percentage increase of 3.8 percent. In 1997, survey measures changed to capture more detailed aspects of asthma prevalence, and estimates before and after the change cannot be directly compared. The measure most comparable to the pre-1997 asthma period prevalence estimate is current asthma prevalence, which had remained stable (at 7.4 percent) since it first became available in 2001 but recently began increasing so that overall, the annual percentage increase from 2001 to 2009 was 1.2 percent. Asthma attack prevalence remained level between 3.9 percent and 4.3 percent from 1997 to 2009.

Asthma Prevalence Differs by Demographic Characteristics

Significant differences in current asthma prevalence exist between many population subgroups. Figure 5.1 compares 2009 current asthma prevalence between population subgroups. Overall, females have higher current asthma prevalence than males, although among children aged birth to seventeen, boys have a higher prevalence (11.3%) than girls (7.9%). Children have higher current asthma prevalence than adults. Compared with white persons, prevalence is higher among black and lower among Asian persons. Compared with non-Hispanic white and non-Hispanic black persons, current asthma prevalence is higher among Puerto Rican and lower among Mexican persons. Those with family income below the federal poverty level have higher

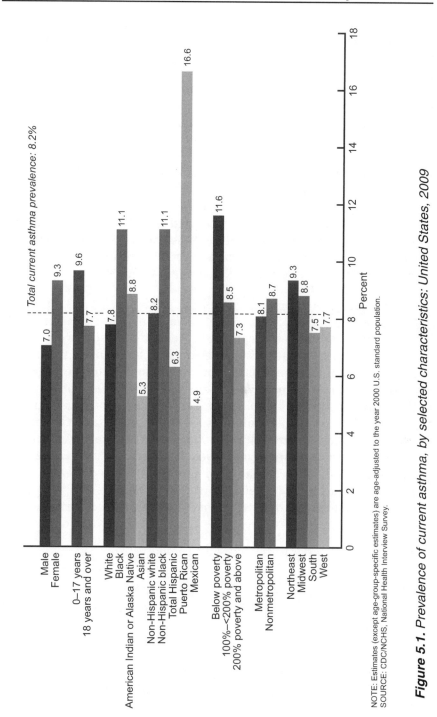

Total current asthma prevalence: 8.2%

	Percent
Male	7.0
Female	9.3
0–17 years	9.6
18 years and over	7.7
White	7.8
Black	11.1
American Indian or Alaska Native	8.8
Asian	5.3
Non-Hispanic white	8.2
Non-Hispanic black	11.1
Total Hispanic	6.3
Puerto Rican	16.6
Mexican	4.9
Below poverty	11.6
100%–<200% poverty	8.5
200% poverty and above	7.3
Metropolitan	8.1
Nonmetropolitan	8.7
Northeast	9.3
Midwest	8.8
South	7.5
West	7.7

NOTE: Estimates (except age-group-specific estimates) are age-adjusted to the year 2000 U.S. standard population.
SOURCE: CDC/NCHS, National Health Interview Survey.

Figure 5.1. *Prevalence of current asthma, by selected characteristics: United States, 2009*

asthma prevalence than those with incomes in the near poor (100 percent to less than 200 percent of poverty) and not poor (200 percent of poverty and above) categories. The near poor also have higher prevalence compared with the not poor. There is no difference in prevalence rates between residents of metropolitan and nonmetropolitan areas, but when examined by geographic region, prevalence is higher in the Northeast than in the West and South and in the Midwest compared with the South.

Figure 5.2 shows sex differences in more detail across lifespan. Boys have higher prevalence than girls throughout most of childhood. During early adolescence, current asthma prevalence declines among males, whereas in females, current asthma prevalence rises steadily through childhood so that between ages fourteen and seventeen years, prevalence rates are similar among boys and girls. This pattern of change continues to early adulthood so that throughout most of adulthood, women report higher current asthma prevalence compared with men.

School and Work Absences Are Common among Persons with Symptomatic Asthma

In 2008, children aged five to seventeen years with at least one asthma attack in the previous year were reported to miss 10.5 million school days in the past year. Nearly 60 percent had at least one asthma absence day in the past year, and 5.5 percent were reported to have an activity limitation due to asthma. An activity limitation is defined as a long-term reduction in a person's capacity to perform the usual kind or amount of activities associated with his or her age group as a result of a chronic condition. Adults aged eighteen and over who had at least one asthma attack in the past twelve months and were currently employed reported missing 14.2 million work days, and nearly 34 percent missed at least one work day due to asthma in the previous year. Among those employed, 6 percent of adults with at least one asthma attack in the previous year reported that a breathing problem caused an activity limitation. Missed work days were also measured among adults with at least one asthma attack in the past twelve months who were not currently employed and included missed days of work around the house. Among those not currently employed, 22 million days of housework or other types of activities were missed, and 27 percent of those with at least one asthma attack in the past twelve months reported an activity limitation caused by a breathing problem. This information is summarized in Table 5.2.

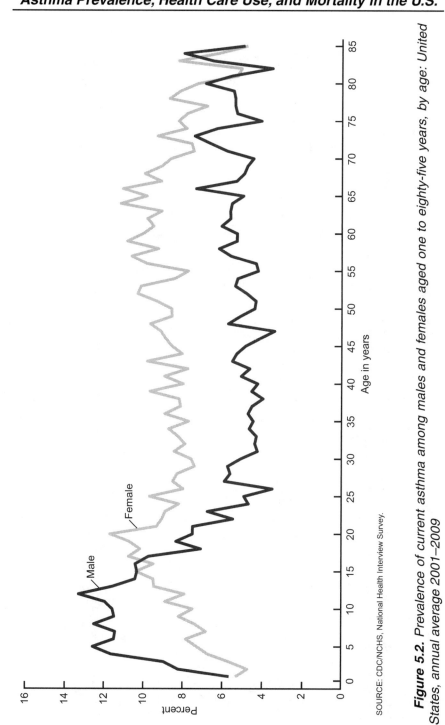

SOURCE: CDC/NCHS, National Health Interview Survey.

Figure 5.2. Prevalence of current asthma among males and females aged one to eighty-five years, by age: United States, annual average 2001–2009

Table 5.2. School and Work Absences and Percentage with Activity Limitation Caused by Asthma among Persons with at Least One Asthma Attack in the Past Year: United States, 2008

Population	Weighted population size, in millions	Total days missed, in millions (standard error)[a]	Percentage with one or more asthma absence days in past year (standard error)[a]	Percentage with activity limitation caused by asthma or breathing problem (standard error)
Children 5–17 years	3.3	10.5 (1.3)	58.7 (3.6)	5.5 (1.2)
Adults 18 years and over, currently employed	4.9	14.2 (4.7)	33.5 (2.8)	6.2 (1.3)
Adults 18 years and over, not currently employed	3.8	22.0 (5.9)	29.1 (3.1)	26.5 (2.7)

Source: CDC/NCHS, National Health Interview Survey.

[a]Records with missing responses for days of school (1 percent among children aged five to seventeen years), work (0.4 percent among adults currently employed), or housework or other activity (25.1 percent among adults not currently employed) missed due to asthma are excluded.

Healthcare Use for Asthma Is High, and Disparities Remain in Asthma Healthcare Use and Mortality

In 2007, 13.9 million visits for asthma were made to private physician offices (7.2 million for adults and 6.7 million for children aged zero to seventeen years) and 1.4 million visits to hospital outpatient departments (0.6 million for adults and 0.8 million for children aged zero to seventeen years). The National Heart, Lung, and Blood Institute guidelines for the clinical management of asthma recommend periodic preventive ambulatory visits for asthma monitoring, and a proportion of visits in nonemergent ambulatory settings may reflect appropriate disease management. In contrast, visits to emergency departments (EDs) and hospital stays for asthma represent adverse outcomes. There were 1.75 million ED visits (1.11 million for adults and 0.64 million for children aged zero to seventeen) and 456,000 asthma hospitalizations (299,000 for adults and 157,000 for children aged zero to seventeen). There were 3,447 deaths due to asthma in 2007 (3,262 among adults and 185 among children aged zero to seventeen).

To account for differing prevalence rates between groups and to focus on the population at risk for these outcomes, healthcare use rates in Table 5.3 were calculated per one hundred persons with current asthma. Because numbers of asthma deaths are smaller, death rates were calculated per ten thousand persons with current asthma. Estimates by income are not available, and less detail is available on healthcare use and mortality by race or ethnicity. Even after accounting for prevalence differences between groups, differences are seen in healthcare use and mortality burdens between groups. Healthcare use is highest among children aged zero to four (rates per one hundred persons with current asthma for total ambulatory visits were 144.9, for ED visits 24.6, and for hospitalizations 8.4). However, deaths from asthma are rare among children aged zero to seventeen, with 174 deaths on average per year from 2005–2007.

To illustrate differences between groups, the rates in Table 5.3 were used to calculate the rate ratios shown in Figure 5.3. A rate ratio of 1.0 indicates equal rates between the groups being compared. The largest differences are seen for race and age groups. The black-to-white rate ratio was nearly 1.0 for total ambulatory visits but was greater than 1.0 for ED visits, hospitalizations, and deaths. The rate ratios for children compared with adults were above 1.0 for all types of health care services but below 1.0 for death.

Table 5.3. Asthma Healthcare Use per 100 Persons with Current Asthma, and Asthma Deaths per 10,000 Persons with Current Asthma, by Selected Characteristics: United States, Annual Average 2005–2007

Characteristics	Office Outpatient Visits per 100 Persons with Asthma	Total Hospital Outpatient Visits per 100 Persons with Asthma	Total Ambulatory Visits per 100 persons with asthma	Emergency Department Visits per 100 persons with asthma	Hospitalizations per 100 persons with asthma	Deaths per 10,000 persons with asthma
	Number (standard error)					
Total	54.8 (5.6)	5.6 (0.7)	60.4 (5.6)	7.5 (0.4)	1.4 (0.2)	1.6 (0.0)
Sex						
Male	61.6 (7.3)	5.8 (0.8)	67.4 (7.3)	7.7 (0.5)	1.3 (0.2)	1.4 (0.1)
Female	50.0 (6.2)	5.5 (0.7)	55.5 (6.2)	7.4 (0.5)	1.4 (0.2)	1.8 (0.0)
Race						
White	57.4 (6.3)	4.6 (0.6)	62.0 (6.3)	5.6 (0.4)	0.9 (0.1)	1.4 (0.0)
Black	49.4 (9.2)	11.5 (2.1)	60.9 (9.4)	18.6 (1.6)	2.0 (0.3)	2.7 (0.1)
Other	38.5 (9.5)	3.4 (0.8)	41.9 (9.5)	4.1 (0.8)	0.8 (0.2)	1.1 (0.1)
Ethnicity						
Hispanic	72.1 (19.8)	11.1 (2.3)	83.2 (19.9)	10.7 (1.2)	— —[a]	0.9 (0.1)
Non-Hispanic	52.4 (5.4)	4.8 (0.6)	57.2 (5.4)	7.1 (0.4)	— —	1.7 (0.1)
Age						
Under 18 years	77.5 (10.3)	9.7 (1.7)	87.2 (10.4)	9.9 (0.9)	1.6 (0.3)	0.3 (0.0)
18 years and over	45.4 (5.4)	3.9 (0.5)	49.3 (5.4)	6.5 (0.4)	1.3 (0.2)	2.1 (0.1)

Sources: CDC/NCHS, National Ambulatory Medical Care Survey, National Hospital Ambulatory Medical Care Survey, National Hospital Discharge Survey, mortality component of the National Vital Statistics System, and National Health Interview Survey (population with current asthma).
[a]Data on Hispanic ethnicity are not available for hospitalization.

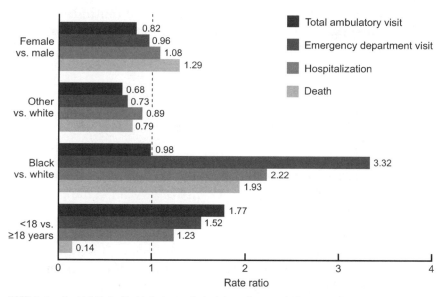

NOTE: A rate ratio of 1.0 (dashed line) indicates equal rates between the groups being compared.
SOURCES: CDC/NCHS, National Ambulatory Medical Care Survey, National Hospital Ambulatory Medical Care Survey, National Hospital Discharge Survey, Mortality component of the National Vital Statistics System, and National Health Interview Survey (population with current asthma).

Figure 5.3. *Relative burden of asthma healthcare use and mortality, adjusted for current asthma prevalence, by sex, race, and age group: United States, annual average 2005–2007*

Summary

Although increases in asthma prevalence have slowed since the mid-1990s, asthma prevalence remains at historically high levels. Current asthma prevalence differs between groups, with higher rates among females, children, non-Hispanic black and Puerto Rican persons, those with family income below the poverty level, and those residing in the Northeast and Midwest regions. Asthma can involve costs related to healthcare use and morbidity, including missed work and school days. Even after accounting for prevalence differences between groups, healthcare use differs among groups. Non-Hispanic black persons have relatively low rates of ambulatory visits compared with their use of urgent healthcare services, which may represent underuse of or lower access to preventive services. In contrast, although children have higher healthcare use than adults, they have much lower death rates. However, because adverse asthma outcomes are theoretically preventable, lowering asthma death rates among people of all ages remains a priority. The large asthma burden and continued adverse outcomes present an ongoing public health challenge, including the effort to enhance uptake of underutilized management strategies to control symptoms.

References

1. *National Asthma Education and Prevention Program. Expert Panel Report 3: Guidelines for the diagnosis and management of asthma.* NIH pub no 07–4051. Bethesda, MD: National Heart, Lung, and Blood Institute, National Institutes of Health. 2007. Available from: http://www.nhlbi.nih.gov/guidelines/asthma/.

2. Botman SL, Moore TF, Moriarity CL, Parsons VL. Design and estimation for the National Health Interview Survey, 1995–2004. National Center for Health Statistics. Vital Health Stat 2(130). 2000. Available from: http://www.cdc.gov/ nchs/data/series/sr_02/sr02_130.pdf.

3. RTI International. SUDAAN language manual, release 10. Research Triangle Park, NC: RTI International. 2008.

4. U.S. Department of Health and Human Services. Tracking Healthy People 2010. Washington, DC: Government Printing Office. 2000.

5   Schenker N, Raghunathan TE, Chiu PL, Makuc DM, Zhang G, Cohen AJ. Multiple imputation of family income and personal earnings in the National Health Interview Survey: Methods and examples. National Center for Health Statistics. 2008. Available from: http://www.cdc.gov/nchs/data/nhis/tecdoc.pdf.

6. Klein RJ, Schoenborn CA. Age adjustment using the 2000 projected U.S. population. Healthy People 2010 statistical notes, no 20. Hyattsville, MD: National Center for Health Statistics. 2001.

7. Joinpoint regression program, version 3.4 [computer software]. Bethesda, MD: National Cancer Institute, National Institutes of Health. 2010. Available from: http://srab.cancer.gov/joinpoint.

8. Xu JQ, Kochanek KD, Murphy SL, Tejada-Vera B. Deaths: Final data for 2007. National vital statistics reports; vol 58 no 19. Hyattsville, MD: National Center for Health Statistics. 2010. Available from: http:// www.cdc.gov/nchs/data/nvsr/ nvsr58/ nvsr58_19.pdf.

Chapter 6

The Global Burden of Asthma

Asthma is a chronic inflammatory lung disease characterized by recurrent breathing problems and symptoms such as breathlessness, wheezing, chest tightness, and coughing.[1] Asthma symptoms vary over time, and also differ in severity from one individual to another. In the most extreme cases, the airways can become so inflamed and constricted that people are unable to breathe. When it is not effectively treated, asthma can lead to hospitalization, missed time from work and school, limitations on physical activity, sleepless nights, and in some cases death.

Causes and Prevalence of Asthma

The causes of asthma are not fully understood, but the disease is a result of interaction between environmental and hereditary factors.[1,2] Up to 90 percent of asthma is classified as allergic[3] and is triggered by allergens such as dust mites (in bedding, carpets etc.), animal dander, pollen, and mould.[3] Tobacco smoke and exposure to chemical irritants in the workplace are also considered risk factors.[4]

Asthma impacts people of all ages and ethnic backgrounds, and it is estimated that as many as three hundred million people worldwide suffer from the disease.[5] In Europe, thirty million people are affected by asthma, and the prevalence in Western Europe has doubled over the last decade.[5] By 2025 it is predicted that a further one hundred million people worldwide will suffer from asthma, mainly due to the increasing number of people living in towns and cities.[5]

Although asthma affects all age groups, it often starts in childhood.[6] Approximately half of the people with asthma have experienced an attack before the age of ten.[6]

Asthma Rates across Europe

The United Kingdom (UK) and Ireland have some of the highest asthma rates in the world—almost double the European average (13.8 percent versus 7.2 percent). The number of asthma attacks has increased by 500 percent in the last twenty-five years and the UK's general practitioners see more than three thousand new cases every day (i.e., twenty thousand per week).[5]

Around 8 percent of the Swiss population now suffer from asthma, compared with only 2 percent twenty-five to thirty years ago.[2]

Table 6.1 shows the highest prevalence rates in Europe.[7]

Table 6.1. Highest Prevalence Rates in Europe (average 7.2%)

Country	Prevalence (%)
UK	13.8
Finland	11.0
Ireland	10.5
Netherlands	8.7
Switzerland	8.0
France	6.9
Spain	5.0
Germany	4.7

Source: Health, Food and Alcohol and Safety, Special Eurobarometer 186 / Wave 59.0, European Opinion Group EEIG, December 2003; *The European Lung White Book: The First Comprehensive Survey on Respiratory Health in Europe* 2003.

Impact of Severe Asthma

Severe asthma has a serious impact on the lives of patients, affecting their relationships, social lives, and work opportunities. It can cause potentially life-threatening asthma exacerbations with debilitating breathlessness, and a constant fear that the next attack could be fatal.

Some patients with severe symptoms are less responsive to standard asthma therapy and have been shown to experience greater morbidity and a lower quality of life than those whose disease is adequately controlled.[8] These patients are at greater risk of experiencing severe asthma attacks, hospitalization, and even death from their asthma.[9,10] According to the World Health Organization, one person dies every hour from asthma-related causes in Western Europe,[11] and experts claim the majority of these deaths are preventable.

Out of the total population of patients with asthma, the proportion with severe disease has been estimated at 18 percent in Western Europe and 32 percent in Central and Eastern Europe.[12,13] This equates to around 1 to 3 percent of the general population,[14] the equivalent of 4.5 to 14 million people in the twenty-five countries of the European Union. Approximately 20 percent of these patients have uncontrolled severe persistent asthma,[13] and approximately 50 percent of these are considered allergic to common aeroallergens.[8] The percentage with severe persistent uncontrolled allergic asthma can therefore be estimated as approximately 2 percent of all asthma patients.

Personal Consequences of Severe Asthma

In 2005 the European Federation of Allergy and Airways Diseases Patients' Associations (EFA) conducted a survey of 1,300 patients with severe asthma in France, Germany, Spain, Sweden, and the UK.[15] The results demonstrate the impact that severe asthma can have on individuals' lives:

- 75 percent of those interviewed suffered disturbed sleep once a week or more, and the same percentage experienced wheezing attacks on a weekly basis.

- Around one in five experienced speech-limiting attacks once a week—especially frightening since they would be unable to cry out for help.

- More than half of respondents said they suffered anxiety and stress because of their asthma, and one in four said they felt their condition was life-threatening. The most common words associated with asthma were "breathlessness," "suffocation," and "fear."

- More than one in three said their social life was restricted. Almost a third said asthma stopped them going on holiday; 38 percent said it stopped them going out with friends; 49 percent could not have pets or visit people with pets; and 70 percent were unable to participate in physical activities.

- One in five felt that they missed out on job opportunities (in Sweden the number rose to one in three), and 9 percent thought their illness has cost them promotion. Some had been forced to change jobs or retire early.

Economic Burden

The social and economic burden of asthma is substantial. In Europe the cost of asthma is estimated at 17.7 billion euros a year, in addition to lost productivity estimated at 9.8 billion euros.[2]

Patients with inadequately controlled severe asthma account for much of the morbidity, mortality, and economic burden associated with the disease.[2,9,10] In the UK, around half of the total cost of asthma is accounted for by the 20 percent of patients with the most severe form of the disease.[5]

Management of Severe Asthma

Asthma is a chronic condition which often requires continuous medical care. Patients with moderate to severe asthma have to take long-term daily medication, such as anti-inflammatory drugs.[4]

Experts are concerned that the level of asthma control in Europe falls short of the goals for long-term disease control outlined in guidelines established by the Global Initiative for Asthma (GINA), including minimal symptoms, no emergency visits, and no limitation on daily activities.[1,16]

References

1. GINA Global Initiative for Asthma. *Pocket Guide for Asthma Management and Prevention.*

2. *The European Lung White Book: The First Comprehensive Survey on Respiratory Health in Europe* 2003.

3. Holt PG, Macaubas C, Stumbles PA, et al. The role of allergy in the development of asthma. *Nature* 1999; 402(Suppl.):B12–17.

4. World Health Organization; www.who.int/mediacentre/factsheets/fs206/en/

5. GINA Global Initiative for Asthma. *The Global Burden of Asthma Report*, 2004.

6. www.ginasthma.com/QandA.asp?intId=114

7. Health, Food and Alcohol and Safety, Special Eurobarometer 186 / Wave 59.0, European Opinion Group EEIG, December 2003.

8. European Network for Understanding Mechanisms of Severe Asthma (2003). The ENFUMOSA cross-sectional European multicentre study of the clinical phenotype of chronic severe asthma. *European Respiratory Journal* 22:470–77.

9. Tough SC, Hessel PA, Ruff M, et al. Features that distinguish those who die from asthma from community controls with asthma. *J Asthma* 1998; 35:657–65.

10. Turner MO, Noertjojo K, Vedal S, et al. Risk factors for near-fatal asthma. A case-control study in hospitalized patients with asthma. *Am J Respir Crit Care Med* 1998; 157:1804–9.

11. The World Health Report 2003, Shaping the Future, the World Health Organization.

12. Rabe KF, Vermeire PA, Soriano JB, et al. Clinical management of asthma in 1999: the Asthma Insights and Reality in Europe (AIRE) study. *Eur Respir J* 2000; 16:802–7.

13. Rabe K F, Adachi M, Lai CK, et al. Worldwide severity and control of asthma in children and adults: the global Asthma Insights and Reality surveys. *J Allergy Clin Immunol* 2004; 114:40–47.

14. Siroux V, Pin I, Pison C, et al. Severe asthma in the general: population: definition and prevalence. *Rev Mal Respir* 2004; 21:961–69.

15. European Federation of Allergy and Airways Diseases Patients' Associations (EFA) survey 'Fighting for Breath,' May 2005.

16. www.ginasthma.com/PressReleaseItem.asp?l1=6&l2=1&intId =893

Part Two

Recognizing and Diagnosing Asthma

Chapter 7

Asthma Attacks

Chapter Contents

Section 7.1

What Is an Asthma Attack and What Triggers It?

"What Is an Asthma Attack" is excepted from "Asthma: Basic Information," Centers for Disease Control and Prevention, April 24, 2009. "What Causes an Asthma Attack" is excerpted from "Asthma Fast Facts for Kids," Centers for Disease Control and Prevention, April 24, 2009.

What Is an Asthma Attack?

An asthma attack happens in your body's airways, which are the paths that carry air to your lungs. As the air moves through your lungs, the airways become smaller, like the branches of a tree are smaller than the tree trunk. During an asthma attack, the sides of the airways in your lungs swell and the airways shrink. Less air gets in and out of your lungs, and mucus that your body produces clogs up the airways even more. The attack may include coughing, chest tightness, wheezing, and trouble breathing. Some people call an asthma attack an episode.

What Causes an Asthma Attack?

An asthma attack is when you have trouble catching your breath. Many different asthma "triggers" can cause this to happen. Some common "triggers" are as follows:

- Dust in your house
- Tobacco smoke
- Dirty air outside
- Cockroach droppings
- Pets
- Mold
- Hard exercise that makes you breathe really fast
- Some medicines

- Bad weather

- Some kinds of food

Things you are worried about can cause an asthma attack. Even getting really excited, or feeling very mad, sad, or scared can cause an asthma attack.

Section 7.2

Signs of an Asthma Attack

Excerpted from "What to Do in an Asthma Emergency," © 2010 Asthma Foundation NSW (www.asthmafoundation.org.au). Reprinted with permission.

Despite controlling your asthma, following your asthma action plan, and taking your medications regularly, you may still experience an asthma flare-up and suffer an asthma attack.

How Do I Know If I'm Having an Attack?

You are having an asthma attack if your asthma symptoms get worse but do not go away when you use your reliever. An asthma attack may develop very rapidly over a few minutes, or it may take a few hours or even days to happen. An asthma attack may be mild, moderate, or severe.

Symptoms of a Mild Asthma Attack

- Cough, wheeze

- Some shortness of breath

- Still able to speak in full sentences between breaths

Symptoms of a Moderate Asthma Attack

- Continual cough, moderate to loud wheeze

- Obvious difficulty breathing

- Only able to speak in short phrases between breaths

Symptoms of a Severe Asthma Attack

- Severe difficulties breathing
- Speak no more than a few words at a time
- Wheeze is often quiet
- Sucking in of the throat and rib muscles
- Pale and sweaty
- May have blue lips
- Very distressed and anxious

Note: If you or someone else is having a severe attack, you should call an ambulance (dial 911) immediately.

As well as experiencing some of the above symptoms, young children may appear restless, unable to settle, and may have problems eating or drinking. They may also have severe coughing or vomiting.

Section 7.3

What to Do During an Asthma Attack

"What Do You Do During an Asthma Attack?" © 2010 West Virginia
Asthma Education and Prevention Program (www.wvasthma.org).
Reprinted with permission.

Common Symptoms of an Asthma Attack

- Coughing

- Chest pain or tightness

- Shortness of or gasping for breath

- Wheezing

- Flushed, pale, ashen, or bluish looking skin

- Speaking in clipped or short bursts of speech

What to Do During an Asthma Attack

1. Have the person *stop* whatever activity he or she is doing.
    Send another person to get help. *Do not* leave the person alone.

2. Follow the person's Asthma Action Plan or emergency plan if
    there is one.

3. If the individual has a rescue inhaler or nebulizer (with medi-
    cines such as albuterol, Proventil, Ventolin, or Xopenex), have
    him or her use it immediately (preferably with a spacer or
    valved holding chamber).

    During an asthma attack an individual should:

    - Prepare inhaler for use by shaking canister for several
      seconds. Exhale or empty all air out of lungs, and follow as
      listed below with or without a spacer.

    - Inhaler with a spacer or holding chamber: Inhale one puff of
      medication by depressing the canister once, breathe in slowly
      and deeply, hold breath for ten seconds, and then exhale.

- Inhaler without a spacer or holding chamber: Place inhaler at the opening of the lips or a distance of one inch from open mouth; depress canister one time and inhale medicine quickly at the same time; hold breath for ten seconds and then exhale.

- Wait thirty seconds to one minute between puffs of inhaled medication.

- Shake inhaler canister between puffs.

- Repeat process, depress canister, inhale another puff, hold breath for ten seconds, and exhale.

- Continue as needed, typically four to eight puffs (depending on severity of symptoms).

  —Have the individual sit up and slowly breathe in through the nose and out through pursed lips (pursed lip breathing). Pursed lip breathing technique is as follows:

- Start by sitting comfortably in a chair. Do not lie down.

- Relax your shoulders and neck. Concentrate on not gasping for air as you drop your shoulders.

- Breathe in slowly through your nose. Concentrate.

- Purse your lips together tightly as if trying to whistle, and blow out slowly through your mouth. Take as much time as possible to exhale in this way.

- Relax. Keep using the pursed-lip breathing until the breathless feeling goes away. Rest between breaths if you feel dizzy.

  —Give sips of room temperature water.

4. Repeat above steps if symptoms continue.

5. If symptoms continue or worsen, seek immediate medical help.

Rescue inhaled medications such as albuterol and Xopenex should provide relief of immediate asthma symptoms (wheezing, shortness of breath, coughing) within five to ten minutes of use.

Per national guidelines (National Heart, Lung, and Blood Institute: Expert Panel Report 3) for "home" management of asthma attacks, up to two treatments (either nebulizer or metered dose inhaler) twenty minutes apart may be administered, assessing condition throughout both treatments to determine if emergency transport/emergency department treatment is necessary. This guideline is for all age groups from infants to adults.

Call 911 if:

- You are not sure what to do;
- Rescue medications are not working (symptoms are getting worse, not better) or meds are unavailable;
- The person's lips or fingernails are blue;
- The individual is having difficulty talking, walking, or drinking liquids;
- The person's nostrils are flaring out;
- You see neck, throat, or chest muscle retractions;
- The person is in obvious distress, there is a change in level of consciousness, or the individual is showing signs of confusion; or
- The individual's condition is deteriorating.

Chapter 8

Diagnosing Asthma

Chapter Contents

Section 8.1

Symptoms of Asthma

"Asthma Symptoms," © 2005 American Association for Respiratory
Care (www.yourlunghealth.org). Reprinted with permission.
Reviewed by David A. Cooke, MD, FACP, May 2011.

Asthma is a disease with many different symptoms that occur in many different ways and combinations. Some people with asthma only have symptoms periodically and they are generally mild. Others have symptoms more often and may also experience symptoms that are more severe. Others still have symptoms every day or symptoms that are so severe they are life threatening.

The most common asthma symptoms include:

- coughing, especially at night;

- wheezing;

- shortness of breath;

- chest tightness, pain, or pressure.

The good news is, most people with asthma will begin to have these and other symptoms early enough to seek appropriate treatment and stop a severe attack from occurring. Symptoms that indicate the onset of an asthma attack include:

- frequent cough, particularly at night;

- shortness of breath or easily losing your breath;

- tiring easily or feeling weak while exercising;

- wheezing or coughing after exercise;

- feeling tired, upset, moody, or grouchy;

- experiencing signs of a cold or allergies;

- sleeping difficulties;

- lung function changes as measured by a peak flow meter.

When early symptoms occur, follow your doctor's instructions for changing and/or increasing your medications. If your doctor has prescribed the proper medications, this will usually stop an attack from occurring or getting worse.

How can you know when an attack is approaching the danger zone? If you've had early symptoms of asthma and medication changes haven't helped—or you have been unable to follow doctor's recommendations on adjusting your doses—you should seek further medical attention if any of the following occur:

- you have a day or nighttime cough that doesn't go away;

- you can't stop coughing;

- you experience very rapid breathing;

- wheezing persists;

- you experience tightness or pressure in your chest;

- you experience ongoing shortness of breath;

- the muscles in your neck and chest tighten;

- you experience feelings of anxiety or panic;

- your face becomes pale or sweaty;

- our bronchodilator medications don't provide immediate relief of symptoms;

- your peak flow readings drop markedly (usually less than 50 percent of predicted).

In extremely severe cases, you may also stop wheezing, a condition known as a "silent chest," your lips or fingernails may turn blue, indicating a lack of oxygen, and you will find it difficult or impossible to talk. These severe symptoms occur when the airways are so tight that air cannot move back and forth and require immediate emergency medical care.

Section 8.2

How Asthma Is Diagnosed

Excerpted from "How Is Asthma Diagnosed?" National Heart,
Lung, and Blood Institute, National Institutes of Health,
February 2011.

Your primary care doctor will diagnose asthma based on your medical and family histories, a physical exam, and test results.

Your doctor also will figure out the severity of your asthma—that is, whether it's intermittent, mild, moderate, or severe. The level of severity will determine what treatment you'll start on.

You may need to see an asthma specialist if any of the following are true:

- You need special tests to help diagnose asthma

- You've had a life-threatening asthma attack

- You need more than one kind of medicine or higher doses of medicine to control your asthma, or if you have overall problems getting your asthma well controlled

- You're thinking about getting allergy treatments

Medical and Family Histories

Your doctor may ask about your family history of asthma and allergies. He or she also may ask whether you have asthma symptoms and when and how often they occur.

Let your doctor know whether your symptoms seem to happen only during certain times of the year or in certain places, or if they get worse at night.

Your doctor also may want to know what factors seem to trigger your symptoms or worsen them.

Your doctor may ask you about related health conditions that can interfere with asthma management. These conditions include a runny nose, sinus infections, reflux disease, psychological stress, and sleep apnea.

Physical Exam

Your doctor will listen to your breathing and look for signs of asthma or allergies. These signs include wheezing, a runny nose or swollen nasal passages, and allergic skin conditions (such as eczema).

Keep in mind that you can still have asthma even if you don't have these signs on the day that your doctor examines you.

Diagnostic Tests

Lung Function Test

Your doctor will use a test called spirometry to check how your lungs are working. This test measures how much air you can breathe in and out. It also measures how fast you can blow air out.

Your doctor also may give you medicine and then test you again to see whether the results have improved.

If the starting results are lower than normal and improve with the medicine, and if your medical history shows a pattern of asthma symptoms, your diagnosis will likely be asthma.

Other Tests

Your doctor may recommend other tests if he or she needs more information to make a diagnosis. Other tests may include the following:

- Allergy testing to find out which allergens affect you, if any.

- A test to measure how sensitive your airways are. This is called a bronchoprovocation test. Using spirometry, this test repeatedly measures your lung function during physical activity or after you receive increasing doses of cold air or a special chemical to breathe in.

- A test to show whether you have another condition with the same symptoms as asthma, such as reflux disease, vocal cord dysfunction, or sleep apnea.

- A chest x-ray or an electrocardiogram (EKG). These tests will help find out whether a foreign object or other disease may be causing your symptoms.

Section 8.3

How Asthma Is Classified

Based on the results of your visit with an asthma specialist, your asthma will be classified in one of the following categories (based on National Heart Blood and Lung Institute guidelines).

Mild Intermittent Asthma

- Symptoms of cough, wheeze, chest tightness, or difficulty breathing less than twice a week

- Flare-ups-brief, but intensity may vary

- Nighttime symptoms less than twice a month

- No symptoms between flare-ups

- Lung function test FEV1 (forced expiratory volume in one second) equal to or above 80 percent of normal values

- Peak flow less than 20 percent variability a.m.-to-a.m. or a.m.-to-p.m., day-to-day

Mild Persistent Asthma

- Symptoms of cough, wheeze, chest tightness, or difficulty breathing three to six times a week

- Flare-ups-may affect activity level

- Nighttime symptoms three to four times a month

- Lung function test FEV1 equal to or above 80 percent of normal values

- Peak flow less than 20 to 30 percent variability

Moderate Persistent Asthma

- Symptoms of cough, wheeze, chest tightness, or difficulty breathing daily
- Flare-ups may affect activity level
- Nighttime symptoms five or more times a month
- Lung function test FEV1 above 60 percent but below 80 percent of normal values
- Peak flow more than 30 percent variability

Severe Persistent Asthma

- Symptoms of cough, wheeze, chest tightness, or difficulty breathing continual
- Nighttime symptoms frequently
- Lung function test FEV1 less than or equal to 60 percent of normal values
- Peak flow more than 30 percent variability

The level of asthma severity will determine what types of medicine you will need to get your asthma under control.

Chapter 9

Tests and Procedures Used to Diagnose Asthma

Chapter Contents

Section 9.1

Lung Function Tests

National Heart, Lung, and Blood Institute,
National Institutes of Health, August 2010.

Understanding Lung Function Tests

Lung function tests, also called pulmonary function tests, measure how well your lungs work. These tests are used to look for the cause of breathing problems, such as shortness of breath.

Lung function tests measure the following things:

- How much air you can take into your lungs. This amount is compared to that of other people your age, height, and sex. This allows your doctor to see whether you're in the normal range.

- How much air you can blow out of your lungs and how fast you can do it.

- How well your lungs deliver oxygen to your blood.

- The strength of your breathing muscles.

Doctors use lung function tests to help diagnose conditions such as asthma, pulmonary fibrosis (scarring of the lung tissue), and chronic obstructive pulmonary disease (COPD).

Lung function tests also are used to check the extent of damage caused by conditions such as pulmonary fibrosis and sarcoidosis. Also, these tests may be used to check how well treatments, such as asthma medicines, are working.

Overview

Lung function tests include breathing tests and tests that measure the oxygen level in your blood. The breathing tests most often used are as follows:

- **Spirometry:** This test measures how much air you can breathe in and out. It also measures how fast you can blow air out.

- **Lung volume measurement:** This test, in addition to spirometry, measures how much air remains in your lungs after you breathe out fully.

- **Lung diffusion capacity:** This test measures how well oxygen passes from your lungs to your bloodstream.

These tests may not show what's causing breathing problems. So, you may have other tests as well, such as a cardiopulmonary exercise test. This test measures how well your lungs and heart work while you exercise on a treadmill or bicycle.

Two tests that measure the oxygen level in your blood are pulse oximetry and arterial blood gas tests. These tests also are called blood oxygen tests.

Pulse oximetry measures the blood oxygen level using a special light. For an arterial blood gas test, your doctor inserts a needle into an artery, usually in your wrist, and takes a sample of blood. The oxygen level of the blood sample is measured.

Outlook

Lung function tests usually are painless and rarely cause side effects. You may feel some discomfort during an arterial blood gas test when the needle is inserted into the artery.

Types of Lung Function Tests

Breathing Tests

Spirometry: Spirometry measures how much air you breathe in and out and how fast you blow it out. This is measured two ways: peak expiratory flow rate (PEFR) and forced expiratory volume in one second (FEV1).

PEFR refers to the amount of air you can blow out as quickly as possible. FEV1 refers to the amount of air you can blow out in one second.

During the test, a technician will ask you to take a deep breath in. Then, you'll blow as hard as you can into a tube connected to a small machine. The machine is called a spirometer.

Your doctor may have you inhale a medicine that helps open your airways. He or she will want to see whether the medicine changes or improves the test results.

Spirometry helps check for conditions that affect how much air you can breathe in, such as pulmonary fibrosis (scarring of the lung tissue). The test also helps detect diseases that affect how fast you can breathe air out, like asthma and chronic obstructive pulmonary disease (COPD).

Lung volume measurement: This test measures the size of your lungs and how much air you can breathe in and out. During the test, you sit inside a glass booth and breathe into a tube that's hooked to a computer.

Sometimes you breathe in nitrogen or helium gas and then blow it out. The gas you breathe out is measured to test how much air your lungs can hold.

Lung volume measurement can help diagnose pulmonary fibrosis or a stiff or weak chest wall.

Lung diffusion capacity: This test measures how well oxygen passes from your lungs to your bloodstream. During this test, you breathe in a type of gas through a tube. You hold your breath for a brief moment and then blow out the gas.

Abnormal test results may suggest loss of lung tissue, emphysema (a type of COPD), very bad scarring of the lung tissue, or problems with blood flow through the body's arteries.

Tests to Measure Oxygen Level

Pulse oximetry and arterial blood gas tests show how much oxygen is in your blood. During pulse oximetry, a small sensor is attached to your finger or ear. The sensor uses light to estimate how much oxygen is in your blood. This test is painless and no needles are used.

For an arterial blood gas test, a blood sample is taken from an artery, usually in your wrist. The sample is sent to a laboratory, where its oxygen level is measured.

Testing in Infants and Young Children

Spirometry and other measures of lung function usually can be done in children older than six years, if they can follow directions well. Spirometry may be tried in children as young as five years. However, technicians who have special training with young children may need to do the testing.

Instead of spirometry, a growing number of medical centers measure respiratory system resistance. This is another way to test lung function in young children.

The child wears nose clips and has his or her cheeks supported with an adult's hands. The child breathes in and out quietly on a mouthpiece, while the technician measures changes in pressure at the mouth. During these lung function tests, parents can help comfort their children and encourage them to cooperate.

Very young children (younger than two years) may need an infant lung function test. This requires special equipment and medical staff. This type of test is available only at a few medical centers.

The doctor gives the child medicine to help him or her sleep through the test. A technician places a mask over the child's nose and mouth and a vest around the child's chest.

The mask and vest are attached to a lung function machine. The machine gently pushes air into the child's lungs through the mask. As the child exhales, the vest slightly squeezes his or her chest. This helps push more air out of the lungs. The exhaled air is then measured.

In children younger than five years, doctors likely will use signs and symptoms, medical history, and a physical exam to diagnose lung problems.

Pulse oximetry and arterial blood gas tests can be used for children of all ages.

Other Names for Lung Function Tests

- Lung diffusion testing; also called diffusing capacity and diffusing capacity of the lung for carbon monoxide, or DLCO

- Pulmonary function tests, or PFTs

Arterial blood gas tests also are called blood gas analyses or ABGs.

Who Needs Lung Function Tests?

People who have breathing problems, such as shortness of breath, may need lung function tests. These tests help find the cause of breathing problems.

Doctors use lung function tests to help diagnose conditions such as asthma, pulmonary fibrosis (scarring of the lung tissue), and chronic obstructive pulmonary disease (COPD).

Lung function tests also are used to check the extent of damage caused by conditions such as pulmonary fibrosis and sarcoidosis. Also, these tests may be used to check how well treatments, such as asthma medicines, are working.

Diagnosing Lung Conditions

Your doctor will diagnose a lung condition based on your medical and family histories, a physical exam, and test results.

Medical and Family Histories

Your doctor will ask you questions, such as the following:

- Do you ever feel like you can't get enough air?
- Does your chest feel tight sometimes?
- Do you have periods of coughing or wheezing (a whistling sound when you breathe)?
- Do you ever have chest pain?
- Can you walk or run as fast as other people your age?

Your doctor also will ask whether you or anyone in your family has ever:

- had asthma or allergies;
- had heart disease;
- smoked;
- traveled to places where they may have been exposed to tuberculosis;
- had a job that exposed them to dust, fumes, or particles (like asbestos).

Physical Exam

Your doctor will check your heart rate, breathing rate, and blood pressure. He or she also will listen to your heart and lungs with a stethoscope and feel your abdomen and limbs.

Your doctor will look for signs of heart or lung disease, or another disease that may be causing your symptoms.

Lung and Heart Tests

Based on your medical history and physical exam, your doctor will recommend tests. A chest x-ray usually is the first test done to find the cause of a breathing problem. This test takes pictures of the organs and structures inside your chest.

Your doctor may do lung function tests to find out even more about how well your lungs work.

Your doctor also may do tests to check your heart, such as an electrocardiogram (EKG) or a stress test. An EKG detects and records your heart's electrical activity. A stress test shows how well your heart works during physical activity.

What to Expect Before Lung Function Tests

If you take breathing medicines, your doctor may ask you to stop them for a short time before spirometry, lung volume measurement, or lung diffusion capacity tests.

No special preparation is needed before pulse oximetry and arterial blood gas tests. If you're getting oxygen therapy, your doctor may ask you to stop using it for a short time before the tests. This allows your doctor to check your blood oxygen level without the added oxygen.

What to Expect During Lung Function Tests

Breathing Tests

Spirometry may be done in your doctor's office or in a special lung function laboratory (lab). Lung volume measurement and lung diffusion capacity tests are done in a special lab or clinic. For these tests, you sit in a chair next to a machine that measures your breathing. For spirometry, you sit or stand next to the machine.

Before the tests, a technician places soft clips on your nose. This allows you to breathe only through a tube that's attached to the testing machine. The technician will tell you how to breathe into the tube. For example, you may be asked to breathe normally, slowly, or rapidly.

The deep breathing done in some of the tests may make you feel short of breath, dizzy, or light-headed, or it may make you cough.

Spirometry: For this test, you take a deep breath and then exhale as fast and as hard as you can into the tube. With spirometry, your doctor may give you a medicine that helps open your airways. Your doctor will want to see whether the medicine changes or improves the test results.

Lung volume measurement: For this test, you sit in a clear glass booth and breathe through the tube attached to the testing machine. The changes in pressure inside the booth are measured to show how much air you can breathe into your lungs.

Sometimes you breathe in nitrogen or helium gas and then exhale. The gas that you breathe out is measured.

Lung diffusion capacity: During this test, you breathe in gas through the tube, hold your breath for ten seconds, and then rapidly blow it out. The gas contains a small amount of carbon monoxide, which won't harm you.

Tests to Measure Oxygen Level

Pulse oximetry is done in a doctor's office or hospital. An arterial blood gas test is done in a lab or hospital.

Pulse oximetry: For this test, a small sensor is attached to your finger or ear using a clip or flexible tape. The sensor is then attached to a cable that leads to a small machine called an oximeter. The oximeter shows the amount of oxygen in your blood. This test is painless and no needles are used.

Arterial blood gas: During this test, your doctor or technician inserts a needle into an artery, usually in your wrist, and takes a sample of blood. You may feel some discomfort when the needle is inserted. The sample is then sent to a lab where its oxygen level is measured.

After the needle is removed, you may feel mild pressure or throbbing at the needle site. Applying pressure to the area for five to ten minutes should stop the bleeding. You'll be given a small bandage to place on the area.

What to Expect After Lung Function Tests

You can return to your normal activities and restart your medicines after lung function tests. Talk with your doctor about when you'll get the test results.

What Do Lung Function Tests Show?

Breathing Tests

Spirometry: Spirometry can show whether you have a blockage (obstruction) in your airways, which may be a sign of asthma, chronic obstructive pulmonary disease [COPD], or another obstructive lung disorder, or smaller than normal lungs (restriction), which may be a sign of heart failure, pulmonary fibrosis (scarring of the lung tissue), or another restrictive lung disorder.

Lung volume measurement: This test shows the size of your lungs. Abnormal test results may show that you have pulmonary fibrosis or a stiff or weak chest wall.

Lung diffusion capacity: This test can show a problem with oxygen moving from your lungs into your bloodstream. This may be a sign of loss of lung tissue, emphysema (a type of COPD), or problems with blood flow through the body's arteries.

Tests to Measure Oxygen Level

Pulse oximetry and arterial blood gas tests measure the oxygen level in your blood. These tests show how well your lungs are taking in oxygen and moving it into the bloodstream. A low level of oxygen in the blood may be a sign of a lung or heart disorder.

What Are the Risks of Lung Function Tests?

Spirometry, lung volume measurement, and lung diffusion capacity tests usually are safe. These tests rarely cause problems.

Pulse oximetry has no risks. Side effects from arterial blood gas tests are rare.

Key Points

- Lung function tests, also called pulmonary function tests, measure how well your lungs work. These tests are used to look for the cause of breathing problems, such as shortness of breath.

- Lung function tests show how much air you can take into your lungs, how much air you can blow out of your lungs and how fast you can do it, how well your lungs deliver oxygen to your blood, and the strength of your breathing muscles.

- Lung function tests can help diagnose conditions such as asthma, pulmonary fibrosis (scarring of the lung tissue), and chronic obstructive pulmonary disease (COPD).

- Lung function tests also are used to check the extent of damage caused by conditions such as pulmonary fibrosis and sarcoidosis. These tests also are used to check how well treatments, such as asthma medicines, are working.

- Breathing tests include spirometry, lung volume measurement, and lung diffusion capacity. Pulse oximetry and arterial blood gas tests measure the oxygen level in your blood.

- If you take breathing medicines, your doctor may ask you to stop them for a short time before spirometry, a lung volume measurement test, or a lung diffusion capacity test. No special preparation is needed before pulse oximetry and arterial blood gas tests.

- For breathing tests, you'll breathe through a tube that's attached to a testing machine. You may be asked to breathe normally, slowly, or rapidly. You also may be asked to breathe in a small amount of gas and then blow it out.

- For the tests that measure oxygen level in the blood, either a small sensor will be attached to your finger or ear to measure the oxygen level, or your doctor will take a small sample of your blood to measure the oxygen level.

- You can return to your normal activities and restart your medicines after lung function tests. Talk with your doctor about when you'll get the test results.

- Lung function tests can show whether you have signs of a lung or heart condition. These tests also can show how well treatments for breathing problems, such as asthma medicines, are working.

- Lung function tests are painless and rarely cause side effects. You may feel some discomfort during the arterial blood gas test when the needle is inserted into the artery.

Section 9.2

Spirometry

Reprinted from "Spirometry," "Who Should Have a Spirometry?" "What Does a Spirometry Tell My Doctor?" "What You Need to Do Before the Test," and "What Happens During the Test?" © 2006 American Association for Respiratory Care (www.yourlunghealth.org). Reprinted with permission. Reviewed by David A. Cooke, MD, FACP, May 2011.

Spirometry

Many people who have lung disease may be unaware there is anything wrong with their lungs. Often lung disease symptoms are ignored or thought to be "just being out of shape" or part of "getting older."

The earlier you know you have lung disease, the earlier you and your doctor can take steps to improve your lung health and to prevent further damage to the airway. Some measures such as smoking cessation and avoiding respiratory irritants can help you stop the damage to your lungs.

Spirometry is effective in diagnosing COPD and asthma, tracking the progression of the disease, and managing medication changes.

Who Should Have a Spirometry?

If you answer yes to any of the following questions you should ask your doctor about having a spirometry test:

- Do you (now) or have you ever smoked?

- Are you short of breath more often than other people?

- Do you have a cough that does not go away? For example: daily coughing or the "morning" cough?

- If you cough, do you cough up mucus?

- Do people around you smoke?

- Do you work around chemicals and dust?

- Does bronchitis or emphysema run in your family?

- Do you wheeze (a whistling or squeaky sound when you breathe)?

What Does a Spirometry Tell My Doctor?

Spirometry is a simple breathing test that can be done in a physician's office that measures the amount of air you can blow out after you have taken in the deepest breath you can. The results of this test give two important numbers that measure airway obstruction.

FVC: Forced vital capacity: This is the total volume of air you can forcefully blow out. It is an assessment of the size of your lungs, how well your lungs expand and contract, and how well the air passages open and close.

Patients with obstructive lung disease usually have a normal or only slightly decreased vital capacity. A reduced FVC is associated with restrictive lung disorders, diseases that may be caused by inflammation or scarring of the lung tissue (interstitial lung disease), or by abnormalities of the muscles or skeleton of the chest wall.

FEV1: Forced expiratory volume: This is the volume of air that you can blow out in the first second of exhalation.

Typically FEV1 is considered "normal" if greater than 80 percent of predicted. FEV1 is reduced in both obstructive and restrictive lung disease.

FEV1/FVC: This ratio compares the volume of air expelled in the first second to the total volume expelled.

In healthy patients the FEV1/FVC is usually around 70 to 80 percent. In patients with obstructive lung disease FEV1/FVC decreases and can be as low as 20 to 30 percent in severe obstructive airway disease. Restrictive disorders have a near normal FEV1/FVC ratio.

What You Need to Do Before the Test

Wear comfortable clothing.

Ideally you should not use your inhalers before your spirometry. There are different types of bronchodilators; some are long acting and others are short acting inhalers so ask your doctor how long you should avoid using your inhaler/s before the test.

If you experience breathing problems before your test, go ahead and use your inhaler/s. Inform the person performing the test the name of the inhaler/s you used, dosage/puffs taken, and the time you used them.

What Happens During the Test?

You will be asked several questions (listed below) that will be used to determine what "normal" lung values would be for you if your lungs were healthy:

- **Age:** Lung function declines with age.

- **Height:** Taller people have larger lungs.

- **Sex:** Women have smaller lung volumes.

- **Race:** African Americans and Asians generally have smaller lung volumes.

You will be asked to sit up straight and uncross your legs or to stand up.

Often you will have a nose plug placed on your nose.

You will be instructed to:

- Take in a big breath.

- Place the mouthpiece into your mouth and seal your lips tightly around the mouthpiece.

- Blast your air into the mouthpiece as hard and fast as you can, squeezing out all the air in your lungs.

- Keep on blowing out the same breath until you are told to stop.

To make sure you understand the directions, ask the technician to demonstrate the procedure.

The test will be repeated several times to make sure that the measurements are correct.

The spirometry may be repeated after you receive a bronchodilator inhaler or nebulizer.

Section 9.3

Bronchoprovocation Challenge Testing

What is a bronchial provocation test?

The bronchial provocation test evaluates how sensitive the airways in your lungs are. A spirometry breathing test is done before and after you inhale a spray. One example of the spray that may be inhaled is methacholine. Other specific agents in your environment may also be used. Spirometry can show how much air you can breathe in and out. It also shows how fast you can breathe in and out. The spirometry results are compared before and after you inhale the spray to see what changes there are in your breathing. You will be given additional information at the time of the test.

A laryngoscopy may be scheduled after the bronchial provocation test. A laryngoscopy is often done to identify if your vocal cords may be causing you to have trouble breathing.

How do you get ready for the test?

Please follow these directions when getting ready for this test. These medicines will affect the results of some of these tests and need to be stopped before the testing is done. If the medicine is not stopped before the test we will not be able to complete the test.

Stop this inhaled medicine for seven days before your appointment:

- Spiriva (tiotropium)

Stop these inhaled medicines for forty-eight hours before your appointment:

- Advair (Serevent and Flovent)
- Serevent (salmeterol)
- Symbicort (Pulmicort and Foradil)
- Dulera (Azmanex and Foradil)
- Foradil (formoterol)
- Perforomist (formoterol)
- Brovana(arformoterol)
- Intal (cromolyn), Tilade (nedocromil)

Stop these inhaled medicines for twenty-four hours before your appointment:

- Atrovent (ipratropium)
- Combivent (albuterol and ipratropium)
- DuoNeb (albuterol and ipratropium)

Stop these oral medicines for twenty-four hours before your appointment:

- Accolate (zafirlukast)
- Zyflo (zileuton)
- Singular (montelukast)

Stop these oral medicines for twenty-four hours before your appointment:

- Volmax, Ventolin, Proventil, Proventil Repetabs (albuterol), Metaprel (metaproterenol), Bricanyl, Brethine (terbutaline)

Stop these inhaled medicines for six to eight hours before your appointment:

- Proventil HFA, Ventolin HFA, ProAir (albuterol), Xopenex (levalbuterol), Maxair (pirbuterol), Alupent, Metaprel (metaproterenol), Primatene Mist

Continue to take all your other medicine as you usually do.

Exercising can drop blood sugar in patients who are taking medications to control diabetes. Bring your glucose meter, test strips, and a source of fast-acting glucose with you (such as glucose tablets or glucose gel).

Adults: If a laryngoscopy is scheduled at the same time, do not eat for two hours before the test is scheduled.

Children: If a laryngoscopy is scheduled at the same time, do not eat for three hours before the test is scheduled.

What is done during the bronchial provocation test?

You will do a number of breathing tests. You will be asked to inhale a spray between the breathing tests. The technician will explain what you need to do during each test. A good effort during the testing is important to get good results. The technician will coach you during each test to help you give a good effort. If you have questions during the tests, please ask the technician.

You may be asked to sit in a Plexiglas booth for some of the testing. This booth is called a body box or plethysmograph. You will do different breathing techniques, blowing into a tube, while in the booth. Each breathing technique is often repeated to make sure the test is reliable.

If your doctor has scheduled you for a laryngoscopy this will be done right after the breathing tests are completed. During the laryngoscopy a doctor will place a small tube (fiber optic probe) in your nose. The tube is passed through your nose to the back of your throat after topical anesthesia is applied. The movement of the vocal cords can be seen with the probe. Please do not eat two to three hours prior to the test if a laryngoscopy has been scheduled.

How long will the test take?

Bronchial provocation testing often takes one-and-a-half to two hours.

Section 9.4

Nitric Oxide Test

For years, physicians have assessed asthma by measuring how much air a patient can exhale. Now, some doctors are beginning to measure what's in that breathed-out air—specifically, nitric oxide (NO). Scientists have discovered that the amount of nitric oxide in a patient's breath indicates the degree of inflammation in the airways.

This is important because airway inflammation sets the stage for noisy asthma symptoms such as coughing and wheezing (bronchospasm). Physicians have found that treating the underlying inflammation with anti-inflammatory medications like inhaled corticosteroids reduces the symptoms and prevents the exacerbations associated with asthma.

Asthma treatment guidelines call for use of the lowest possible dose of inhaled corticosteroids to achieve disease control. By measuring NO, physicians will know if there is inflammation present inside the airways and can better tailor anti-inflammatory medications to treat asthma.

Research studies in patients with asthma show:

- exhaled nitric oxide (eNO) levels may help predict asthma exacerbations before they occur;

- eNO levels can help predict which patients will and will not benefit from inhaled corticosteroids;

- eNO levels can help physicians determine whether allergen exposure is causing inflammation inside the lungs;

- eNO levels can help physicians know if patients are actually taking their anti-inflammatory medications as prescribed.

Nitric oxide tests do not replace spirometry and other lung function measurements. However, combined with lung function tests and medical history, nitric oxide measurements can help physicians determine the severity of asthma more accurately, especially among those patients whose asthma symptoms are subtle or inconsistent.

The tests are noninvasive and simple enough for people of all ages, including children, to carry out accurately. In the NIOX MINO monitoring system, approved by the U.S. Food and Drug Administration, patients first exhale thoroughly to clear their lungs as much as possible, then inhale filtered air through the MINO machine and exhale (breathe out) into the monitor. The resulting exhaled breath is thus clean of nitric oxide that might have been in the environment. Patients control the strength of their exhalation by watching images on a screen and listening for sounds that direct them to blow more or less forcefully. The MINO measures eNO according to guidelines set by the American Thoracic Society.

Some medical researchers look forward to eNO measuring devices that will be so inexpensive that they become available for home use—like a peak flow meter. Then patients and physicians can work together to monitor and manage asthma symptoms with greater precision.

Section 9.5

Allergy Testing

Many people with asthma are allergic to things that they breathe in. These tiny particles that can cause allergic reactions are called "allergens" (pronounced AL'-ER-GENZ). Examples of airborne allergens are the pollens of grasses, trees, and weeds, spores of molds, danders of cats and dogs and other furry animals, debris from cockroaches, and house dust mites. People with a tendency to allergies will usually be allergic to some but not all such allergens; different people are allergic to different things.

Breathing in Allergens Can Make Your Asthma Worse and Can Cause Asthmatic Attacks

Day to day inhalation of allergens to which you are sensitive can worsen the inflammation of the bronchial tubes in asthma. It can make your asthma more active (meaning that you are more likely to be troubled by cough, wheeze, shortness of breath, chest tightness, or nighttime awakenings from asthma symptoms) and make you more likely to have a serious attack of asthma. In addition, heavy exposure to an allergen to which you are sensitive can bring on a sudden attack of asthma or an attack that develops a few hours after the exposure.

It May Be Helpful to Determine the Allergens to Which You Are Sensitive

You and your doctor may decide that it would be helpful to know to which allergens you are sensitive. This information is used less often for the purpose of initiating "allergy shots" (also called desensitization injections) and more often to help reduce your exposure to those things that may specifically worsen your asthma. For instance, if you are strongly allergic to the house dust mite, simple actions can be taken in the home, and especially in the bedroom, that will decrease the amount of allergen from dust mites that you breathe in, causing a likely improvement in your asthma.

Reviewing Your Own Experiences with Allergic Exposures

The process of determining your particular allergies to inhaled allergens begins by considering those exposures that have caused you to have asthmatic reactions in the past: Is your asthma worse in the spring or fall? Does it come on when you dust or vacuum? Does a damp, mildewy room cause you to have symptoms of asthma? These and similar questions are important to determining your asthmatic allergies and to interpreting the results of allergy testing.

Tests for Allergic Sensitivity

Besides reviewing your own past experiences, there are two principal methods to test for your sensitivity to various allergens. One involves a blood test to analyze for antibody proteins that your body may have made in reaction to particular allergens; the other involves testing for reactions in your skin to the same allergens that you might breathe in. Some physicians rely primarily on the latter (allergy skin tests) because they are more sensitive, less expensive, give immediate results, and can test a larger number of different allergens than the blood tests. This section discusses the details of this process of allergy skin testing.

How Allergy Skin Testing Is Done

To test your reaction to an allergen, a drop of liquid containing the allergen in placed on your skin (generally the inside of your forearms is used). A small lance with a pinpoint is poked through the liquid into the top layer of skin. This type of skin test is called a "prick test." If you are allergic to the allergen, after about two minutes the skin begins to form a reaction. It becomes red, slightly swollen, and itchy: it makes a hive. The size of the hive is measured and recorded. The larger the hive, the more likely it is that you are allergic to the allergen tested.

Different Types of Allergy Skin Tests

Sometimes, if a very intense allergic sensitivity is suspected, then only a light scratch is made through the liquid that contains the allergen ("scratch test"). This way only a very little bit of the allergen is introduced into the skin. Other times, when it is particularly important to investigate sensitivity to a specific allergen, a small amount of the liquid is injected under the surface of the skin with a skinny needle ("intra-dermal test"). This method puts a little greater amount of the allergen into the skin.

The usual practice in allergy skin testing is to test all at once a group of common allergens to which one might be sensitive. Generally twenty-five to thirty prick tests are done at one time. The twenty-five to thirty drops of liquid containing the various allergens are lined up in two rows on each forearm, then a prick is made through each one. Within about five minutes the results of the test are known.

What Are Some Possible Bad Reactions to Allergy Skin Tests?

Bad reactions to allergy skin tests are rare, but they can happen. In particular, it is possible for the small amount of allergen in the skin to set off an attack of asthma, and, even more rarely, a period of dangerously low blood pressure, called an anaphylactic reaction. Because allergy skin testing involves these risks, although very small, you will be asked to give written permission on a "consent form" prior to the testing, and you will be asked to stay under medical observation for one to two hours after testing to ensure that no delayed reactions occur.

Interpreting the Results of Your Allergy Skin Tests

Interpretation of the results of the allergy skin tests will involve your doctor. The idea on which allergy skin testing for asthma is based is that if you make a reaction in your skin to a particular allergen (a "positive" result), you probably also will make a similar allergic reaction in the bronchial tubes of your lungs if you were to breathe in the same allergen. Although this is not always the case, it often is; and it is especially likely to be true if you have ever experienced asthmatic symptoms when exposed to the allergen. The opposite is also true and may provide you with equally useful information. If you do not make a reaction in your skin to the allergen (a "negative" result) and have not experienced asthmatic symptoms when you breathe in the allergen, you almost certainly do not have asthmatic sensitivity to that allergen.

Medications to Avoid Before Your Allergy Skin Testing

Finally, it is possible to get a false result on the allergy skin test if you have taken certain medications before the test that can interfere with the reaction in your skin. These medications are the group called antihistamines. Common examples of antihistamines are Benadryl, Chlor-Trimeton, Claritin, Zyrtec, Clarinex, and Allegra. Some of these medications can affect the results of allergy skin tests for several days after you take them. As a result, you will be asked to avoid all antihistamines for several hours or days before the skin tests.

Section 9.6

Chest X-Rays

"Chest X-Ray," National Heart, Lung, and Blood Institute,
National Institutes of Health, August, 2010.

What Is a Chest X-Ray?

A chest x-ray is a painless, noninvasive test that creates pictures of the structures inside your chest, such as your heart, lungs, and blood vessels. "Noninvasive" means that no surgery is done and no instruments are inserted into your body.

This test is done to find the cause of symptoms such as shortness of breath, chest pain, chronic cough (a cough that lasts a long time), and fever.

Overview

X-rays are electromagnetic waves. They use ionizing radiation to create pictures of the inside of your body.

A chest x-ray takes pictures of the inside of your chest. The different tissues in your chest absorb different amounts of radiation.

Your ribs and spine are bony and absorb radiation well. They normally appear light on a chest x-ray. Your lungs, which are filled with air, normally appear dark. A disease in the chest that changes how radiation is absorbed also will appear on a chest x-ray.

Chest x-rays help doctors diagnose conditions such as pneumonia, heart failure, lung cancer, lung tissue scarring, and sarcoidosis. Doctors also may use chest x-rays to see how well treatments for certain conditions are working. Also, doctors often use chest x-rays before surgery to look at the structures in the chest.

Chest x-rays are the most common x-ray test used to diagnose health problems.

Outlook

Chest x-rays have few risks. The amount of radiation used in a chest x-ray is very small. A lead apron may be used to protect certain parts of your body from the radiation.

A chest x-ray gives out a radiation dose similar to the amount of radiation you're naturally exposed to over ten days.

Other Names for a Chest X-Ray

- Chest radiography
- CXR

Who Needs a Chest X-Ray?

Doctors may recommend chest x-rays for people who have symptoms such as shortness of breath, chest pain, chronic cough (a cough that lasts a long time), or fever. The test can help find the cause of these symptoms.

Chest x-rays look for conditions such as pneumonia, heart failure, lung cancer, lung tissue scarring, or sarcoidosis. The test also is used to check how well treatments for certain conditions are working.

Chest x-rays also are used to evaluate people who test positive for tuberculosis exposure on skin tests.

Sometimes, doctors recommend more chest x-rays within hours, days, or months of an earlier chest x-ray. This allows them to follow up on a condition.

People who are having certain types of surgery also may need chest x-rays. Doctors often use the test before surgery to look at the structures inside the chest.

What to Expect Before a Chest X-Ray

You don't have to do anything special to prepare for a chest x-ray. However, you may want to wear a shirt that's easy to take off. Before the test, you'll be asked to undress from the waist up and wear a gown.

You also may want to avoid wearing jewelry and other metal objects. You'll be asked to take off any jewelry, eyeglasses, and metal objects that might interfere with the x-ray picture. Let the x-ray technician (a person specially trained to do x-ray tests) know if you have any body piercings on your chest.

Let your doctor know if you're pregnant or may be pregnant. In general, women should avoid all x-ray tests during pregnancy. Sometimes, though, having an x-ray is important to the health of the mother and fetus. If an x-ray is needed, the technician will take extra steps to protect the fetus from radiation.

What to Expect During a Chest X-Ray

Chest x-rays are done at doctors' offices, clinics, hospitals, and other healthcare facilities. The location depends on the situation. An x-ray technician oversees the test. This person is specially trained to do x-ray tests.

The entire test usually takes about fifteen minutes.

During the Test

Depending on your doctor's request, you'll stand, sit, or lie for the chest x-ray. The technician will help position you correctly. He or she may cover you with a heavy lead apron to protect certain parts of your body from the radiation.

The x-ray equipment usually consists of two parts. One part, a boxlike machine, holds the x-ray film or a special plate that records the picture digitally. You'll sit or stand next to this machine. The second part is the x-ray tube, which is located about six feet away.

Before the pictures are taken, the technician will walk behind a wall or into the next room to turn on the x-ray machine. This helps reduce his or her exposure to the radiation.

Usually, two views of the chest are taken. The first is a view from the back. The second is a view from the side.

For a view from the back, you'll sit or stand so that your chest rests against the image plate. The x-ray tube will be behind you. For the side view, you'll turn to your side and raise your arms above your head.

If you need to lie down for the test, you'll lie on a table that contains the x-ray film or plate. The x-ray tube will be over the table.

You'll need to hold very still while the pictures are taken. The technician may ask you to hold your breath for a few seconds. These steps help prevent a blurry picture.

Although the test is painless, you may feel some discomfort from the coolness of the exam room and the x-ray plate. If you have arthritis or injuries to the chest wall, shoulders, or arms, you may feel discomfort holding a position during the test. The technician may be able to help you find a more comfortable position.

When the test is done, you'll need to wait while the technician checks the quality of the x-ray pictures. He or she needs to make sure that the pictures are good enough for the doctor to use.

What to Expect After a Chest X-Ray

You usually can go back to your normal routine right after a chest x-ray.

A radiologist will analyze, or "read," your x-ray images. This doctor is specially trained to supervise x-ray tests and look at the x-ray pictures.

The radiologist will send a report to your doctor (who requested the x-ray test). Your doctor will discuss the results with you.

In an emergency, you'll get the x-ray results right away. Otherwise, it may take twenty-four hours or more. Talk with your doctor about when you should expect the results.

What Does a Chest X-Ray Show?

Chest x-rays show the structures in and around the chest. The test is used to look for and track conditions of the heart, lungs, bones, and chest cavity. For example, chest x-ray pictures may show signs of pneumonia, heart failure, lung cancer, lung tissue scarring, or sarcoidosis.

Chest x-rays do have limits. They only show conditions that change the size of tissues in the chest or how the tissues absorb radiation. Also, chest x-rays create two-dimensional pictures. This means that denser structures, like bone or the heart, may hide some signs of disease. Very small areas of cancer and blood clots in the lungs usually don't show up on chest x-rays.

For these reasons, your doctor may recommend other tests to confirm a diagnosis.

What Are the Risks of a Chest X-Ray?

Chest x-rays have few risks. The amount of radiation used in a chest x-ray is very small. A lead apron may be used to protect certain parts of your body from the radiation.

The test gives out a radiation dose similar to the amount of radiation you're naturally exposed to over ten days.

Key Points

- A chest x-ray is a painless, noninvasive test that creates pictures of the structures inside your chest, such as your heart, lungs, and blood vessels.

- Chest x-rays are done to find the cause of symptoms such as shortness of breath, chest pain, chronic cough (a cough that lasts a long time), and fever.

- Chest x-rays help doctors diagnose conditions such as pneumonia, heart failure, lung cancer, lung tissue scarring, and sarcoidosis. Doctors also may use chest x-rays to see how well treatments for certain conditions are working. Also, doctors often use chest x-rays before some types of surgery to look at the structures in the chest.

- X-rays use ionizing radiation to create pictures of the inside of your body. Chest x-rays are the most common x-ray test used to diagnose health problems.

- Chest x-rays have few risks. The amount of radiation used in a chest x-ray is very small. Sometimes, a lead apron may be used to protect certain parts of your body from the radiation.

- You don't have to do anything special to prepare for a chest x-ray. However, you may want to wear a shirt that's easy to take off. You also may want to avoid wearing jewelry and other metal objects.

- Before the test, let your doctor know if you're pregnant or may be pregnant. In general, women should avoid all x-ray tests during pregnancy. Sometimes, though, having an x-ray is important to the health of the mother and fetus. If an x-ray is needed, the x-ray technician will take extra steps to protect the fetus from radiation.

- A chest x-ray usually takes about fifteen minutes. You'll sit, stand, or lie for the test. Usually, two views of the chest are taken. The first view is from the back. The second view is from the side. You'll need to hold very still while the pictures are taken. The technician may ask you to hold your breath for a few seconds. These steps help prevent blurry pictures.

137

- You usually can go back to your normal routine right after a chest x-ray. In an emergency, you'll get the x-ray results right away. Otherwise, it may take twenty-four hours or more. Talk with your doctor about when you should expect the results.

- Chest x-rays do have limits. They only show conditions that change the size of tissues in the chest or how the tissues absorb radiation. Also, chest x-rays create two-dimensional pictures. This means that denser structures, like bone or the heart, may hide some signs of disease. Very small areas of cancer and blood clots in the lungs usually don't show up on chest x-rays. For these reasons, your doctor may recommend other tests to confirm a diagnosis.

Chapter 10

Types of Asthma

Chapter Contents

Section 10.1

Adult-Onset Asthma

Many adults with asthma were first diagnosed as a child, and have either managed their asthma all their life, or the asthma seemed to disappear for a number of years and came back later. There is, however, a significant group of people who develop asthma for the first time in their lives as adults. This is called adult-onset asthma.

It is important that the diagnosis of asthma as an adult is done carefully to make sure other illnesses such as heart disease are not the cause of symptoms. Your doctor will ask about your family and medical history, and check your lungs with tests like a spirometry test.

Symptoms

The symptoms of adult-onset asthma are:

- shortness of breath;
- wheeze;
- coughing, especially at night or early in the morning;
- chest tightness.

Management

The management of adult-onset asthma is the same as for all people who have asthma:

- regular medical reviews;
- medication;
- healthy lifestyle;
- a written asthma action plan.

What Causes Adult-Onset Asthma?

What causes asthma, regardless of age, remains unclear. We do not understand why symptoms develop at a certain age or why they might seem to "disappear" even though the airways are still sensitive and inflamed. The important thing to remember is asthma can be managed with:

- good control;
- appropriate, prescribed medication;
- regular check-ups with your doctor; and
- a written asthma action plan.

Asthma Triggers

For most people with asthma, triggers are only a problem when their asthma is not well controlled. To manage asthma symptoms and reduce the risk of a severe attack, you have to treat the underlying airway inflammation with medication. This is the best way to reduce asthma symptoms and the risk of needing to go to the hospital or dying from asthma.

Appropriate use of medication also reduces the chance you will get any symptoms in response to something that previously triggered your sensitive airways. Triggers that are more often an issue for those that develop adult-onset asthma are:

- **Smoking:** Both active and passive smoking can cause chronic bronchitis and emphysema, which are lung diseases that belong to a group of illnesses known as chronic obstructive pulmonary disease (COPD). Although there is no cure for COPD, research has shown that if you quit smoking, you may stop your symptoms from getting worse.

- **Colds and Flu:** Everyone gets colds or the flu from time to time, and these can easily make your asthma worse. It is important to recognize when your asthma is getting worse, and know what to do about it. Having a written asthma action plan can help you monitor your asthma.

- **Other Medications:** As you get older you might need to take regular medications for different conditions. Some medications can interact with asthma medications, or can make asthma worse. You should always talk to your doctor or pharmacist before starting any new medication, whether it is prescription, over the counter, or herbal medicine to ensure it won't have any negative effects on your asthma.

Section 10.2

Allergic Asthma

What Is Allergic Asthma?

Allergic (extrinsic) asthma is characterized by symptoms that are triggered by an allergic reaction. Allergic asthma is airway obstruction and inflammation that is partially reversible with medication. Allergic asthma is the most common form of asthma, affecting over 50 percent of the twenty million asthma sufferers. Over 2.5 million children under age eighteen suffer from allergic asthma. Many of the symptoms of allergic and non-allergic asthma are the same (coughing, wheezing, shortness of breath or rapid breathing, and chest tightness). However, allergic asthma is triggered by inhaled allergens such as dust mite allergen, pet dander, pollen, mold, etc. resulting in asthma symptoms.

Allergic Asthma FAQs

What Is Allergic Asthma?

Allergic asthma is how doctors describe a particular type of asthma. In people with this common condition, certain types of allergens can trigger asthma attacks and symptoms such as coughing, wheezing, and shortness of breath.

How Common Is It?

The National Institutes of Health estimates that 60 percent of the people in the United States with asthma have allergic asthma.

What Triggers Allergic Asthma?

You are probably aware of many things that can trigger your asthma. Mold, dust mites, cockroaches, and pet dander are common examples of year-round allergens. What you may not know is how something as simple as visiting a friend who has a pet can lead to an asthma attack. The reason, in part, is a substance produced by the body called immunoglobulin E (IgE).

What Is IgE?

IgE is short for immunoglobulin E, which is a type of antibody produced by the immune system. Its major purpose appears to be to fight parasite infections. When IgE comes in contact with a parasite, it sticks tight, and sends signals telling white blood cells to attack.

However, IgE also plays an important role in allergic asthma. People with allergic asthma produce IgE molecules that react to allergens like pollen or dust, rather than just parasites. If you have allergic asthma, breathing in an allergen will cause IgE molecules to activate.

Activation of IgE can cause a series of chemical reactions known as the allergic-inflammatory process in allergic asthma. It can result in two things: (1) the muscles that surround the airways in your lungs begin to tighten (this is known as constriction of the airways); and, (2) your airways become irritated and swell up (this is known as inflammation of the airways).

Together, constriction and inflammation of the airways make it harder for you to breathe. This can lead to an asthma attack.

How Can I Tell If I Have Allergic Asthma?

Only a doctor can confirm a diagnosis of allergic asthma. This is typically done using a skin or blood test to see if your asthma is triggered by year-round allergens in the air.

Allergic Asthma A to Z

Are you taking a proactive role in managing your allergic asthma? Knowing the terminology is the first step to helping you better communicate with your healthcare provider to keep your allergic asthma under control. Here are some of the most common terms.

Allergic asthma is a disease of the lungs in which an allergic reaction to inhaled allergens causes your asthma symptoms to appear.

Common inhaled allergens include dust mite allergen, pet dander, pollen, and mold spores.

Blood tests done by your doctor can help determine if you have allergic asthma. Knowing if you have allergic asthma or non-allergic asthma is very important to help you doctor develop the right management and treatment plan for you.

Cascade, often called the "allergic cascade," is the name for the series of reactions your immune system goes through after you've been exposure to an allergen. At the end of this "cascade," your allergy or asthma symptoms appear. That's why it's important to know what things trigger your personal "allergic cascade" so you can avoid and prevent the cascade from ever starting.

Diagnosis of allergic asthma begins with a discussion with your doctor about your medical history, a physical exam that includes a lung function test, and, in some cases, a chest or sinus x-ray.

Extrinsic asthma is just another name for "allergic asthma," the most common form of asthma, affecting over ten million people in the United States.

Family history of asthma or allergies is something that doctors look at to help determine if you might have allergic asthma. This disease tends to be more common among people who have a family history of allergies or asthma.

Genetics play a role in asthma. People whose brothers, sisters, or parents have asthma are more likely to develop the illness themselves. If only one parent has asthma, chances are one in three that each child will have asthma. If both parents have asthma, chances are seven in ten that their children will also.

Home environment is a critical factor in managing your allergic asthma. If pet dander, smoke, mold, or other triggers are all over your house, your asthma symptoms are likely to be much worse than if you eliminated these from your home environment.

Immunoglobulin E (IgE) is the name of the antibody that plays a major role in allergic diseases. IgE antibodies detect allergens and cause the "allergic cascade" to begin.

Keeping track of your asthma symptoms can help determine your triggers and prevent future attacks. Create an "asthma management plan" with your doctor.

Long-term control medicines, or anti-inflammatory drugs, make airways less sensitive. These important medicines help reduce coughing, wheezing, and allow you to live an active "life without limits!"

Mortality rates (death rates) among African Americans who have asthma are three times higher than others. If you're in this high-risk group, talk to your doctor about more ways to recognize and prevent asthma symptoms so you don't become a statistic.

Non-allergic asthma (also called intrinsic asthma) is triggered by irritants, not allergens. Many of the symptoms of allergic and non-allergic asthma are the same (coughing, wheezing, shortness of breath or rapid breathing, and chest tightness), but, with non-allergic asthma, symptoms are not caused by an allergic reaction.

Occupational asthma is when asthma symptoms are triggered by things related to conditions at your workplace. Symptoms are the same as other types of asthma, but some of the irritants that cause symptoms may be unique to your workplace, such as exposure to certain chemicals, dirt or dust, vapors, etc. People who work in factories, manufacturing plants, and even bakers who are exposed to airborne flour may show symptoms of asthma.

Peak flow meter is a diagnostic tool to measure how well your lungs are able to expel air. During an asthma flare-up, the large airways in the lungs slowly begin to narrow. A peak flow meter will show the speed of air leaving the lungs to measure the peak expiratory flow (PEF).

Quick-reliever medications should only be used in emergency situations, such as during an asthma attack. If you are taking long-term controller medications properly, you should almost never need these emergency medicines.

Rhinitis—sneezing, runny nose—may be caused by irritants or allergens, and, if not treated, it can lead to difficulty breathing. Nearly half of all those who have asthma also have "allergic rhinitis," so make sure you talk with your doctor about avoidance of rhinitis triggers and prevention of symptoms.

Sinusitis is sinus inflammation caused by a bacterial or viral infection, or an allergic reaction. More than 50 percent of people with moderate to severe asthma also have chronic sinusitis.

Triggers are different substances that can cause your asthma to act up. Allergic triggers can cause a series of chemical reactions resulting in the constriction and inflammation of the airways in your lungs. Common allergic triggers include pollen, dust mites, mold spores, and pet dander.

Understanding your asthma triggers is a key to controlling your condition. Knowing your triggers can help your healthcare professional make better prevention and treatment recommendations.

Viral respiratory infections—such as head or chest colds—are common among people with asthma; in fact, it's the number one asthma trigger among kids. Studies show that viral respiratory infections can make asthma symptoms worse for kids and adults. That's why it's important to get a flu shot and to protect against cold and flu every year.

Weather changes, cold air, or dry wind can sometimes trigger asthma symptoms. During the hot weather season, outdoor ground-level ozone can be a problem and people with asthma and allergies should drink plenty of fluids.

eXtrinsic asthma is another term for the type of asthma that can be triggered by allergens or irritants in your external environment at home, work, school, or outdoors.

You're in control! Don't let asthma control you. With proper prevention, treatment, and management of your asthma you can live "life without limits!"

Zoom! Traveling with asthma just means that you have to put a little extra thought and preparation into your trip.

Section 10.3

Exercise-Induced Asthma

Reprinted with permission of the American College of Sports Medicine (www.acsm.org). Copyright © 2005 American College of Sports Medicine. Editor's note added by David A. Cooke, MD, FACP, April 2011.

"Out of Shape?" Maybe Not . . .

Many people incorrectly believe that they are "out of shape," when in fact they may have exercise-induced asthma (EIA). Because the symptoms of EIA are similar to poor fitness, shortness of breath and a tight feeling in the chest, it is difficult to tell the difference between them. Increased training does not stop the problem, and for some, the symptoms of EIA may deter them from exercising. Exercise-induced asthma may not be life threatening, but it is uncomfortable. EIA affects more people than was originally believed. Clinicians estimate that up to 15 percent of the general population may suffer from this easily overlooked condition. Approximately 11 percent of the 1984 United States Olympic Team had symptoms of exercise-induced asthma. The good news is that EIA is controllable.

What Is Exercise-Induced Asthma?

Exercise-induced asthma is a reaction of the passages of the lunges that is caused by exercise. The bronchial tubes become irritated during exercise and begin to constrict. The bronchial muscles around the tube go into spasm, thus the term "broncho spasm." Mucus builds up in the tubes, and the cells that line the airways also start to swell, closing the airways even more. Thus, you have problems getting air in and out of your lungs.

Probable Cause

What triggers an EIA attack is not yet completely known. Your airway warms and moistens incoming air, which is usually cooler and drier. In the process the airways can cool down and dry out, which can irritate sensitive tissues. The amount of air moved in and out of the lungs increases during exercise, thus increasing the amount of cooling and drying. The bronchial tubes react to this process with EIA. Although chronic asthma sufferers are more likely to have EIA, the presence of EIA does not lead to chronic asthma.

Symptoms of Exercise-Induced Asthma

The symptoms of EIA include: shortness of breath during or after exercise, chest tightness or pain, coughing, and wheezing. These symptoms start a few minutes into exercise and may last for thirty to sixty minutes. In contrast, if the problem is poor fitness, the symptoms will usually disappear a few minutes after stopping exercise.

What to Do

You should speak with your doctor if you think you have exercise-induced asthma. Only a doctor can decide whether you have EIA. An exercise test can be used to determine EIA. However, this test will not be positive for everyone with EIA. Many doctors will base their diagnosis on your history and symptoms, and may have you use a trial of bronchodilator therapy prior to exercise. Although chest pain is a symptom of EIA, it is important for your doctor to rule out cardiovascular disease.

You can take several simple steps to reduce the chance of having an EIA attack. Breathing through your nose will help warm and moisten the air before it reaches the bronchial tubes, though it's not very easy during anything but a mild workout. Staying out of cold, dry air may be the best course of action, but if you do exercise outdoors, wear a face mask or scarf, which enriches inhaled air with heat and moisture from your skin. If you exercise inside, such as on an indoor track, on a treadmill, or in the warm, moist air of an indoor swimming pool, you are less likely to have an EIA episode. Lower-intensity sports, such as golf, baseball, or weightlifting are less likely to stimulate EIA (though they provide fewer cardiovascular benefits). And no matter what your activity, if high amounts of airborne irritants like pollen increase your chance of an attack, it makes good sense to exercise indoors on days when those pollutants are high.

Most Importantly—you should continue to exercise. Exercise training will improve fitness so that a lower level of breathing is needed at a given exercise level. Good cardiovascular fitness will enable you to exercise at a higher intensity before causing an EIA attack.

Tips to train by:

- Exercise indoors
- Cover mouth and nose when outdoors
- Warm up forty-five to sixty minutes before training
- Interval training

Additional Workout Strategies

Nature has created an EIA loophole called the "refractory period." The refractory period lasts up to two hours after an exercise-induced asthma attack. During this time your lungs are less likely to react as strongly. If you warm up forty-five minutes to an hour before your workout you may be able to exercise without too many symptoms. In addition, EIA usually starts several minutes into a workout. Some athletes have found they can exercise easier by using alternating work and rest periods (interval training).

Medicines for EIA

Though some people can keep their exercise-induced asthma under control with simple workout strategies, you may need medication. There are two broad types of medications that your physician might prescribe.

Bronchodilators work to keep the airways relaxed and open, and are used before or during exercise. A relatively new class of drugs called leukotriene inhibitors blocks the chemical the body uses to constrict the bronchial muscles. The other main categories of medicines are the anti-inflammatories. These include inhaled corticosteroids, which reduce the sensitivity to airways.

While most available medications are inhaled, some are taken in pill form. No one medicine works best for everyone, and you may need a combination for best control. Table 10.1 lists the generic medicines, indicating how they work and for how long. Side effects, in cases where they exist, are possible tremors, nausea, or heart palpitations. If you are an athlete, it is important to check that the medication suggested for you is legal, as several of these have been on the list of banned medications for different sports.

Table 10.1. Medicines for Exercise-Induced Asthma

Medication	How Long Before Exercise?	Lasts How Long?
Short-acting beta agonists (B)	15–30 minutes	2 hours
Salmeterol (B)	30–60 minutes	12 hours
Cromolyn sodium or nedocromil sodium (A)	10–20 minutes	2 hours
Inhaled corticosteroids (A)	Ongoing therapy	Ongoing therapy
Ipratropium bromide (B)	1 hour	2–3 hours
Oral theophylline (B)	Ongoing therapy	Ongoing therapy
Leukotriene inhibitors (B)	Ongoing therapy	Ongoing therapy

Note: A = Anti-inflammatory; B = Bronchodilator

Editor's Note

All of the above medications are effective for exercise-induced asthma. However, theophylline is now rarely used, due to the development of safer and more effective medications. Salmeterol is recommended only for patients who also take an inhaled corticosteroid, as studies found a higher risk of death when salmeterol was used alone.

Section 10.4

Occupational Asthma

Up to 15 percent of newly diagnosed asthma cases in adults are related to exposure to agents encountered at work. If you experience asthma symptoms at work, and these symptoms improve when you are away from work, e.g. during holidays or on weekends, you may have what is called work-related or occupational asthma. Occupational asthma can occur in many types of workplaces, but is most commonly reported where people are working with flour and isocyanates (chemicals which are found in paints as hardening agents).

Work-aggravated asthma is different from occupational asthma, which occurs when there is sensitization to a substance encountered at work. Work-aggravated asthma occurs when people who already have asthma are exposed to factors such as gases or fumes, smoke, dust, or cold dry air, which irritate the airways, causing asthma symptoms to occur and make a preexisting condition worse.

What causes occupational asthma?

Over four thousand substances in the workplace (known as sensitizers) may cause asthma. Repeated exposure to these sensitizers over a period of time (usually years) may produce permanent asthma symptoms identical to non-occupational asthma. This usually takes weeks or years to develop.

What are the symptoms of occupational asthma?

Symptoms include wheezing and coughing, shortness of breath, and tightness across the chest. Often these symptoms will develop after irritation is noticed in the nose and eyes. Other workers may be affected or may have left the job because of these symptoms.

Symptoms may vary during the working week or shift. In the early stages of exposure, symptoms tend to improve when the worker is away from work. However, once the airways are sensitized, continued exposure even in small amounts can produce symptoms. Continued exposure may also lead to more symptoms and eventually to permanent asthma in some people.

How do I know if I have occupational asthma?

If you suspect something is affecting your breathing at work, go and see your doctor. They will ask you questions about your symptoms and your work, and carry out tests such as a spirometry test to decide if you might have occupational asthma. They may also ask you to keep a diary of your symptoms to compare with your working hours.

It can be very difficult to distinguish between true occupational asthma and work-exacerbated asthma, and it may be necessary for your doctor to refer you to a respiratory specialist with expertise in this area.

Note: If you are working with known sensitizers, it is the responsibility of your employer to ensure that there is adequate ventilation and respiratory protection (e.g., a mask).

Table 10.2. Common Sensitizers and Occupations Where Workers May Be Exposed

Agent	Example occupations
Wood dust (e.g., western red cedar, redwood, oak)	Carpenters, builders, sawmill workers, sanders, model builders
Isocyanates	Automotive industry, mechanics, painters, adhesive workers, chemical industry, polyurethane foam workers
Formaldehyde	Cosmetics industry, embalmers, foundry workers, hairdressers, laboratory staff, medical personnel, paper industry, plastics industry, rubber industry, tanners
Platinum salts	Chemists, dentists, electronics industry, photographers, metallurgists
Latex	Healthcare workers, textile industry, toy manufacturers
Flour and grain dust	Bakers, cooks, pizza makers, grocers, farmers, combine harvester drivers
Animal allergens (e.g., urine, dander)	Veterinary surgery workers, animal care workers, laboratory workers, jockeys, animal breeders, pet shop employees

Table adapted from Hoy, R., Abramson, M., Sim, M. (2010). Work related asthma. Diagnosis and management. *Australian Family Physician*, 39 (1/2), 39–42.

What is the treatment for occupational asthma?

Early diagnosis and management by removing any exposure to irritants in the workplace is the best way to treat occupational asthma and prevent it becoming a permanent condition. Otherwise, treatment with the usual asthma inhalers is usually effective.

Note: Occupational asthma does not always mean having to leave your workplace, as workplace strategies can be developed. For example, if exposure cannot be minimized or ceased, then employers must provide adequate respiratory protection and/or substitute the irritant substance with a known non-irritant.

If you develop asthma symptoms at work, or your existing asthma gets worse, it is essential that you visit your doctor for tests and an accurate diagnosis. If you did not already have a diagnosis of asthma and/or a written asthma action plan, then this should be provided to you.

What if I only had temporary symptoms?

If you have inhaled a high dose of a substance that causes damage to the airways, possibly as part of an industrial accident or spillage, you may temporarily experience breathlessness and wheeze similar to asthma. This is called reactive airways dysfunction syndrome (RADS). Symptoms usually occur within twenty-four hours of a single exposure to very high concentrations of a chemical spill, irritant gases, corrosive mists, or solvent vapors. Usually, symptoms will gradually improve as your airways heal, but occasionally workers can be left with permanent symptoms. It is very important to have a medical check if this does happen, and to make sure your work environment is safe.

Section 10.5

Aspirin-Induced Asthma

What Is Aspirin-Induced asthma?

Aspirin-induced asthma is characterized by aggressive and continuous inflammation of the airways leading to worsening of asthma after ingestion of aspirin and other nonsteroidal anti-inflammatory drugs (NSAIDs). There are many other terms for this condition, including:

- ASA-induced asthma;
- aspirin triad;
- ASA sensitivity;
- ASA-intolerant asthma;
- ASA-exacerbated respiratory disease.

However, aspirin-induced asthma has the most widespread use and acceptance in clinical medicine. As in asthma, this is a disease that occurs in the lungs.

Statistics on Aspirin-Induced Asthma

The case of aspirin-induced asthma is common among patients with asthma as a disease. A Finland study concluded that the prevalence of aspirin-induced shortness of breath or asthma attacks was 1.2 percent. Also a study from Poland concluded that the prevalence was 4.3 percent in patients with a diagnosis of asthma. In Perth, Western Australia, the prevalence of chest symptoms triggered by aspirin was 10 to 11 percent among patients with asthma.

Risk Factors for Aspirin-Induced Asthma

The predisposing factors for this disease remain vague. Age is important, as the disease usually begins at thirty to fifty years old.

However, all ages can be affected. Studies have indicated the possibility of genetic risk factors for this disease.

Progression of Aspirin-Induced Asthma

Aspirin-induced asthma develops following a characteristic sequence of events. At an average age of thirty years old, persistent rhinitis (hay fever) will appear, followed by asthma, aspirin sensitivity, and nasal polyps. The triad of asthma, aspirin sensitivity, and nasal polyps is termed Samter triad. The exact mechanism of this disease remains unknown, however continuing research has shed some light. It is thought that certain biochemical compounds in the body are either overproduced or underproduced, leading to imbalance of these compounds. This disease is thought to have an allergic component to the mechanism.

How Is Aspirin-Induced Asthma Diagnosed?

If the patient needs to be admitted to the hospital and the disease is severe enough, routine tests will be acquired. This includes looking at the blood function, liver function, kidney function, lung function, and blood electrolytes. Usually an "arterial blood gas" will be done to assess the concentration of oxygen and carbon dioxide in the blood.

Prognosis of Aspirin-Induced Asthma

Aspirin-induced asthma does not lead to high death rates on its own and is not life-threatening. However it can lead to significant inconvenience if left untreated. Symptoms of asthma attack can be debilitating.

How Is Aspirin-Induced Asthma Treated?

Treatment of this disease consists of the following:

- **NSAID avoidance:** As in other allergic disease, it is important to avoid the medications known to cause the asthma attack. Aside from aspirin, other NSAIDs should bee avoided as well. NSAIDs are a group of drugs usually used as painkillers, including ibuprofen, naproxen, diclofenac, etc. Although acetaminophen (Tylenol, paracetamol) is a generally safe substitute for pain relief, it does have weak cyclooxygenase inhibitory properties. As many as 7 percent of the patients who are sensitive to aspirin may react to acetaminophen if taken at high doses. Hence it is wise to avoid acetaminophen as well.

- **Using COX-2 inhibitors:** COX-2 inhibitors are drugs commonly used as pain relief as well, but slightly different from NSAIDs. Current studies suggest that COX-2 inhibitors such as celecoxib do not induce asthma attack in patients with aspirin-induced asthma.

- **Aspirin desensitization:** Desensitization involves using a protocol that requires one to three days of in-patient treatment with daily aspirin ingestion. This treatment is especially useful in patients who require aspirin or other NSAIDs regularly for pain relief, such as patients with concurrent joint condition. Aspirin or NSAIDs must be used daily after desensitization, or the aspirin sensitivity may recur.

- **Sinus disease:** Patients with inflammation of the sinuses should be treated with oral or nasal steroids. Sinus rinses are also helpful, and antibiotics may be useful if there is evidence of infection. If nasal polyps are found, they should be treated accordingly. Nasal steroids and rinses are the usual first-line treatments for polyps. Current research is underway regarding new treatment for this, including leukotriene modifiers such as montelukast and zileuton.

References

1. Eneli, I, Sadri, K, Camargo, C Jr, Barr, RG. Acetaminophen and the risk of asthma: the epidemiologic and pathophysiologic evidence. *Chest* 2005; 127:604.

2. Hedman J, Kaprio J, Poussa T, Nieminen MM. Prevalence of asthma, aspirin intolerance, nasal polyposis and chronic obstructive pulmonary disease in a population-based study. *Int J Epidemiol* 1999; 28:717–22.

3. Kasper L, Sladek K, Duplaga M, Bochenek G, Liebhard J, Gladysz U, et al. Prevalence of asthma with aspirin hypersensitivity in the adult population of Poland. *Allergy* 2003 Oct; 58(10):1064–66.

4. Szczeklik A. Aspirin-induced asthma: advances in pathogenesis, diagnosis, and management. *Allergy Clin Immunol* 2003 May; 111(5):913–21.

5. Up to Date: Aspirin induced asthma [online]. 2005. [Cited 2005 October 17th]. Available from: URL: http://www.utdol.com/appli cation/topic.asp?file=asthma/10092&type=A&selectedTitle=1~7.

6. Vally H, Taylor ML, Thompson PJ. The prevalence of aspirin-intolerant asthma (AIA) in Australian asthmatic patients. *Thorax* 2002; 57:569–74.

Section 10.6

Cough-Variant Asthma

While cough may accompany the usual symptoms associated with asthma, in cough-variant asthma, cough alone may be a precursor to or the sole symptom in an asthmatic. When cough is the only asthma symptom, this is known as cough-variant asthma (CVA).

What is cough-variant asthma?

The main symptom of CVA is a chronic, nonproductive cough. These asthma patients have cough as the main or only symptom of their asthma. These patients are a small percentage of total asthma patients. CVA patients are, however, a distinct group rather than merely being thought of as "coughing asthmatics."

CVA patients have some differences from patients with typical asthma. For example, while normal asthmatics do not differ from healthy volunteers in their cough reflex, CVA patients have a more sensitive cough reflex. Interestingly, CVA patients have a smaller reaction to methacholine challenge testing compared to other asthmatics.

How is cough-variant asthma diagnosed?

Because cough is a common symptom for asthma, your provider may order spirometry. If spirometry demonstrates reversible obstruction, your provider may start a therapeutic trial for asthma. However, asthmatics may have a normal lung exam and spirometry, creating a "diagnostic dilemma," where your doctor may suspect, but is unable to prove, you have asthma.

In this case, your provider may perform methacholine challenge testing in order to demonstrate bronchial hyperresponsiveness and diagnose asthma. If a methacholine challenge test does not produce hyperresponsiveness, it is unlikely that asthma is the cause of a cough. A definitive diagnose can be made if the cough symptoms respond after asthma treatment.

How is cough-variant asthma treated?

Treatment of CVA is virtually the same as for asthma. Partial improvement of cough may be seen as quickly as one week with bronchodilators like albuterol, but may not completely resolve for up to eight weeks after starting an inhaled steroid like Flovent.

If the cough only partially resolves, your provider may try a more potent steroid like oral prednisone. Alternatively, your provider may do special tests to identify eosinophils, a marker of inflammation, in your lung. If eosinophils are present in the lung, zafirlukast has been shown to improve cough among patients with CVA and has been beneficial in CVA patients without a good response to inhaled steroids.

A small group of patients may experience worsening of the cough with inhaled steroids due to the aerosols used in the inhaler device. Alternatively, if the cough worsens, it is important that it is not another condition, like gastroesophageal reflux disease (GERD), causing the symptoms.

Section 10.7

Nocturnal Asthma

Perhaps this scenario sounds familiar. You (or your child) go to bed feeling well. Maybe during the day you had some mild asthma symptoms, used your inhaler in the evening, and fell asleep that night without difficulty. But at three or four in the morning, you suddenly wake from your sleep short of breath. You feel a tight band squeezing your chest. A short, dry cough emanates from high in your throat. You sit up and look for your quick-acting bronchodilator inhaler. Where did you put it? Did you leave it under your pillow, as you routinely do, or on top of the bedside table? You know that you will feel much better if you can use your medication to open the breathing tubes quickly.

This episode is an example of nocturnal asthma, a common event for many people with asthma. In one study of more than one thousand children with mild-moderate asthma, over a one-month period of observation, nighttime awakenings due to asthma occurred at least once in 35 percent of the children (who were being treated with bronchodilator medication only during this period). Nighttime awakenings are even more common in adults and in persons with severe asthma.

Biorhythms to Our Breathing

In asthma, lung function varies over time. The bronchial tubes may narrow during the day, causing daytime symptoms of asthma. Why shouldn't they narrow at night, causing nocturnal asthma? While it is true that one should not necessarily expect sleep to protect against bronchial tube narrowing, there does seem to be something special about the early morning hours that predisposes to symptoms at that time. If you could measure lung function around the clock, you would find that airways are commonly at their narrowest near 4:00 a.m. There is a natural daily biorhythm that puts us at greatest risk for asthmatic symptoms around this early morning hour. Our cortisol and adrenaline blood levels are at their lowest levels then; histamine levels tend to be high. In patients prone to develop nocturnal asthma, the flux of inflammatory cells into their airways tends to be greatest around that time.

More mundane explanations may account for your waking at night with asthma. Perhaps it is that pet cat or dog, curled up inches from your head, that triggers an allergic reaction at night. Perhaps it is the accumulation of dust mite allergens in your pillow and mattress, spread into the air every time you or your bedmate turn over in bed. Perhaps the nasal mucus from your allergic rhinitis tends to drip into the back of your throat while you sleep on your back, or perhaps stomach acid tends to regurgitate up into your chest when you lie down shortly after a big meal. Or perhaps the weight of all those extra pounds around your midriff, pushing up on your breathing muscles (the diaphragm) when you lie supine, compromises your breathing just enough to cause you symptoms overnight. In addition, the quick-acting bronchodilator that you took earlier in the evening exerts its beneficial effects for only a few hours. It is no longer acting on your bronchial tubes at 4:00 a.m.

A Warning Sign?

For many people, starting to wake at night due to asthma is a warning sign that your asthma is becoming less well controlled. It is evidence that the bronchial tubes are becoming more twitchy, that the system of bronchial tubes is becoming more unstable, with a greater tendency to constrict.

If you are having nighttime awakenings from your asthma, it is a useful clue—for you and for your doctor—that it is time to: 1) do some detective work into the possible causes of your asthma symptoms, and 2) intensify your treatment. Highly effective treatments are available, both anti-inflammatory medications that will subdue the twitchiness of the airways and long-acting bronchodilators that will prevent constriction of the bronchial muscles throughout the night.

Laryngospasm

There is another condition that sounds in many ways like nocturnal asthma but is, in fact, unrelated. In this condition the blockage to breathing occurs not in the bronchial tubes, but at the level of the vocal cords. It occurs in people with or without asthma, and is properly diagnosed as laryngospasm (spasm of the larynx or vocal cords).

Nighttime awakenings due to laryngospasm are utterly frightening. Patients report that they wake unable to breathe at all. It may sound like an exaggeration, but in truth for a few seconds the vocal cords at the base of the neck shut closed, blocking any movement of air in or out of the lungs. For a few seconds there is no air passing in or out, no ability to talk or call out. The best thing to do is not to panic. Within moments, the vocal cords begin to relax, and a small amount of air can pass between them. At this phase the breathing makes a noise that you might call "wheezing," but it is different. It occurs only when you breathe in, it has only one note or pitch, and it clearly originates in the throat area. Within seconds, this inspiratory noise (properly referred to as stridor) lessens and stops. The whole episode is over in less than a minute, although your heart may keep pounding from the fright!

Spasm of the vocal cords of this sort is probably triggered when some saliva or mucus or coughed liquid hits the nerve endings that densely surround this area. It is an uncontrollable reflex, meant to protect your windpipe from the aspiration of foreign material. The vocal cords will always begin to relax on their own. There is no need (or time) to reach for any medication. Continue to try to breathe calmly, and in a few seconds you will find that you can do so again.

Section 10.8

Cardiac Asthma: An Asthma Mimic

Excerpted from "Bronchial Asthma and Cardiac Asthma."
Reprinted with permission from www.mydr.com.au. © 2010 UBM
Medica Australia. All rights reserved.

Bronchial asthma is another name for the common form of asthma. The term "bronchial" is occasionally used to differentiate it from what doctors sometimes call "cardiac" asthma, which is not true asthma but breathing difficulties caused by heart failure. Although the two conditions have similar symptoms, including shortness of breath and wheezing (a whistling sound in the chest), they have quite different causes.

Cardiac Asthma

In cardiac asthma, the reduced pumping efficiency of the left side of the heart leads to a buildup of fluid in the lungs (pulmonary edema). This fluid buildup can cause breathlessness and wheezing. Cardiac asthma has very similar symptoms to bronchial asthma. The main symptoms and signs of cardiac asthma are:

- shortness of breath with or without wheezing;
- cough;
- rapid and shallow breathing;
- an increase in blood pressure and heart rate; and
- a feeling of apprehension.

The pattern of shortness of breath helps doctors determine which type of asthma you have—people with bronchial asthma tend to experience shortness of breath early in the morning, whereas people with heart failure and cardiac asthma often find they wake up breathless a few hours after going to bed, and have to sit upright to catch their breath. This is because in people with heart failure, lying down for prolonged periods will cause fluid to accumulate in the lungs, leading to shortness of breath.

Both bronchial and cardiac asthma can make people short of breath when they exert themselves. In bronchial asthma, symptoms are usually brought on by vigorous exercise and tend to be worse after the exercise than during it. On the other hand, cardiac asthma tends to happen during less vigorous exertion—someone with heart failure can find themselves short of breath while climbing stairs, or in severe cases, while getting dressed.

People with heart failure also often have problems with swollen ankles that worsen during the course of the day. They may also feel very tired, put on weight, and have to urinate frequently.

Cardiac asthma can be a life-threatening condition, and you should consult your doctor if you think you have symptoms of cardiac asthma.

Section 10.9

Status Asthmaticus

Status Asthmaticus, or SA for short, is a severe asthma attack usually of long duration or abruptly sudden in onset. In SA, asthma symptoms persist and respiratory function declines, despite standard treatments.

SA can lead to respiratory failure, prolonged hospitalization, and even death, and it signifies a medical emergency that requires immediate and aggressive treatments. As many as 10 percent of people who experience SA will die.

Of the total population, asthma affects approximately 8 percent of adults and 10 percent of children. Of these, 5 percent to 10 percent have a severe form of asthma and are at greater risk for status asthmaticus.

What Happens During a Severe Asthma Attack?

During a severe asthma attack, the way the body normally processes gases is impaired. This leads to lower oxygen levels and higher carbon dioxide levels in the blood, which, in extreme cases, can cause coma and death.

Asthma also creates air trapping in the lungs, a condition that causes increased pressure in the chest. This can cause lung collapse and even cardiac arrest.

Two Types of Status Asthmaticus

There are two types of SA. The first and more common type is a slow-onset attack. This may take a long time to unfold and usually results because of inadequate treatment. The person with this type of SA will experience days or weeks of worsening symptoms, punctuated by moments of relief, and ending in symptoms that cannot be reversed with medications in the home.

The second type of severe attack is a sudden-onset attack. The person experiencing this type of SA has not experienced any worsening symptoms in the preceding weeks, but is struck with sudden and severe bronchospasm, breathlessness, wheezing, and cough. This type of asthma attack is often brought on by a large exposure to trigger substances, such as pollen, dust, or food allergens.

How Doctors Diagnose Status Asthmaticus

The following are signs and symptoms that doctors use to diagnose SA:

- Breathlessness at rest
- Inability to speak in sentences or not being able to speak at all
- High respiratory rate (greater than thirty breaths per minute)
- Elevated pulse (greater than 120 beats per minute)
- Agitation (although as the attack progresses, sleepiness is more worrisome)
- Low levels of oxygen in the blood
- Diminished breathing capacity, as measured by peak expiratory flow (PEF)

How Doctors Treat Status Asthmaticus

Standard treatment of status asthmaticus in the emergency room includes:

- oxygen by mask;

- measurement of PEF;

- inhaled medications that relax and open the airways (beta-agonists);

- steroids (such as prednisone) given either by mouth or intravenously;

- inhaled anticholinergic medications (such as Atrovent).

Other medications that may be used during an acute episode include:

- beta-agonists injected under the skin (such as terbutaline);

- magnesium sulfate intravenously;

- leukotriene modifiers (such as zafirlukast or zileuton) by mouth.

Mechanical ventilation is a treatment of last resort because of the risk of trauma to the lungs and other serious complications that can occur. About 4 percent of emergency room visits for asthma will result in the patient needing mechanical ventilation.

People with Asthma Should Know Their PEF Measurement

There are more than five thousand deaths from asthma in the United States each year. Often the severity of symptoms for a person with asthma are not closely related to the severity of his or her lung dysfunction. Therefore, it is important for all asthmatics to measure their PEF regularly. This is done by using a peak flow meter, which is a small plastic device that is exhaled into forcefully, which measures the PEF.

The PEF measurement gives information about respiratory status, any decline from the person's own normal (baseline) condition, and the need to increase medications or seek medical treatment. Any person with asthma who has a decline of 30 percent or more in PEF, particularly if rescue inhalers are not being effective, should seek medical attention without hesitation.

Part Three

Medications and Asthma Management

Chapter 11

Treating Asthma Symptoms

Chapter Contents

Section 11.1

Basic Principles for Asthma Control

Excerpted from "How Is Asthma Treated and Controlled?"
National Heart, Lung, and Blood Institute, National Institutes of Health,
February 2011.

Asthma is a long-term disease that can't be cured. The goal of asthma treatment is to control the disease. Good asthma control will do the following things:

- Prevent chronic and troublesome symptoms, such as coughing and shortness of breath

- Reduce your need for quick-relief medicines

- Help you maintain good lung function

- Let you maintain your normal activity level and sleep through the night

- Prevent asthma attacks that could result in an emergency room visit or hospital stay

To control asthma, partner with your doctor to manage your asthma or your child's asthma. Children aged ten or older—and younger children who are able—also should take an active role in their asthma care.

Taking an active role to control your asthma involves the following:

- Working with your doctor to treat other conditions that can interfere with asthma management.

- Avoiding things that worsen your asthma (asthma triggers). However, one trigger you should not avoid is physical activity. Physical activity is an important part of a healthy lifestyle. Talk with your doctor about medicines that can help you stay active.

- Working with your doctor and other healthcare providers to create and follow an asthma action plan.

An asthma action plan gives guidance on taking your medicines properly, avoiding asthma triggers (except physical activity), tracking your level of asthma control, responding to worsening asthma, and seeking emergency care when needed.

Asthma is treated with two types of medicines: long-term control and quick-relief medicines. Long-term control medicines help reduce airway inflammation and prevent asthma symptoms. Quick-relief, or "rescue," medicines relieve asthma symptoms that may flare up.

Your initial treatment will depend on the severity of your asthma. Follow-up asthma treatment will depend on how well your asthma action plan is controlling your symptoms and preventing asthma attacks.

Your level of asthma control can vary over time and with changes in your home, school, or work environments. These changes can alter how often you're exposed to the factors that can worsen your asthma.

Your doctor may need to increase your medicine if your asthma doesn't stay under control. On the other hand, if your asthma is well controlled for several months, your doctor may decrease your medicine. These adjustments to your medicine will help you maintain the best control possible with the least amount of medicine necessary.

Asthma treatment for certain groups of people—such as children, pregnant women, or those for whom exercise brings on asthma symptoms—will need to be adjusted to meet their special needs.

Follow an Asthma Action Plan

You can work with your doctor to create a personal asthma action plan. The plan will describe your daily treatments, such as which medicines to take and when to take them. The plan also will explain when to call your doctor or go to the emergency room.

If your child has asthma, all of the people who care for him or her should know about the child's asthma action plan. This includes babysitters and workers at daycare centers, schools, and camps. These caretakers can help your child follow his or her action plan.

Avoid Things That Can Worsen Your Asthma

Many common things (sometimes called asthma triggers) can set off or worsen your asthma symptoms. Once you know what these things are, you can take steps to control many of them.

For example, exposure to pollens or air pollution may make your asthma worse. If so, try to limit time outdoors when the levels of these substances in the outdoor air are high. If animal fur triggers your asthma symptoms, keep pets with fur out of your home or bedroom.

One asthma trigger you should not avoid is physical activity. Physical activity is an important part of a healthy lifestyle. Talk with your doctor about medicines that can help you stay active.

If your asthma symptoms clearly are related to allergens, and you can't avoid exposure to those allergens, your doctor may advise you to get allergy shots for the specific allergens that trigger your asthma symptoms.

You may need to see a specialist if you're thinking about getting allergy shots. These shots may lessen or prevent your asthma symptoms, but they can't cure your asthma.

Several health conditions can make asthma harder to manage. These conditions include runny nose, sinus infections, reflux disease, psychological stress, and sleep apnea. Your doctor will treat these conditions as well.

Medicines

Your doctor will consider many things when deciding which asthma medicines are best for you. Doctors usually use a stepwise approach to prescribing medicines. Your doctor will check to see how well a medicine works for you; he or she will adjust the dose or medicine as needed.

Asthma medicines can be taken in pill form, but most are taken using a device called an inhaler. An inhaler allows the medicine to go directly to your lungs.

Not all inhalers are used the same way. Ask your doctor or another healthcare provider to show you the right way to use your inhaler. Ask your doctor to review the way you use your inhaler at every visit.

Track Your Asthma

To track your asthma, keep records of your symptoms, check your peak flow number using a peak flow meter, and get regular asthma checkups.

Record Your Symptoms

You can record your asthma symptoms in a diary to see how well your treatments are controlling your asthma.

Asthma is "well controlled" if the following are true:

- You have symptoms no more than two days a week, and these symptoms don't wake you from sleep more than one or two nights a month.

- You can do all your normal activities.

- You take quick-relief medicines no more than two days a week.

- You have no more than one asthma attack a year that requires you to take corticosteroids by mouth.

- Your peak flow doesn't drop below 80 percent of your personal best number.

If your asthma isn't well controlled, contact your doctor. He or she may need to change your asthma action plan.

Use a Peak Flow Meter

This small, hand-held device shows how well air moves out of your lungs. You blow into the device and it gives you a score, or peak flow number. Your score shows how well your lungs are working at the time of the test.

Your doctor will tell you how and when to use your peak flow meter. He or she also will teach you how to take your medicines based on your score.

Your doctor and other healthcare providers may ask you to use your peak flow meter each morning and keep a record of your results. You may find it very useful to record peak flow scores for a couple of weeks before each medical visit and take the results with you.

When you're first diagnosed with asthma, it's important to find out your "personal best" peak flow number. To do this, you record your score each day for a two- to three-week period when your asthma is well controlled. The highest number you get during that time is your personal best. You can compare this number to future numbers to make sure your asthma is under control.

Your peak flow meter can help warn you of an asthma attack, even before you notice symptoms. If your score shows that your breathing is getting worse, you should take your quick-relief medicines the way your asthma action plan directs. Then you can use the peak flow meter to check how well the medicine worked.

Get Asthma Checkups

When you first begin treatment, you'll see your doctor about every two to six weeks. Once your asthma is under control, your doctor may want to see you anywhere from once a month to twice a year.

During these checkups, your doctor or nurse will ask whether you've had an asthma attack since the last visit or any changes in symptoms or peak flow measurements. You also will be asked about your daily activities. This will help your doctor or nurse assess your level of asthma control.

Your doctor or nurse also will ask whether you have any problems or concerns with taking your medicines or following your asthma action plan. Based on your answers to these questions, your doctor may change the dose of your medicine or give you a new medicine.

If your control is very good, you may be able to take less medicine. The goal is to use the least amount of medicine needed to control your asthma.

Emergency Care

Most people who have asthma, including many children, can safely manage their symptoms by following their asthma action plans. However, there may be times when you need medical attention.

Call your doctor for advice if either of the following are true:

- Your medicines don't relieve an asthma attack
- Your peak flow is less than half of your personal best peak flow number

Call 9–1–1 for emergency care if either of the following are true:

- You have trouble walking and talking because you're out of breath
- You have blue lips or fingernails

At the hospital, you'll be closely watched and given oxygen and more medicines, as well as medicines at higher doses than you take at home. Such treatment can save your life.

Asthma Treatment for Special Groups

The treatments described above generally apply to all people who have asthma. However, some aspects of treatment differ for people in certain age groups and those who have special needs.

Children

It's hard to diagnose asthma in children younger than five years. Thus, it's hard to know whether young children who wheeze or have other asthma symptoms will benefit from long-term control medicines. (Quick-relief medicines tend to relieve wheezing in young children whether they have asthma or not.)

Doctors will treat infants and young children who have asthma symptoms with long-term control medicines if the child's asthma health assessment indicates that the symptoms are persistent and likely to continue after six years of age.

Inhaled corticosteroids are the preferred treatment for young children. Montelukast is an alternative option. Treatment may be given for a trial period of one month to six weeks. The treatment usually is stopped if benefits aren't seen during that time and the doctor and parents are confident the medicine was used properly.

Inhaled corticosteroids can possibly slow the growth of children of all ages. If slowed growth occurs, it usually is apparent in the first several months of treatment, is generally small, and doesn't get worse over time. Poorly controlled asthma also may reduce a child's growth rate.

Most experts think the benefits of inhaled corticosteroids for children who need them to control their asthma far outweigh the risk of slowed growth.

Older Adults

Doctors may need to adjust asthma treatment for older adults who take certain other medicines, such as beta blockers, aspirin and other pain relievers, and anti-inflammatory medicines. These medicines can prevent asthma medicines from working properly and may worsen asthma symptoms.

Be sure to tell your doctor about all of the medicines you take, including over-the-counter medicines.

Older adults may develop weak bones from using inhaled corticosteroids, especially at high doses. Talk with your doctor about taking calcium and vitamin D pills, as well as other ways to help keep your bones strong.

Pregnant Women

Pregnant women who have asthma need to control the disease to ensure a good supply of oxygen to their babies. Poor asthma control increases the risk that a baby will be born early and have a low birth weight. Poor asthma control can even risk the baby's life.

Studies show that it's safer to take asthma medicines while pregnant than to risk having an asthma attack.

Talk with your doctor if you have asthma and are pregnant or planning to get pregnant. Your level of asthma control may get better or it may get worse while you're pregnant. Your healthcare team will check your asthma control often and adjust your treatment as needed.

People Whose Asthma Symptoms Occur with Physical Activity

Physical activity is an important part of a healthy lifestyle. Adults need physical activity to maintain good health. Children need it for growth and development.

In many people, however, physical activity may trigger asthma symptoms. If this happens to you or your child, talk with your doctor about the best ways to control asthma so you can stay active.

The following medicines may help prevent asthma symptoms caused by physical activity:

- Short-acting beta$_2$-agonists (quick-relief medicine) taken shortly before physical activity can last two to three hours and prevent exercise-related symptoms in most people who take them.

- Long-acting beta$_2$-agonists can be protective for up to twelve hours. However, with daily use, they'll no longer give up to twelve hours of protection. Also, frequent use for physical activity may be a sign that asthma is poorly controlled.

- Leukotriene modifiers are taken several hours before physical activity. They help relieve asthma symptoms brought on by physical activity in up to half of the people who take them.

- Long-term control medicines are sometimes used to help prevent exercise-related symptoms. Frequent or severe symptoms due to physical activity may indicate poorly controlled asthma and the need to either start or increase long-term control medicines that reduce inflammation.

Easing into physical activity with a warm-up period may be helpful. You also may want to wear a mask or scarf over your mouth when exercising in cold weather.

If you use your asthma medicines as your doctor directs, you should be able to take part in any physical activity or sport you choose.

People Having Surgery

Asthma may add to the risk of having problems during and after surgery. For instance, having a tube put into your throat may cause an asthma attack.

Tell your surgeon about your asthma when you first consult him or her. The surgeon can take steps to lower your risk, such as giving you asthma medicines before or during surgery.

Section 11.2

Stepwise Approach to Treatment

The goal of asthma care is to ensure that your asthma is well controlled, by which we mean infrequent symptoms (day and night), the ability to exercise without limitation due to your breathing, good lung function (as measured, for instance, with a peak flow meter), and rare exacerbations of your asthma ("asthma attacks"). In this section we review how to go about achieving this goal—in accordance with the recommendations of the Expert Panel of the National Asthma Education and Prevention Program in their most recent (third) set of guidelines, released in August 2007.

The National Guidelines lay out a six-step approach to treating asthma, from occasional use of quick-acting bronchodilators like albuterol (Pro-Air, Proventil, or Ventolin) for intermittent asthma to daily use of oral corticosteroids like prednisone for severe persistent asthma refractory to all other therapies. However, their treatment recommendations do not begin with medications. First, they explore other important strategies for bringing asthma under control, aspects of care that go hand-in-hand with the pharmacologic treatments of asthma:

- Make sure that the diagnosis of asthma is correct. Other diseases of the chest can cause wheezing, cough, and shortness of breath. If you have emphysema or recurrent bouts of bronchitis or heart failure, you will need a different approach to treatment than what is outlined in the recommendations of the Expert Panel.

- Make frequent assessments of your asthma control. Asthma can be a dynamic condition, varying from season to season, one location to another, or changing simply as a result of growing older. The treatments appropriate for the way your asthma used to be may no longer be appropriate for your asthma as it is now. Be attentive to your asthma symptoms and keep in touch with your doctor about your asthma.

- Avoid those things that make your asthma worse. It makes no sense to take more and more medications for your asthma while sleeping with the pet cat to which you are allergic. Your child's asthma control will improve if he or she is no longer exposed to secondhand cigarette smoke; and your asthma will likewise improve if you quit smoking cigarettes. By identifying those things that aggravate your asthma and making an effort to avoid them as much as possible, especially in your home, you can often achieve better asthma control without escalating your medication use.

- Attend to medical conditions that may adversely impact your asthma. Asthma may not be your only medical problem. To get your asthma under good control it may be important to address these other conditions simultaneously. Common examples include sinusitis, allergic rhinitis, gastroesophageal reflux disease, obesity, depression, anemia, and many other common problems.

- Be prepared to deal with an asthma attack, should one occur. Your medical treatment is meant to prevent asthma attacks, but it may fail to do so, even under the best of circumstances. It is estimated that as many as 20 percent of persons with asthma will have suffered an asthmatic attack requiring urgent care within the past year. So be prepared: know what works and what doesn't work in reversing an asthma attack, and know when to get help in treating your asthma attack.

In choosing medications to treat asthma, you and your doctor will want to find the least amount of medication needed to keep you symptom-free and safe from asthmatic attacks. In the lingo of the current asthma Guidelines, the goals of asthma therapy are to achieve current control and reduce future risk. If you are feeling well and have had at most one serious asthmatic attack over the past year, your current asthma therapy may be sufficient. If you are frequently using your quick-relief bronchodilator, are waking at night with asthmatic symptoms, have a low peak flow value, or are limited in your activities because of your asthma, then it is probably time to "step up" your asthma therapy. By "stepping up," we mean taking a more powerful medication or combination of medications likely to bring your asthma under good control. Here (with some minor Partners Asthma Center modifications) is how the national Expert Panel views the process of "stepping up" asthma medications . . . in six steps:

- **Step 1:** Use your quick-acting inhaled bronchodilator, such as albuterol, metaproterenol (Alupent), levalbuterol (Xopenex), or pirbuterol (Maxair), as needed for relief of symptoms and, if needed, prior to exercise.

- **Step 2:** Add daily use of an inhaled corticosteroid, such as beclomethasone (Qvar), budesonide (Pulmicort), fluticasone (Flovent), mometasone (Asmanex), and others, in addition to your quick-acting bronchodilator taken as needed. You can use a low dose of inhaled corticosteroid and some can be taken once daily. An alternative option is a leukotriene blocker, such as montelukast (Singulair) or zafirlukast (Accolate).

- **Step 3:** Two options are offered at this step: increase the dose of your daily steroid inhaler (using a higher strength inhaler or taking more puffs per day) or continue a low dose of inhaled steroid and add a long-acting inhaled bronchodilator like formoterol (Foradil) or salmeterol (Serevent). Two combination inhalers are available that combine an inhaled steroid and long-acting bronchodilator into one device: Advair (fluticasone plus salmeterol) and Symbicort (budesonide plus formoterol). Another option for stepping up care at this level is to add a leukotriene blocker (Singulair or Accolate) to an inhaled steroid.

- **Step 4:** Daily use of both an inhaled steroid (now at moderate doses) and a long-acting inhaled bronchodilator is recommended. Convenient examples are the combination inhalers, Symbicort 160/4.5, taken two puffs twice daily, or Advair 250/50, taken one inhalation twice daily.

- **Step 5:** Persistent asthma of this severity requires high doses of inhaled steroids plus a long-acting inhaled bronchodilator. Other options that might be tried as well include the oral leukotriene modifier called zileuton (Zyflo) and the anti-IgE monoclonal antibody omalizumab (Xolair), given as injections to patients with documented severe allergic asthma.

- **Step 6:** Everything in Step 5 remains appropriate for Step 6, plus use of oral steroids such as prednisone or prednisolone taken daily or perhaps every other day. Also appropriate for patients at this level of asthma severity: consultation with an asthma expert.

Section 11.3

Understanding the Different Types of Asthma Medications

"Asthma Medications," reprinted with permission from the Asthma and Allergy Foundation of America, www.aafa.org, © 2005. All rights reserved. Revised by David A. Cooke, MD, FACP, May 2011.

Can medicine cure my asthma?

No, there is no cure for asthma. Although asthma cannot be cured it can be controlled. There are many medicines that help people with asthma. Some are preventive medicines and others are known as quick relievers. The preventive medicines are used for long-term control of the disease and work to make asthma attacks less frequent and less severe. Quick-reliever medicines offer short-term relief of symptoms when asthma episodes occur.

Unless your asthma is very mild, chances are you have prescriptions for at least two different medicines. That can be confusing. The more you understand about what those medicines do and why they help, the more likely you are to use them correctly.

Although there are some potential unfavorable side effects from taking asthma medications, the benefit of successfully controlling your asthma outweighs the risks. It is important to discuss each of your asthma medications with your physician to learn more about their effects.

As just discussed, there are two kinds of asthma medications: long-term controllers and quick relievers.

Long-term control medicines: Standard asthma treatment begins with long-term relief from anti-inflammatory drugs. These drugs make the airways less sensitive, and keep them from reacting as easily to triggers. They reduce coughing, wheezing, and the struggle for breath, and they allow you to live an active life. To have long-term control of your asthma depends on you. Anti-inflammatory drugs must be taken exactly as they are prescribed.

Inhaled corticosteroids (AeroBid, Alevsco, Azmacort, Flovent, Pulmicort, QVAR) prevent and reduce airway swelling and decrease the amount of mucus in the lungs. These are usually the first choice long-term control medications, and reduce symptoms and risk of death from asthma. They are generally safe when taken as directed. They are not the same as anabolic steroids, which some athletes take to build muscles.

If you are taking an inhaled anti-inflammatory medicine and you feel your asthma symptoms getting worse, talk with your doctor about continuing or increasing the medicine that you are already taking. You may also need to add an oral corticosteroid or a short-acting beta antagonist (bronchodilator) for relief.

Oral corticosteroids (Pills or tablets: Aristocort, Celestone, Decadron, Medrol, Prednisone, Sterapred; Liquid for children: Pediapred, Prelone) are used as short-term treatment for severe asthma episodes or as long-term therapy for some people with very severe asthma. Again, these are not the same as anabolic steroids.

Long-acting beta agonists (Inhaled: Brovana, Foradil, Serevent) can be taken to help control daily symptoms, including nighttime asthma. They should not be used without an anti-inflammatory medication, as they increase risk of asthma death if used alone. This type of medicine can also prevent asthma triggered by exercise.

Because long-acting beta agonists cannot relieve symptoms quickly, they should not be used for an acute attack. You also need a short-acting, inhaled beta agonist for acute symptoms.

Long-acting, inhaled beta agonists are not a substitute for anti-inflammatory medicine. You should not decrease or stop taking your anti-inflammatory medicine without talking to your doctor, even if you feel better.

Leukotriene modifiers (Tablets: Accolate, Singulair, Zyflo) are a newer type of long-term control medication. They prevent airway inflammation and swelling, decrease the amount of mucus in the lungs, and open the airways.

Cromolyn sodium (Inhaled: Intal) and Nedocromil sodium (Inhaled: Tilade) prevent airways from swelling when they come in contact with asthma triggers. They are less effective than inhaled corticosteroids, but can be used to prevent asthma caused by exercise.

Combined therapy medicine (inhaled) contains both a controller and reliever medicine. This combination of a long-acting bronchodilator and corticosteroid is used for long-term control. Combinations include Advair, Dulera, and Symbicort.

Omalizumab (Xolair) is an Anti-IgE (immunoglobulin E) therapy (injected) treatment for people with moderate or severe allergic asthma. It attempts to eliminate IgE antibodies involved in asthma. This drug is not inhaled, but rather injected by your doctor on a regular basis. It does not eliminate your need for other asthma medications, but it can help to reduce your use of them. Due to its significant cost, this form of therapy is currently reserved for moderate to severe cases requiring multiple medications.

Quick-relief medicines: These medicines ease the wheezing, coughing, and tightness of the chest that occurs during asthma episodes.

Short-acting bronchodilators are one type of quick-relief medicines. They open airways by relaxing muscles that tighten in and around the airways during asthma episodes.

Short-acting beta agonists (Inhaled: Albuterol, Alupent, Brethine, Maxair, ProAir HFA, Proventil HFA, Ventolin HFA, Xopenex) relieve asthma symptoms quickly and some prevent asthma caused by exercise.

If you use one of these medicines every day, or if you use it more than three times in a single day, your asthma may be getting worse, or you may not be using your inhaler correctly. Talk with your doctor right away about adding or increasing a medication, and about your inhaler technique.

Oral beta agonists (Syrup, tablets, and long-acting tablets: Alupent, Brethine, Bricanyl, Proventil, Proventil Repetabs, Ventolin, Volmax). Syrup may be used for children, while long-acting tablets may be used for nighttime asthma. Oral preparations generally cause more side effects than the inhaled form.

Theophylline (Oral, slow acting: Aerolate, Elixophyllin, Quibron-T, Resbid, Slo-Bid, T-Phyl, Theolair, Theo-24, Theo-Dur, Theo-X, Uni-Dur, Uniphyl) can be used for persistently symptomatic asthma, and especially to prevent nighttime asthma. Theophylline must remain at a constant level in the bloodstream to be effective. Too high a level can be dangerous. Your doctor will do regular blood tests. Once a first-line drug, theophylline is rarely used for asthma today, and has been largely replaced by inhaled corticosteroids and leukotriene modifiers. However, it can be effective in selected patients.

The job of these medicines is to control your asthma in both normal and stressful situations so that your airways remain open and your lungs operate properly. This enables you to live an active life free from fear of struggling for breath. But for the medicines to do their best work, you must understand your condition, know what your medicines can and cannot do, and use them exactly as instructed by your doctor. Your intelligent use of asthma medicines is as important as the medicines themselves!

Can medicine alone help my asthma?

No. Although medicines help a lot, you cannot expect them to do the job alone. You have to help. You have to avoid the things that cause (or trigger) your asthma symptoms as much as you can, even if they are things you like. In planning to avoid these triggers, you need to think about outdoor exposure as well as the things at home and at work that cause your problem.

Will I always have to take the same amount of medicine?

Not necessarily. You will probably take most when you begin treatment, while your doctor learns what causes your asthma, which medicine(s) control it most effectively, and at what doses. Once this is completed, your medications may be reduced in number, frequency, or dose. The goal of this "step-down" method is to gain control of your asthma as quickly as possible, then maintain effective control with as little medication as necessary. Once long-term, anti-inflammatory therapy has begun, proper monitoring requires examination by a doctor every one to six months.

Will I have to take medicine all the time?

Not necessarily. Because asthma is a chronic condition that is controllable but currently cannot be cured, you will have asthma all the time even if your are symptom free much of the time. Your medical treatment will take into consideration the severity and frequency of your symptoms. If you have little inflammation between episodes, and if the episodes are infrequent, your treatment will emphasize quick relief from acute symptoms, particularly if they are mild.

If your symptoms occur at certain times and from a known and predictable cause, you will be treated accordingly. If, for example, you have "seasonal asthma" because of an allergy to a specific pollen, you may take medicines only when that pollen is in the air. But asthma so specific is uncommon, and most people with asthma take some form of medication most or all of the time.

Will medicine help me sleep better?

Yes. It is common for asthma symptoms to occur at night, and many people tell of the panic of awakening in a struggle for breath. These nighttime symptoms can be controlled with asthma medicines taken on a regular basis.

In addition, some bedding materials may be among your allergens, and must be replaced with non-allergenic materials. Air filters in your bedroom may also help to maximize the benefits of your medicines if you have nighttime symptoms of asthma.

Will medicines help me breathe better when I exercise?

Yes. Physical activity, especially when combined with an irritant like cold air, may cause your airways to open and close irregularly. This is called exertion-induced bronchospasm (EIB). The short-term-relief asthma medicines, taken before and during exercise, usually control this. Thanks to these medicines, many Olympic and professional athletes enjoy successful sports careers despite their asthma.

Do asthma drugs have side effects?

Yes, as do all drugs. No medicine is so exact that it can do its intended job without having unintended side effects as well. It is important, therefore, that you give your doctor accurate information about your entire health condition, not just your asthma symptoms. Doing away with some asthma drugs on the basis of other health problems, like high blood pressure, is one important way of reducing your risks.

For most people with asthma, long-term control of inflammation of the airways is the key to successful treatment. Prescribing drugs based on information you supply is your doctor's responsibility. Faithful reporting of changes and reactions is yours. And only you can make sure that you take your medication exactly as it is prescribed.

The greatest danger for most people taking asthma medicine, especially by inhaler, is overuse. Don't give in to "just another puff," or "if two puffs work, three must be better," or "half a dose between doses." Overuse of these medications over a period of years may prove to be very harmful.

Your doctor, your pharmacist, and the medicine's label will tell you exactly the frequency and amount of your doses. Do not exceed them without your doctor's instructions. If either your doctor or pharmacist says that "you are going through this awfully quickly," you are almost certainly overusing. Overusing is overdosing.

Section 11.4

Treating Asthma-Related Conditions

Excerpted from "Asthma in Adults, " © 2011 A.D.A.M., Inc.
Reprinted with permission.

Immunizations

Patients with asthma should get an annual flu vaccine, and they should receive the vaccination against pneumococcal pneumonia at least once.

Treating Seasonal Allergies and Sinusitis

Patients with asthma and chronic allergic rhinitis may need to take medications daily. Patients with severe seasonal allergies may need to start medications a few weeks before the pollen season, and to continue medicine until the season is over.

Immunotherapy ("allergy shots") may help reduce asthma symptoms, and the use of asthma medications, in patients with known allergies. They may also help prevent the development of asthma in children with allergies. Immunotherapy poses some risk for severe allergic reactions, however, especially for children with poorly controlled asthma.

Treatment of allergies and sinusitis can help control asthma.

Preventing and Treating Respiratory Infections

Respiratory infections, including the common cold, can interact with allergies to worsen asthma. People with asthma should try to minimize their risk for respiratory tract infections. Washing hands is a very simple but effective preventive measure.

Treating Gastroesophageal Reflux Disease (GERD)

Patients with obvious symptoms of reflux (heartburn) may consider the following lifestyle changes:

• Avoiding heavy meals and meals with fried food.

- Avoiding caffeine, chocolate, onions, and garlic.
- Avoiding eating or drinking at least three hours before bedtime.
- Elevating the head of the bed by six inches.
- Taking medications treating gastroesophageal reflux. Be sure to talk to your doctor before taking these medicines.

Managing Hormonal-Related Asthma

Women who suspect that menstrual-related changes may influence asthma severity should keep a diary of their menstrual dates and times of asthma attacks. Sometimes, adjusting medications in anticipation of menstruation may help prevent attacks.

Chapter 12

Mild Asthma: Experts Differ on Best Course of Action

Chapter Contents

Section 12.1

Research Reveals Regular Treatment for Mild Asthma Improves Lung Function

A study by the Woolcock Institute of Medical Research in Sydney, Australia, is the first to demonstrate that in patients with very mild or well-controlled asthma, regular treatment with low-dose inhaled corticosteroids (ICS) leads to significantly better day–to-day lung function.

The study published in *Primary Care Respiratory Journal*, was conducted over an eleven-month period, and compared the effects of inhaled corticosteroids (ICS) and placebo on asthma control in mild asthmatics.

The results of the study raise questions about the current emphasis in asthma treatment which is based largely on controlling symptoms, and which does not advocate ICS treatment for patients with symptoms two days a week or less.

Results showed significant and clinically important treatment benefits on markers such as lung function, airway hyperresponsiveness and exhaled nitric oxide, which are all predictors of the risk of future adverse outcomes such as exacerbations.

Results indicated that a "ceiling" effect for lung function, often assumed to prevail in mild asthma, does not exist. Even patients whose lung function is over 90 percent of predicted normal value may have room to further improve their personal best with treatment.

The study also demonstrated subjects receiving placebo were nearly three times more likely to experience a mild exacerbation.

"In recent years the emphasis in asthma treatment has been on how well a patient's symptoms are controlled," says Woolcock research leader Associate Professor Helen Reddel.

"The patients in this study had asthma that was so mild, with symptoms once a week or less, that they themselves didn't see any benefit in regular preventer treatment," she said.

"However for those participants receiving ICS during the study, their lung function was better, they had less airway inflammation and less airway twitchiness. All of these things are predictors of reduction in risk of future adverse outcomes

"While we're not advocating that every patient with mild asthma should be on preventer medication, the study shows that when we are discussing the risks and benefits of treatment with these patients, we should talk about their risk of future exacerbations as well as whether they will notice any difference in their current symptoms."

"In the same way, for patients with high blood pressure, we talk about giving treatment to reduce their risk of stroke in the future rather than whether they will feel any different here and now."

Dr. Reddel explains that while the study sample size was small, the measurement of airway twitchiness, airway inflammation, and daily spirometry provided information about future risk that is often not possible in larger groups.

Section 12.2

Study Challenges Current Treatment for Mild Asthma

"Study Challenges Current Treatment for Mild Asthma," University of California–San Francisco News Office, April 13, 2005. Reprinted with permission. This University of California at San Francisco News Release is based upon the following published manuscript: "Daily versus As-Needed Corticosteroids for Mild Persistent Asthma," by Homer A. Boushey, MD, et al., *New England Journal of Medicine*, April 14, 2005; *Proceedings of the National Academy of Sciences*, December 7, 2004; 352(15): 1519–1528, http://www.nejm.org/doi/pdf/10.1056/NEJ Moa042552. Editor's notes added by David A. Cooke, MD, FACP, May 2011.

People with "mild persistent asthma"—about a quarter of all asthma sufferers—appear to gain adequate relief by inhaling anti-inflammatory steroids only during periods of bad symptoms, rather than daily as current guidelines recommend, a new study shows.

Symptoms of mild, persistent asthma are wheezing, coughing, or chest tightness two to six days of the week, or awakening due to asthma two or three times a month. Conventional treatment usually requires two prescribed drugs: a "beta agonist" for immediate relief, and daily use of inhaled corticosteroids to reduce airway inflammation and minimize risk of severe asthma attacks and airway scarring that might permanently reduce lung capacity.

But the year-long controlled study shows that adult asthma sufferers fare about as well whether they take a steroid drug every day or only during asthma attacks. Changes in lung function, overall frequency of symptoms, and the number of severe attacks were about the same, whichever regimen was followed.

According to one of the study's authors, if the estimated four million people with mild persistent asthma took inhaled steroids only when symptoms flared, the annual medication costs would be about $2 billion lower—or up to $150 a month per patient less—than if they took the steroids every day as current National Institutes of Health (NIH) guidelines recommend.

The multi-center study, known as the Improving Asthma Control Trial (IMPACT), was funded by the National Heart, Lung and Blood

Institute, and led by scientists at the University of California–San Francisco (UCSF) and Harvard Medical School.

The results were published in the April 14, 2005, issue of the *New England Journal of Medicine*. The issue also includes an editorial on the study and its likely impact on treatment for asthma.

"There is no question that use of inhaled corticosteroids or other anti-inflammatory drugs known as anti-leukotrienes are effective—and necessary—for patients with moderate or severe asthma, but our findings suggest that the NIH guidelines for treating asthma may have gone a little too far in requiring patients with truly mild asthma to take these anti-inflammatory drugs every day," said Homer Boushey, MD, professor of medicine at UCSF and study co-leader.

"This study will need confirmation before the findings should change the standard of practice, but it suggests that adults with mild asthma may do about as well if they have the medication on hand and are advised to take them for a week or two just when their symptoms flare up."

About twenty million Americans suffer from asthma, with most experiencing symptoms that are considered "mild intermittent" or "mild persistent"—requiring occasional use of beta agonists to relieve symptoms but causing few emergency department visits or hospitalizations. Opinion has been divided among experts as to how best to treat these conditions. In 1997, an expert NIH panel recommended daily use of inhaled steroids to prevent attacks, and theoretically, to counter the possibility of permanent, debilitating airway scarring which would further aggravate breathing. But only about 30 percent of patients who are prescribed inhaled steroids refill their prescriptions.

"The steroids do not provide immediate relief; that's the job of the beta agonists such as albuterol," Boushey explained. "Either because patients experience no obvious, immediate benefit, or because they are concerned about using inhaled steroids—or some combination of reasons—most people discontinue steroid use for asthma. Our study shows that for mild asthma, at least for the short term, this 'folk wisdom' is a safe practice.

"We can't say for sure though that inhaled corticosteroid treatment might not be good for preventing airway 'scarring' and progressive loss of pulmonary function in the long run. What we can say is that the patients in our study, who all had mild asthma, did not have many severe attacks, and did not seem to be losing pulmonary function rapidly."

[Editor's Note: The theory that inhaled corticosteroids could prevent permanent loss of pulmonary function has been disproven. However, it remains clear that inhaled steroids greatly improve symptoms and reduce the risk of severe asthma exacerbations and death.]

The researchers noted that patients who used the corticosteroids daily did experience some benefits: "They had more symptom-free days and less bronchial inflammation. But daily use of the steroids did not significantly reduce the risk of severe attacks or prevent loss of pulmonary function," Boushey stressed

The six-city study involved 225 adult patients with mild persistent asthma. During the one-year study, participants took daily doses of either a placebo or one of two anti-inflammatory medications—inhalant corticosteroids or anti-leukotrienes. All participants also had use of clearly labeled inhalant steroid sprays to take for short periods for mild worsening of asthma, and prednisone tablets for more severe episodes. In this way, the study not only compared the two anti-inflammatory drugs against each other and a placebo, but also tested intermittent versus continual medication, since those in the placebo group ended up taking the anti-inflammatory mediations only during flare-ups. All three groups experienced about the same degree of relief, the researchers report.

All those enrolled in the study were taught how to recognize symptoms of worsening asthma and how to treat themselves with short courses of therapy. Many patients found that simply learning how to take care of themselves made a big difference in their ability to live with their asthma after the study ended, the researchers note.

"One of the most important things we did during this study was to work closely with the participants to help them effectively manage their asthma symptoms," said Audrey Plough, RN, the nurse coordinator for the UCSF site of the study.

After one year, the three groups not only showed similar lung function and severity of symptoms, but also similar "quality of life" scores—measures of physical, social, and emotional impairments due to asthma.

"The results of IMPACT suggest that for the type of patients with mild persistent asthma included in this study, choosing not to take daily medications may be okay, but this choice should be made in consultation with the patient's healthcare provider," said Elliot Israel, MD, co-leader of the study at Brigham and Women's Hospital in Boston.

"People with more severe asthma must follow recommendations for daily medications, and all asthma patients—even those with mild asthma—should adequately treat their symptoms," he added.

The National Asthma Education and Prevention Program which had recommended the daily anti-inflammatory regimen for patients with mild, persistent asthma, is expected to consider the results of the new IMPACT study and others in developing updated guidelines for treatment next year, the researchers note.

"The results of IMPACT will have tangible benefits for both asthma patients and providers," said James Kiley, PhD, director of the NHLBI Division of Lung Diseases. "We established the Asthma Clinical Research Network several years ago for just this purpose—to generate meaningful data on new therapeutic approaches."

Participating centers in the trial, in addition to UCSF and Harvard, were: Columbia Presbyterian Medical Center and Harlem Lung Center, New York; National Jewish Medical and Research Center, Denver; University of Wisconsin, Madison; and Thomas Jefferson Medical College, Philadelphia, Pennsylvania.

[Editor's Note: Despite the results of the IMPACT trial, the 2007 update of the National Asthma Education and Prevention Program, developed by the National Institutes of Health, continues to recommend daily inhaled steroids for most patients with persistent asthma.]

Chapter 13

Reliever and Controller Medications Play Different Roles in Asthma Care

Chapter Contents

Section 13.1

Reliever (Rescue) vs. Controller Medications

The two main types of asthma medicine are controller medications and rescue medications:

- Rescue medications, also called quick-relief or fast-acting medications, work immediately to relieve asthma symptoms when they occur. They're often inhaled directly into the lungs, where they open up the airways and relieve symptoms such as wheezing, coughing, and shortness of breath, often within minutes. But as effective as they are, rescue medications don't have a long-term effect.

- Controller medications, also called preventive or maintenance medications, work over a period of time to reduce airway inflammation and help prevent asthma symptoms from occurring. They may be inhaled or swallowed as a pill or liquid.

Rescue Medications

The most-prescribed rescue medications are quick-acting bronchodilators (usually given through an inhaler or a nebulizer), which loosen the tightened muscles around inflamed airways. The most common of these, beta$_2$-agonists, are related to adrenaline and usually work within minutes to provide temporary relief of symptoms.

If a bronchodilator alone doesn't resolve a severe flare-up, other medications may be given by mouth or injection to help treat it.

If you have been prescribed rescue medication, it's important to keep it on hand. That means at home, at the mall, at sports practice, and even on vacation.

Rescue medications, although an important part of asthma treatment, can be overused. Talk with your doctor about how often you use the rescue medication. If it's too often, the doctor also might prescribe a controller medicine, designed to prevent asthma flare-ups from happening.

Controller Medications

Because airways can be inflamed even in between flare-ups, controller medications might be needed to prevent unexpected asthma flare-ups. Slower-acting controller medicines can take days to weeks to start working, but when they do, they prevent airway inflammation and keep the lungs from making too much mucus.

There are a variety of controller medications, but inhaled corticosteroids are most common. They're usually given through an inhaler or nebulizer. Despite their name, corticosteroids are not the same as performance-enhancing steroids used by athletes. They're a safe and proven form of treatment for asthma.

In fact, inhaled corticosteroids are the preferred long-term treatment for people with frequent asthma symptoms. Research shows that they improve asthma control and their risk of causing long-term negative effects is minimal. (But corticosteroids that are swallowed in liquid or pill form can cause side effects if used daily over a long period of time.)

Long-acting bronchodilators also can be used as controller medications. These relax the muscles of the airways for up to twelve hours, but can't be used for quick relief of symptoms because they don't start to work immediately.

Even if you take controller medicine regularly, rescue medication will still be needed to handle flare-ups when they occur.

Working with the Doctor

Your doctor will determine which type of medicine you need based on the frequency and severity of asthma symptoms. Be sure to report any concerns or changes in the symptoms to help your doctor select the best course of treatment. Both the type and dosage of medication needed are likely to change to continue giving you the best quality of life and prevent flare-ups.

You're an important player in your asthma treatment. For example, you can track how well the medicine is working by using a peak flow meter. You also can record information in an asthma diary and ask your doctor to create an asthma action plan, if you don't already have one.

Section 13.2

Reliever Medications

"Quick-Relief Medications Used to Treat Asthma,"
reprinted with permission from www.getasthmahelp.org, the
website of the Asthma Initiative of Michigan, © 2010.

Quick-relief medications give fast relief for tight, narrowed airways and the symptoms of coughing, wheezing, and chest tightness that happen with asthma.

Examples of quick-relief medications: Proventil HFA, ProAir HFA, Ventolin HFA, albuterol, Maxair, and Xopenex.

Quick-relief medications (listed in alphabetical order):

- **Anticholinergics:** Inhibit muscarinic cholinergic receptors and reduce intrinsic vagal tone of the airway. Ipratropium bromide provides additive benefit to short-acting beta-agonist (SABA) in moderate-to-severe asthma exacerbations. May be used as an alternative bronchodilator for patients who do not tolerate SABA.

- **Short-acting beta$_2$-agonists (SABAs):** Albuterol, levalbuterol, and pirbuterol are bronchodilators that relax smooth muscle. Therapy of choice for relief of acute symptoms and prevention of exercise-induced bronchospasm (EIB).

- **Systemic corticosteroids:** Although not short acting, oral systemic corticosteroids are used for moderate and severe exacerbations as adjunct to SABAs to speed recovery and prevent recurrence of exacerbations.

Short-Acting Beta$_2$-Agonists

Inhaled short-acting beta$_2$-agonists are the drug of choice for treating acute asthma symptoms and attacks, or flare-ups.

When Is It Used?

For relief of acute symptoms and to prevent exercise-induced bronchospasm.

How Does It Work?

Bronchodilation: relax bronchial smooth muscle following adenylate cyclase activation and increase in cyclic adenosine monophosphate (AMP), producing functional antagonism of bronchoconstriction, usually within five to ten minutes of administration (opens up the airways by working on a cellular level).

Possible Side Effects

- Increased heart rate, shakiness, hypokalemia, increased lactic acid, headache, high blood sugar. Inhaled route, in general, causes few side effects.

- Patients who already have heart disease, especially the elderly, may have harmful cardiovascular reactions with inhaled therapy.

Other Information about Using This Type of Medication

- Inhaled route starts working faster, has fewer side effects, and works better than oral medication. The less beta$_2$-selective agents (isoproterenol, metaproterenol, isoetharine, and epinephrine) are not recommended due to their potential for excessive cardiac stimulation, especially in high doses. Albuterol liquid is not recommended.

- For patients with intermittent asthma, regularly scheduled daily use neither harms nor benefits asthma control. Regularly scheduled daily use is not generally recommended.

- If the medication does not seem to be working, or if it needs to be used too often (more than one canister/month) this means that the asthma is not under control, and a doctor needs to evaluate and possibly increase (or start) long-term control therapy. Use of greater than two canisters/month poses additional adverse risks.

Oral (Systemic) Corticosteroids

Used for moderate to severe exacerbations to speed recovery and prevent recurrence of exacerbations.

When Is It Used?

- Usually requires short-term (three to ten days) "burst," broad anti-inflammatory effects.

- Broad anti-inflammatory effects—to stop an asthma flare-up, reverse inflammation, speed recovery, and reduce rate of relapse.

How Does It Work?

- Anti-inflammatory. Blocks late reaction to allergen and reduces airway sensitivity. Inhibits cytokine production, adhesion protein activation, and inflammatory cell migration and activation at the cellular level.

- Reverses beta$_2$-receptor down-regulation. Inhibits microvascular leakage.

Possible Side Effects

- Short-term use: reversible changes in sugar metabolism, increased appetite, fluid retention, weight gain, mood alteration, hypertension, peptic ulcer, and rarely aseptic necrosis of femur.

- Consideration should be given to coexisting conditions that could be worsened by systemic corticosteroids, such as herpes virus infections, varicella, tuberculosis, hypertension, peptic ulcer, and *Strongyloides*.

Other Information about Using This Type of Medication

- Short-term therapy should continue until patient achieves 80 percent peak expiratory flow personal best or symptoms resolve. This usually requires three to ten days, but may require longer.

- There is no evidence that tapering the dose following improvement prevents relapse.

Anticholinergics (Ipratropium Bromide)

May provide some additive benefit to inhaled beta$_2$-agonists in severe asthma attacks. May be an alternative bronchodilator for patients who do not tolerate inhaled beta$_2$-agonists.

When Is It Used?

For relief of acute bronchospasm.

How Does It Work?

- Bronchodilation. Competitive inhibition of muscarinic cholinergic receptors (opens the airways by working at the cellular level).

- Reduces intrinsic vagal tone to the airways. May block reflex bronchoconstriction secondary to irritants or to reflux esophagitis.

- May decrease mucus gland secretion (so body makes less mucus).

Possible Side Effects

Drying of mouth and respiratory secretions, increased wheezing in some people, blurred vision if sprayed in eyes.

Other Information about Using This Type of Medication

- Reverses only cholinergically mediated bronchospasm; does not modify reaction to antigen. Does not block exercise-induced bronchospasm.

- May provide additive effects to beta$_2$-agonist but has slower onset of action.

- Is an alternative for patients with intolerance to beta$_2$-agonists.

- Treatment of choice for bronchospasm due to beta-blocker medication.

Section 13.3

Controller Medications

Excerpted from "Asthma in Adults," © 2011 A.D.A.M., Inc.
Reprinted with permission.

These medications are taken on a regular basis to prevent asthma
attacks and control chronic symptoms.

Inhaled Corticosteroids

Corticosteroids, also called glucocorticoids or steroids, are powerful
anti-inflammatory drugs. Steroids are not bronchodilators (they do
not relax the airways) and have little short-term effect on symptoms.
Instead, they work over time to reduce inflammation and prevent
permanent injury in the lungs. They can also help prevent asthma
attacks from occurring. The use of inhaled corticosteroids in patients
with moderate-to-severe asthma reduces the risk of rehospitalization
and death from asthma.

Taking a corticosteroid drug through an inhaler makes it possible
to provide effective local anti-inflammatory activity in the lungs with
very few side effects elsewhere in the body. (By contrast, steroids taken
by mouth have considerable side effects throughout the body.) Inhaled
corticosteroids are recommended as the primary therapy for any patient needing long-term control medications for persistent asthma.

Examples of inhaled corticosteroids include the following:

- The most recent generation of inhaled steroids include fluticasone (Flovent), budesonide (Pulmicort), triamcinolone (Azmacort
  and others), flunisolide (AeroBid), mometasone furoate (Asmanex), and ciclesonide (Alvesco). These steroids are sometimes combined with a long-acting beta$_2$-agonist in a single inhaler, such
  as budesonide-formoterol (Symbicort) and fluticasone-salmeterol
  (Advair).

- The older corticosteroid inhalants are beclomethasone (Beclovent, Vanceril) and dexamethasone (Decadron Phosphate
  Respihaler and others).

Optimal timing of the dose is important and may vary depending on the medication.

Inhaled steroids are generally considered safe and effective and only rarely cause any of the more serious side effects reported with prolonged use of oral steroids. The following are side effects of inhaled steroids:

- The most common side effects are throat irritation, hoarseness, and dry mouth. Using a spacer device and rinsing the mouth after each treatment can minimize or prevent these effects.

- Rashes, wheezing, facial swelling (edema), fungal infections (thrush) in the mouth and throat, and bruising are also possible but not common with inhalators.

- Inhaled corticosteroids are associated with a higher risk for cataracts in patients over age forty, particularly with higher dosages. (No higher risk is observed in younger people.)

- Some studies report a higher risk for bone loss in patients who take inhaled steroids regularly, a side effect known to occur with oral steroids.

Long-Acting Beta$_2$-Agonists

Long-acting beta$_2$-agonists (LABAs) are used for preventing an asthma attack (not for treating attack symptoms). These drugs should never be used alone in the treatment of asthma in adults or children. They can be dangerous when used alone, because they can mask asthma symptoms, and they can increase the risk of asthma death unless paired with an inhaled steroid. LABAs should only be used in combination with an asthma controller medication, such as an inhaled corticosteroid. LABAs should be used for the shortest time possible, and should only be used by patients whose asthma is not adequately controlled by asthma controller medications.

Salmeterol-fluticasone (Advair) and formoterol-budesonide (Symbicort) are long-acting beta$_2$ agonists products combined with a steroid in a single inhaler that are used for treatment of moderate to severe asthma. The LABA-only versions of these drugs are salmeterol (Serevent Diskus) and formoterol (Foradil Aerolizer).

Doctors are still trying to determine when long-acting beta$_2$-agonists should be added to an asthma treatment plan. If your symptoms do not improve or if symptoms worsen with this type of drug, your doctor will recommend discontinuing it. Do not, however, stop taking this drug or other asthma medications without first talking with your doctor.

Cromolyn

Cromolyn sodium (Intal) is both an anti-inflammatory drug and has antihistamine properties that block asthma triggers, such as allergens, cold, or exercise. A cromolyn nasal spray called NasalCrom has been approved for over-the-counter purchase, but only to relieve nasal congestion caused by allergies. Patients should not use it for self-medication without the advice of a doctor.

Side effects of cromolyn include nasal congestion, coughing, sneezing, wheezing, nausea, nosebleeds, and dry throat.

Leukotriene Antagonists

Leukotriene antagonists (also called anti-leukotrienes or leukotriene modifiers) are pills that block leukotrienes. Leukotrienes are powerful immune system factors that, in excess, produce a battery of damaging chemicals that can cause inflammation and spasms in the airways of people with asthma. As with other anti-inflammatory drugs, leukotrienes are used for prevention, *not* for treating acute asthma attacks.

Leukotriene antagonists include montelukast (Singulair), zafirlukast (Accolate), and zileuton (Zyflo). These drugs are considered an alternative for long-term control of asthma, but inhaled corticosteroids should always be used first. Other potential uses include preventing exercise-induced asthma.

Gastrointestinal distress (stomach upset or pain) is the most common side effect of leukotriene antagonists. Zafirlukast may cause liver injury when taken at higher than standard doses. No adverse effects on the liver have been reported to date with montelukast.

Mental health disturbances and behavioral changes have been associated with these medications. These mood problems include agitation, aggression, anxiousness, dream abnormalities, hallucinations, depression, insomnia, irritability, restlessness, tremor, and suicidal thinking and behavior. Patients who take a leukotriene antagonist drug should be monitored for signs of behavioral and mood changes. Doctors should consider discontinuing the drug if patients exhibit any of these symptoms.

Omalizumab

Omalizumab (Xolair) is FDA-approved for patients age twelve and older who have moderate-to-severe persistent asthma related to allergies. Omalizumab is a biologic drug that targets and blocks the antibody immunoglobulin E (IgE), a chemical trigger of the inflammatory events associated with an allergic asthma attack.

Omalizumab is given by injection every two to four weeks. It is used only to treat patients who have moderate-to-severe persistent asthma related to allergies whose symptoms are not controlled by inhaled corticosteroids.

About one in one thousand patients who take omalizumab develop anaphylaxis (a life-threatening allergic reaction). Patients can develop anaphylaxis after any dose of omalizumab, even if they had no reaction to a first dose. Anaphylaxis may occur up to twenty-four hours after the dose is given.

Omalizumab should always be injected in a doctor's office, and healthcare providers should observe patients for at least two hours after an injection. Patients should also carry emergency self-treatment for anaphylaxis (such as an Epi-Pen) and know how to use it. With an Epi-Pen, or similar auto-injector device, patients can quickly give themselves a life-saving dose of epinephrine.

Anaphylaxis symptoms include the following:

- Difficulty breathing
- Chest tightness
- Dizziness
- Fainting
- Itching and hives
- Swelling of the mouth and throat

The U.S. Food and Drug Administration (FDA) is currently reviewing whether omalizumab may be associated with increased risk for heart and vascular problems (ischemic heart disease, arrhythmias, cardiomyopathy, heart failure, pulmonary hypertension, and blood clots).

Theophylline

Theophylline relaxes the muscles around the bronchioles and also stimulates breathing. Since the introduction of inhaled corticosteroids and long-acting beta$_2$-agonists, theophylline is not used as often for asthma treatment. It may still be used in some circumstances, such as for treating nocturnal asthma. Theophylline is available in tablet, liquid, and injectable forms. Theophylline should not be used by people with peptic ulcers, and should be used with caution by anyone with heart disease, liver disease, high blood pressure, or seizure disorders.

Chapter 14

Inhaled Corticosteroids

Chapter Contents

Section 14.1

What You Need to Know about Inhaled Corticosteroids

What are some common inhaled steroids?

Common inhaled steroids include:

- Asmanex (mometasone);
- Alvesco (ciclesonide);
- Flovent (fluticasone);
- Pulmicort (budesonide);
- Qvar (beclomethasone HFA);
- AeroBid (flunisolide);
- Azmacort (triamcinolone).

How are inhaled steroids typically prescribed?

An inhaled steroid is typically prescribed as a long-term control medicine. This means that it is used every day to maintain control of your lung disease and prevent symptoms. An inhaled steroid prevents and reduces swelling inside the airways, making them less sensitive. It may also decrease mucus production. An inhaled steroid will not provide quick relief for asthma symptoms. In addition, inhaled steroids may help reduce symptoms associated with other chronic lung conditions. Inhaled steroids are the most effective long-term control medicine currently available for asthma. They improve asthma symptoms and lung function. They have also been shown to decrease the need for oral steroids and hospitalization.

How is the dosage of steroids determined?

Your healthcare provider may adjust the dosage of your inhaled steroid based on your symptoms, how often you use your quick relief medicine to control symptoms, and your peak flow results. You still may need a short burst of oral steroids when you have more severe symptoms.

What about side effects and inhaled steroids?

The most common side effects with inhaled steroids are thrush (a yeast infection of the mouth or throat that causes a white discoloration of the tongue), cough, or hoarseness. Rinsing your mouth (and spitting out the water) after inhaling the medicine and using a spacer with an inhaled metered-dose inhaler reduces the risk of thrush. When a dose is prescribed that is normal or higher than the normal dose in the package insert, some systemic side effects may occur. Keep in mind, however, that an inhaled steroid has much less potential for side effects than steroid pills or syrups. There have been concerns regarding the possibility of growth suppression in children. Recent studies have not shown growth suppression over several years of treatment.

What are some recommendations to minimize or prevent steroid side effects?

- Take your long-term control medicines as prescribed to keep your chronic lung disease under good control. This will help decrease the steroid pills to the lowest possible dose.

- Monitor your lung disease. If you notice your peak flow numbers are decreasing or you are having increased symptoms, call your healthcare provider. A short burst of steroid pills given early may prevent the need for a longer burst if treated later.

Section 14.2

Pros and Cons of Inhaled Corticosteroids

"Inhaled Corticosteroids," © 2010 Children's Asthma Education Centre (www.asthma-education.com). Reprinted with permission.

Steroid Facts

- Steroids are hormones that your body makes and uses every day.
- Steroids used to treat asthma are called corticosteroids.
- These steroids are not the same as those banned for athletes.
- The International Olympic Committee approves the use of corticosteroids when prescribed by a doctor to treat asthma.
- Corticosteroids can be pills, syrups, creams, or can be given by needle. Most often they are inhaled into the lungs.
- Inhaled corticosteroids (ICS) are used for asthma and allergic rhinitis (inflammation of the nose). Corticosteroid creams are used to treat eczema (a skin rash).
- Oral corticosteroids (e.g., Pediapred, Prednisone) may be needed to treat severe asthma attacks.
- If needed, oral corticosteroids should only be used for a few days.

Benefits of Inhaled Corticosteroids (ICS)

- Inhaled corticosteroids (ICS) used to treat asthma are called controller medicine.
- For asthma, ICS work on the inside of the airways to decrease swelling and mucous.
- ICS are usually the best medicine to control asthma long term.
- ICS go directly to the lungs, so only small doses of steroids are needed.
- ICS take a few days to start working. It may take a few weeks before the airway swelling is decreased.

- If needed ICS can be used safely for years.

Risks of Inhaled Corticosteroids

- At low doses, side effects are rare.
- In a few children, ICS may cause a hoarse voice or yeast infection in the mouth or throat called "thrush."
- In some children, there may be a short-term effect on growth (height).
- For most children, height is not affected by normal doses of ICS.
- Poor asthma control will also affect growth.

Examples of Inhaled Steroids

Fluticasone:

- Flovent
- Advair (contains Flovent and Serevent)

Budesonide:

- Pulmicort
- Symbicort (contains Pulmicort and Oxeze)

Beclomethasone:

- QVAR

Ciclesonide:

- Alvesco

Instruction for Use of Inhaled Steroids for Asthma

- It is important to know how to use your inhaler properly. Review how to use your inhaler with your doctor, asthma educator, or pharmacist.
- Using a spacer device will help to prevent thrush and allow more medicine to reach the lungs.
- Gargle with water and spit or take a drink after inhaling the corticosteroids to prevent thrush.
- Do not stop inhaled corticosteroids without your doctor's advice.
- Follow your asthma action plan. Review your plan with your doctor at least twice a year.

Section 14.3

Side Effects of Inhaled Corticosteroids

In 1935, the Mayo Clinic reported a research breakthrough that
would affect millions of lives. Doctors had isolated the hormone cortisone from the adrenal glands, the walnut-sized glands sitting on
top of the kidneys. Cortisone produced by the adrenal glands reduces
inflammation in the body.

The Mayo Clinic physicians first used cortisone to treat people
with severe rheumatoid arthritis. Improvements were so dramatic in
soothing swollen joints that patients crippled from the disease were
actually able to walk again.

Pharmaceutical companies have since produced corticosteroids medications that mimic the hormone cortisone. For people with asthma,
corticosteroids literally can be lifesavers by preventing or reversing
inflammation in the airways, making them less sensitive to triggers.
The drugs, sometimes referred to as "preventive" or "long-term control"
medicines, work effectively to keep asthma episodes in check. They are
not the same as anabolic steroids, which some athletes take illegally
to build muscle mass.

Are Corticosteroids Safe?

Oral, or systemic, corticosteroids quickly help out-of-control asthma,
but more than two weeks of daily use may sometimes lead to serious side effects. Inhaled corticosteroids are considered much safer for
lengthier treatment. Unlike the oral forms that must travel throughout
your body to reach your lungs, inhaled corticosteroids are delivered
directly to the airways in small doses with less chance of reaching
other parts of the body. The National Institutes of Health (NIH) calls
inhaled corticosteroids "the most effective long-term therapy available
for patients with persistent asthma. In general [they] are well tolerated
and safe at the recommended dosages."

You have probably read or heard varying reports about the risks of corticosteroid use. The bottom line is that the relatively few side effects are usually balanced by the good they do for your asthma. Steroids are definitely safe when used in the lower dosage range. Problems generally arise with high doses over long periods of time. As consumers and patients, it's important to know what specific side effects may occur and how we can work with our physicians to control them and our asthma.

Localized Risks

Oral candidiasis (thrush): Only 10 to 30 percent of inhaled steroid doses actually reach the lungs. The remainder is left in the mouth or throat or is swallowed, sometimes resulting in thrush, a fungal infection that produces milky white lesions in the mouth. Clinical thrush is far less common in lower dosages and affects more adults than children.

Physicians recommend using a spacer or holding chamber with your inhaler and rinsing your mouth with water after each treatment to reduce the amount of the inhaled steroid deposited in the mouth and throat. If you develop thrush, your doctor may also prescribe a less frequent dose and/or topical or oral antifungal medication.

Dysphonia (hoarseness): This condition is associated with increasing dosages of inhaled corticosteroids and vocal stress. Treatment may include using a spacer/holding chamber, less frequent dosing, and/or temporarily decreasing medication.

Systemic Risks

Slowed growth in children: Some studies have shown that medium-dose inhaled corticosteroids may affect a child's growth. It is not certain that this results in shorter stature in adulthood, but in general, the higher the dose, the greater the risk.

In a 1995 study of seven- to nine-year-olds treated daily with 400 mcg of beclomethasone for seven months, growth was significantly decreased in both boys and girls. There was no evidence of catch-up growth after a five-month period without medication. Yet a 1994 study of inhaled beclomethasone found no significant adverse effects on achieving adult height. Several additional studies have shown similar results, so it appears that inhaled steroids slow growth, but don't affect adult height.

The NIH advises physicians to carefully monitor a young patient's height and to "step down" therapy when possible. NIH notes that even high doses of inhaled corticosteroids with children experiencing severe, persistent asthma create less risk of delayed growth than treatment with oral systemic corticosteroids (pills or capsules).

Osteoporosis (bone disease): In some people, high corticosteroid usage can reduce bone mineral density, leading to osteoporosis. Links have been found between steroid use and inhibiting bone formation, calcium absorption, and the production of sex hormones that help keep bones vital. Brief courses of systemic corticosteroids or low-dose inhaled steroids are not dangerous, but inhaling 1,500 micrograms of beclomethasone per day can lead to bone loss. The doses of other inhaled steroids, which may constitute a risk for osteoporosis, have not been studied.

Even if you need to take steroids for your asthma, you can take measures to protect yourself against osteoporosis. Here are some recommendations:

- Take the lowest dose possible and use inhaled steroids rather than oral preparations.

- Get about 1,500 mg of calcium daily through nutrition or supplements. Because vitamin D helps the body absorb calcium, it may help to take 800 international units (IU) daily of vitamin D.

- Receive replacement female hormone therapy unless prohibited for medical reasons. There are nonhormonal drugs available (bisphosphonates, zolendronic acid, teriparatide, and calcitonin) that work similarly.

Disseminated varicella (chicken pox): The U.S. Food and Drug Administration (FDA) reported that long-term or high-dose oral corticosteroid treatment might place people exposed to chicken pox or measles at increased risk of unusually severe infections or even death. That's because some doses suppress the immune system. "Children who are on immunosuppressant drugs are more susceptible to infections than healthy children," said the FDA. Yet, the NIH Guidelines said there is no evidence that recommended doses of inhaled corticosteroids suppress the immune system.

NIH advises that children who have not had chicken pox and periodically take oral corticosteroids should receive the varicella vaccine after they've been steroid-free for at least one month. Kids who have finished a short course of prednisone may receive the vaccine immediately. For un-immunized adults and children who are exposed to chicken pox while being treated with immunosuppressive levels of steroids, there are immunoglobulin and acyclovir.

Cataracts: The risk of cataracts in patients taking systemic corticosteroids has been well identified, but reports among those taking inhaled steroids are rare. In a notable exception, the *New England Journal of Medicine* published findings of a recent Australian study of inhaled corticosteroid users between the ages of forty-nine and ninety-seven. The authors concluded that the use of inhaled steroids is associated with an increased risk for development of cataracts. Patients taking moderate to high doses of inhaled corticosteroids especially should have regular eye exams.

Table 14.1. What Are Considered Low, Medium, and High Dosages?

Drug		Low	Medium	High
Beclomethasone dipropionate	A	168–504	504–840	840+
	C	84–336	336–672	672+
Budesonide	A	200–400	400–600	600+
Turbuhaler	C	100–200	200–400	400+
Flunisolide	A	500–1,000	1,000–2,000	2,000+
	C	500–750	1,000–1,250	1,250
Fluticasone	A	88–264	264–660	660+
	C	88–176	176–440	440+
Triamcinolone acetonide	A	400–1,000	1,000–2,000	2,000
	C	400–800	800–1,200	1,200

Note: A= adult; C=child; all dosages are daily, in micrograms (MCG).

Source: NIH Guidelines of the Diagnosis and Management of Asthma, April 1997.

Other Risks

The NIH Guidelines also list a few other rare but potential risks of high-dose corticosteroid use. In some cases, oral steroid use has been linked with adrenal suppression, effects on glucose metabolism, and hypertension. Serious medical complications have also been recorded in people on high doses of oral steroids with tuberculosis.

None of the above risks have been reported with inhaled corticosteroids. However, their use in moderate to high doses has been found to contribute to thinning and bruising of the skin, especially among women.

Oral (Systemic) Corticosteroids

- Generally for short-term use
- Quickly controls persistent asthma
- Forms: pills, tablets, or liquid (for children)
- Medications: methylprednisolone, prednisolone, prednisone

Inhaled Corticosteroids

- For long-term asthma prevention; suppress, control, and reverse inflammation
- Forms: dry powder or aerosol
- Medications: beclomethasone dipropionate, budesonide, flunisolide, fluticasone propionate, triamcinolone acetonide

Chapter 15

Nonsteroidal Long-Term Control Medications

Chapter Contents

Section 15.1

Long-Acting Beta Agonists

Long-Acting Beta$_2$-Agonists

Long-acting beta$_2$-agonists help prevent asthma symptoms by relaxing the smooth muscles around the airways. Unlike control medications, long-acting beta$_2$-agonists do not reduce the swelling in the airways themselves, but instead prevent bronchospasm by keeping the airway muscles relaxed. One dose of a long-acting beta$_2$-agonist will be effective for about twelve hours. Inhaled long-acting beta$_2$-agonists are often used to prevent exercise-induced asthma.

Types of Long-Acting Beta$_2$-Agonists

There are two ways patients may take long-acting beta$_2$-agonists:

- **Inhaled long-acting beta$_2$-agonists:** Salmeterol (Serevent, Serevent Diskus) is an inhaled form of long-acting beta$_2$-agonist that begins to take effect one to two hours after administration. It is often used in conjunction with control anti-inflammatory medications and has been shown to have positive effects on quality of life. Inhaled long-acting beta$_2$-agonists are often used for exercise-induced asthma.

- **Oral long-acting beta$_2$-agonists:** Albuterol (Proventil Repetab, Volmax) is taken orally and begins to take effect about thirty minutes after ingestion. It has a peak action at three to four hours and a span of twelve hours. The oral forms of long-acting beta$_2$-agonists are not often prescribed, as there may be additional side effects such as insomnia and jitters.

Side Effects of Long-Acting Beta₂-Agonists

Long-acting beta$_2$-agonists speed the cardiovascular system so users may experience increased heartbeat, muscle tremors or cramps, anxiety, and/or headaches. The side effects from salmeterol are less common than the long-acting oral albuterol preparations.

FDA Announces New Safety Controls for Long-Acting Beta Agonists

The U.S. Food and Drug Administration (FDA) announced in February 2010 that drugs in the class of long-acting beta agonists (LABAs) should never be used alone in the treatment of asthma in children or adults. Manufacturers will be required to include this warning in the product labels of these drugs, along with taking other steps to reduce the overall use of these medications.

These new requirements are based on FDA analyses of clinical trials showing that use of these long-acting medicines is associated with an increased risk of severe worsening of asthma symptoms, leading to hospitalization in both children and adults and death in some patients with asthma. The drugs involved include the single agent products Serevent and Foradil and combination medications Advair and Symbicort that also contain inhaled corticosteroids. These medications improve a patient's ability to breathe freely and reduce the symptoms of asthma by relaxing muscles in the lung's airways.

The FDA will now require that the product labels reflect the following:

- The use of LABAs is contraindicated without the use of an asthma controller medication such as inhaled corticosteroid. Single-agent LABAs should only be used in combination with an asthma controller medication; they should not be used alone.

- LABAs should only be used long-term in patients whose asthma cannot be adequately controlled on asthma controller medications.

- LABAs should be used for the shortest duration of time required to achieve control of asthma symptoms and discontinued, if possible, once asthma control is achieved. Patients should then be maintained on an asthma controller medication.

- Pediatric and adolescent patients who require a LABA in addition to an inhaled corticosteroid should use a combination product containing both an inhaled corticosteroid and a LABA to ensure compliance with both medications.

"Although these medicines play an important role in helping some patients control asthma symptoms, our review of the available clinical trials determined that their use should be limited, whenever possible, due to an increased risk of asthma exacerbations, hospitalizations and death," said Badrul Chowdhury, M.D., director of the Division of Pulmonary and Allergy Products in the FDA's Center for Drug Evaluation and Research.

"The risks of hospitalization and poor outcomes are of particular concern for children; parents need to know that their child with asthma should not be on a LABA alone," said Dianne Murphy, M.D., director of the FDA's Office of Pediatric Therapeutics.

LABAs are approved to treat both people with asthma or with chronic obstructive pulmonary disease (COPD). The new recommendations only apply to the use of LABAs in the treatment of asthma.

The FDA will be requiring the manufacturers of LABAs to conduct additional studies to further evaluate the safety of LABAs when used in combination with inhaled corticosteroids. The FDA will seek input on the design of these studies at a public advisory committee meeting in March 2010.

In addition to these actions, FDA will work with public and private partners under the agency's ongoing Safe Use Initiative to study LABA prescribing practices.

"We will collaborate with our Safe Use partners to evaluate whether prescribing patterns adjust to the new recommendations for this class of asthma drugs. If prescribing patterns don't adjust, we will determine the reasons and consider additional steps to support safe prescribing," said Janet Woodcock, M.D., director of the FDA's Center for Drug Evaluation and Research.

The Safe Use Initiative, launched in November 2009, strives to reduce preventable harm by identifying specific, preventable medication risks and developing, implementing, and evaluating cross-sector interventions with public and private partners who are committed to safe medication use.

Advair and Serevent are marketed by Collegeville, Pennsylvania–based GlaxoSmithKline.

Foradil is marketed by Lebanon, Pennsylvania–based Novartis AG.

Symbicort is marketed by Wilmington, Delaware–based AstraZeneca.

Section 15.2

Leukotriene Modifiers

"Leukotriene Modifiers (Accolate®, Singulair®, Zileuton)," © 2007 University of Utah Asthma Center and the Utah Department of Health Asthma Program (www.health.utah.gov/asthma). Reprinted with permission.

What Are They?

Leukotriene modifiers reduce swelling and inflammation in the airways to prevent asthma symptoms. You may not notice a change in your asthma symptoms for one to two weeks after starting to use them.

These medicines will not stop a sudden asthma attack. Albuterol should be used for sudden asthma attacks.

Only regular daily use of the leukotriene modifiers will prevent asthma symptoms.

It is important that you do not stop or decrease the dose of these medications without contacting your doctor.

How Should They Be Used?

Zafirlukast (Accolate): Zafirlukast is a tablet that is taken by mouth twice a day on an empty stomach (one hour before you eat or two hours after you eat). It is very important to take this medicine on an empty stomach.

Zafirlukast must be taken every day even if you don't have asthma symptoms. If you forget to take your dose on time, do not take twice as much the next time. Take the regularly scheduled dose as soon as you remember, then get back to your regular schedule.

Side effects:

- Zafirlukast (Accolate) causes very few side effects.

- Some people may have headaches, nausea, or diarrhea. Although these side effects are quite uncommon, it is important for you to let your doctor know if you are experiencing any of these while taking zafirlukast.

219

Montelukast (Singulair): Montelukast is a tablet that is taken once a day at nighttime.

You can take Montelukast with or without food.

Montelukast must be taken every day even if you don't have asthma symptoms. If you forget to take your dose on time, do not take twice as much the next time. Take the regularly scheduled dose as soon as you remember, then get back to your regular schedule.

Side effects:

- Montelukast (Singulair) causes very few side effects. Some people may have headaches, stomach upset, or feel extra tired. Even though these side effects are rare, it is important for you to let your doctor know if you are experiencing any of these while taking montelukast.

Zileuton (Zyflo): Zileuton is a tablet that is taken four times a day.

You can take zileuton with or without food. An easy way to remember to take zileuton is to take one tablet with each meal (breakfast, lunch, and dinner) and at bedtime.

Zileuton must be taken every day even if you don't have asthma symptoms.

If you forget to take your dose on time, do not take twice as much the next time. Take the regularly scheduled dose as soon as you remember, then get back to your regular schedule.

Zileuton also comes in a form that is longer acting (Zyflo CR), which can be taken twice daily. This should be taken within one hour of the morning and evening meal.

Zileuton (Zyflo and Zyflo CR) can cause the following side effects:

- Headaches.

- Upset stomach.

- Liver function changes. You will need to have blood tests every month for the first three months, then every two to three months for the next nine months, and then periodically while you are taking zileuton. Symptoms that occur when your liver tests change can include: pain in your right side, extreme tiredness, itching, yellowing of skin or eyes, and nausea. Contact your doctor immediately if these symptoms develop and last for more than one day.

Special Instructions

It is important to remember that leukotriene modifiers will not stop a sudden asthma attack. Albuterol should be used for sudden asthma attacks. The leukotriene modifiers are often used in combination with your other asthma medications. It is important to take the medications as prescribed by your doctor.

Zafirlukast (Accolate) is safe to take with most of your asthma medications. However, if you are currently taking theophylline or a blood thinning medicine like warfarin (Coumadin), make sure that you tell your doctor and pharmacist about it before starting zafirlukast. Be sure to tell your doctor and pharmacist if you start taking any new medications, herbal products, vitamins, or over-the-counter medications.

Montelukast (Singulair) is safe to take with your asthma medications. Be sure to tell your doctor and pharmacist if you start taking any new medications, herbal products, vitamins, or over-the-counter medications.

Zileuton (Zyflo) is safe to take with most of your asthma medications. However, if you are currently taking theophylline, or a blood thinning medicine like warfarin (Coumadin), make sure that you tell your doctor and pharmacist before starting zileuton. Be sure to tell your doctor and pharmacist if you start taking any new medications, herbal products, vitamins, or over-the-counter medications.

Section 15.3

Theophylline

Why Is This Medication Prescribed?

Theophylline is used to prevent and treat wheezing, shortness of
breath, and difficulty breathing caused by asthma, chronic bronchitis,
emphysema, and other lung diseases. It relaxes and opens air passages
in the lungs, making it easier to breathe.

This medication is sometimes prescribed for other uses; ask your
doctor or pharmacist for more information.

How Should This Medicine Be Used?

Theophylline comes as a tablet, capsule, solution, and syrup to take
by mouth. It usually is taken every six, eight, twelve, or twenty-four
hours. Follow the directions on your prescription label carefully, and
ask your doctor or pharmacist to explain any part you do not understand. Take theophylline exactly as directed. Do not take more or less
of it or take it more often than prescribed by your doctor.

Take this medication with a full glass of water on an empty stomach, at least one hour before or two hours after a meal. Do not chew or
crush the extended-release (long-acting) tablets; swallow them whole.
Extended-release capsules (e.g., Theo-Dur Sprinkles) may be swallowed whole or opened and the contents mixed with soft food and
swallowed without chewing.

Theophylline controls symptoms of asthma and other lung diseases
but does not cure them. Continue to take theophylline even if you feel
well. Do not stop taking theophylline without talking to your doctor.

Other Uses for This Medicine

Theophylline is sometimes used to treat breathing problems in
premature infants. Talk to your doctor about the possible risks of using
this drug for your baby's condition.

What Special Precautions Should I Follow?

Before taking theophylline:

- Tell your doctor and pharmacist if you are allergic to theophylline or any other drugs.

- Tell your doctor and pharmacist what prescription medications you are taking, especially allopurinol (Zyloprim), azithromycin (Zithromax), carbamazepine (Tegretol), cimetidine (Tagamet), ciprofloxacin (Cipro), clarithromycin (Biaxin), diuretics ("water pills"), erythromycin, lithium (Eskalith, Lithobid), oral contraceptives, phenytoin (Dilantin), prednisone (Deltasone), propranolol (Inderal), rifampin (Rifadin), tetracycline (Sumycin), and other medications for infections or heart disease.

- Tell your doctor and pharmacist what nonprescription medications and vitamins you are taking, including ephedrine, epinephrine, phenylephrine, phenylpropanolamine, or pseudoephedrine. Many nonprescription products contain these drugs (e.g., diet pills and medications for colds and asthma), so check labels carefully. Do not take these medications without talking to your doctor; they can increase the side effects of theophylline.

- Tell your doctor if you have or have ever had seizures, ulcers, heart disease, an overactive or underactive thyroid gland, high blood pressure, or liver disease or if you have a history of alcohol abuse.

- Tell your doctor if you are pregnant, plan to become pregnant, or are breast-feeding. If you become pregnant while taking theophylline, call your doctor.

- Tell your doctor if you use tobacco products. Cigarette smoking may decrease the effectiveness of theophylline.

What Special Dietary Instructions Should I Follow?

Drinking or eating foods high in caffeine, like coffee, tea, cocoa, and chocolate, may increase the side effects caused by theophylline. Avoid large amounts of these substances while you are taking theophylline.

What Should I Do If I Forget a Dose?

Take the missed dose as soon as you remember it. However, if it is almost time for the next dose, skip the missed dose and continue your regular dosing schedule. Do not take a double dose to make up for a missed one. If you become severely short of breath, call your doctor.

What Side Effects Can This Medication Cause?

Theophylline may cause side effects. Tell your doctor if any of these symptoms are severe or do not go away:

- Upset stomach
- Stomach pain
- Diarrhea
- Headache
- Restlessness
- Insomnia
- Irritability

If you experience any of the following symptoms, call your doctor immediately:

- Vomiting
- Increased or rapid heart rate
- Irregular heartbeat
- Seizures
- Skin rash

If you experience a serious side effect, you or your doctor may send a report to the Food and Drug Administration's (FDA) MedWatch Adverse Event Reporting program online [at http://www.fda.gov/Safety/MedWatch] or by phone [800-332-1088].

What Storage Conditions Are Needed for This Medicine?

Keep this medication in the container it came in, tightly closed, and out of reach of children. Store it at room temperature and away from excess heat and moisture (not in the bathroom). Throw away any medication that is outdated or no longer needed. Talk to your pharmacist about the proper disposal of your medication.

In Case of Emergency/Overdose

In case of overdose, call your local poison control center at 800-222-1222. If the victim has collapsed or is not breathing, call local emergency services at 911.

What Other Information Should I Know?

Keep all appointments with your doctor and the laboratory. Your doctor will order certain lab tests to check your response to theophylline.

Do not change from one brand of theophylline to another without talking to your doctor.

Do not let anyone else take your medication. Ask your pharmacist any questions you have about refilling your prescription.

It is important for you to keep a written list of all of the prescription and nonprescription (over-the-counter) medicines you are taking, as well as any products such as vitamins, minerals, or other dietary supplements. You should bring this list with you each time you visit a doctor or if you are admitted to a hospital. It is also important information to carry with you in case of emergencies.

Brand Names

- Aquaphyllin
- Asmalix
- Bronkodyl
- Elixophyllin
- Quibron-T
- Slo-Phyllin
- Theoclear-80
- Theolair
- Theosol-80
- Truxophyllin

Brand Names of Combination Products

- Ami-rax (containing ephedrine, hydroxyzine, theophylline)
- Asbron G (containing guaifenesin, theophylline)
- Broncodur (containing guaifenesin, theophylline)
- Broncomar GG (containing guaifenesin, theophylline)
- Elixophyllin KI (containing potassium iodide, theophylline)
- Elixophyllin-GG (containing guaifenesin, theophylline)
- Equibron G (containing guaifenesin, theophylline)

- Hydrophed (containing ephedrine, hydroxyzine, theophylline)
- Marax (containing ephedrine, hydroxyzine, theophylline)
- Primatene Dual Action (containing ephedrine, guaifenesin, theophylline)
- Quadrinal (containing ephedrine, phenobarbital, potassium iodide, theophylline)
- Quibron (containing guaifenesin, theophylline)
- Slo-Phyllin GG (containing guaifenesin, theophylline)
- Tedrigen (containing ephedrine, phenobarbital, theophylline)
- Theo G (containing guaifenesin, theophylline)
- Theocon (containing guaifenesin, theophylline)
- Theodrine (containing ephedrine, phenobarbital, theophylline)
- Theolate (containing guaifenesin, theophylline)
- Theomar G.G. (containing guaifenesin, theophylline)
- Theomax (containing ephedrine, hydroxyzine, theophylline)
- Theophyll-GG (containing guaifenesin, theophylline)
- Uni Bronchial (containing guaifenesin, theophylline)

Section 15.4

Anti-Immunoglobulin E (Anti-IgE) Therapy

Anti-immunoglobulin E (Anti-IgE) is a form of treatment for allergic conditions that has been approved for the treatment of asthma. Anti-IgE interferes with the function of IgE. IgE is an antibody in the immune system.

How does anti-IgE work?

IgE tells immune cells to initiate allergic reactions. This may bring on symptoms such as coughing, wheezing, nasal congestion, hives, and swelling. Anti-IgE attaches to IgE in the blood and helps prevent the allergic reaction.

What anti-IgE medicine is available now?

Xolair (omalizumab) is the anti-IgE medicine now available. Xolair is approved by the U.S. Food and Drug Administration (FDA) for use with patients over twelve years of age who:

- have poorly controlled moderate to severe persistent asthma;

- have year-round allergies; and

- are taking routine inhaled steroids.

Xolair has been shown to decrease asthma episodes in some of these patients.

Xolair is given by a shot (injection) one to two times a month. The shots are given in the doctor's office. The dosage varies, depending on the person's weight and IgE blood level. Xolair is a long-term control medicine. This means it is given routinely to prevent asthma symptoms. It is not a quick relief medicine. Some patients improve quickly. Some patients show a gradual benefit. Xolair does not appear to work for all patients.

Are there any side effects or adverse reactions to Xolair?

Common side effects of Xolair include a reaction at the injection site, viral infections, upper respiratory tract infection, sinusitis, headache, and sore throat. These side effects were about as common in patients who received placebo injections.

Several rare, yet severe side effects were reported in the original studies. They include malignancy and anaphylaxis.

In the initial studies, malignancies were seen in 0.5 percent of patients treated with Xolair. The rate was 0.2 percent in patients treated with the placebo dose.

In the initial studies, anaphylaxis was seen in less than 0.1 percent of the patients treated with Xolair. Since Xolair was approved in June 2003 additional reports of anaphylaxis have been reported to the FDA. Information was gathered from about 39,500 patients treated with Xolair. The serious reactions occurred in at least 1 of every 1,000 patients. The reactions these patients had included combinations of symptoms of anaphylaxis.

Symptoms of anaphylaxis include:

- increased trouble breathing, coughing, chest tightness or wheezing;

- dizziness, fainting, rapid or weak heartbeat;

- swelling in the mouth and throat or trouble swallowing;

- flushing, itching, hives or a feeling of warmth;

- vomiting, diarrhea, or stomach cramping.

Although rare, an anaphylaxis reaction can be serious and life-threatening. An anaphylactic reaction may occur with the first dose or after any dose of Xolair. The reaction may occur soon after the shot is given. It may also occur twenty-four hours or more after the shot is given.

What's the safest way to get anti-IgE injections?

Although anaphylaxis is rare, several steps improve the patient's safety when receiving Xolair:

- The Xolair shots are given in the doctor's office.

- The patient will need to stay at the doctor's office for two hours after the initial three shots are given. After the initial three shots the patients will need to stay in the doctor's office for one hour after the shot is given.

- The doctor's office should be ready to treat an anaphylactic reaction.

- The patient will be instructed in the use of an epinephrine auto-injector. This is an easy-to-give shot that the patient can use if having an anaphylactic reaction after leaving the doctors office.

- The patient should wear a Medic-Alert bracelet.

- If you feel you are having an anaphylactic reaction, you need to get medical help right away.

Although anaphylaxis is very rare, these are a number of steps that can increase the patient's safety when receiving anti-IgE treatment. Remember to talk with your doctor if you have any questions.

Section 15.5

Combination Therapies

"Combination Medications," reprinted with permission from the Asthma Society of Canada, © 2011. All rights reserved. For additional information, please visit http://www.asthma.ca.

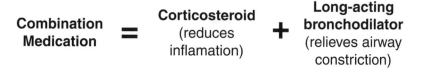

Figure 15.1. *Combination Medications*

Some pharmaceutical manufacturers have combined two controller medications into one inhaler. These inhalers are referred to as "combination medications."

Combination medications contain both an inhaled long-acting bronchodilator (LABA) and an inhaled corticosteroid. This means that two areas of asthma can be effectively treated at the same time: (1) the bronchodilator works by widening your airways, making it easier for you to breathe, and (2) the inhaled steroid reduces and prevents inflammation of your airways.

Recent studies show that many people with asthma find that combination medications give them better control and are convenient to use.

Examples of combination medications are given in Table 15.1:

Table 15.1. Types of Combination Medications

Combination Medications	Corticosteroids	Long-Acting Bronchodilators
Symbicort	Budesonide (Pulmicort)	Formoterol (Oxeze)
Advair	Fluticasone (Flovent)	Salmeterol (Serevent)

Possible side effects of combination medications include:

- rapid heart beat;

- tremor or nervousness;

- cough, throat irritation, or hoarseness.

Chapter 16

Asthma Medication Delivery Mechanisms

Chapter Contents

Section 16.1

Nebulizers

Ivory-tower research studies say that metered-dose inhalers (when used correctly either with or without a valved holding chamber) are just as effective as nebulizers at getting medication deep into your airways. However, many of you have told us otherwise: Inhalers are great when you're out and about, but if you're under the weather and feeling short of breath, there's nothing more therapeutic than inhaling the cool, medicated mist of your trusty nebulizer. Nebulizers have changed a lot through the years. No longer do you have to measure out doses with a syringe, mix with sterile saline, then sit with a loud, bulky machine and inhale and exhale for twenty minutes. Today's medications come in easy-to-use sterile, unit-dose vials and some machines are small enough for dorm rooms and quiet enough for silent nights. But do you know how to use them safely? Used incorrectly, nebulizer medication can cause respiratory symptoms to worsen. Take the Allergy and Asthma Network Mothers of Asthmatics (AANMA) challenge and maximize the mist.

Challenge goals:

- Identify U.S. Food and Drug Administration (FDA)–approved nebulizer medications

- Match the right nebulizer to your medication

- Make nebulizer accessories and machines work in your favor

Step 1: Check Your Medication

Before you begin, take a look at your medicine:

- Has it expired?

- Is the vial crushed or damaged?

- Does the medicine look discolored?

- Has it been exposed to any extremely hot or cold temperatures?

If you answer "yes" to any of these, replace it.

Next, make sure you're using an FDA-approved name-brand or generic medication.

Step 2: Wash Your Hands

To keep your nebulizer—and your lungs—free of germs, always wash your hands before handling the medication and equipment.

Step 3: Gather Your Equipment

Jet compressors force air into the nebulizer cup that holds the liquid medication, breaking the liquid into an aerosol. They come in all sizes and are much quieter than they used to be. The nebulizer cup design determines how consistently the system can produce droplets that are the right size to travel deep into the airways. This is no time to skimp—use quality equipment, keep it meticulously clean, and replace it as recommended. You won't notice the droplet size, but your lungs certainly will. Breath-enhanced and breath-actuated units allow less medication to escape into the air.

Very young children, as well as handicapped or elderly patients unable to hold a mouthpiece in their mouths dependably should always use a mask. Choose one that is soft and pliable enough to fit snugly on the face and large enough to cover the mouth and nose.

Step 4: Pour Medication into Nebulizer Cup

Unit-dose vials are a snap to use; just twist off the top and pour. To avoid spills, choose a nebulizer cup that will sit flat. Take a sniff as you pour and throw out any medication that smells foul, spoiled, or like it may contain rubbing alcohol. (If it smells of alcohol, it's illegal—it's not FDA-approved.)

Step 5: Sit Back and Relax

Put the mask in place or place the mouthpiece over your tongue and close your teeth and lips tightly around it, then turn on the machine. Breathe normally. If you start to cough, turn the machine off until you can breathe freely again. Continue the breathing treatment until the cup is empty. If the medication foams or bubbles, stop the treatment; you may have defective or contaminated medicine or equipment.

Step 6: Wash Up

Follow manufacturer's instructions to keep your nebulizer cup, mouthpiece, and tubing clean. Be fastidious; whatever gets into your cup—from your hands, medication, or house dust—will get into your lungs. When everything is clean and dry, store the system where it will stay dust-free. Nebulizer cup/mouthpiece units and tubing don't last forever. You may not notice, but the plastic will break down over time. Replace them as recommended—and don't forget to clean or change the air filter (most machines have one).

New Technology

Some nebulizing systems use vibration or ultrasound to break down the liquid instead of forced air. These are small, battery-powered, and quiet, but not all medications are suited to the new technology. Check with your healthcare provider to make sure you're using the right system for your medicine.

Fakes and Frauds

Some home health companies and large pharmacies mix and package their own nebulizer medications and market them directly to patients as cheaper and more convenient ("delivered straight to your home!"). These medications may not be manufactured under sterile conditions and may contain bacteria, irritating preservatives, or substandard ingredients.

Section 16.2

Types of Inhalers

Several different kinds of asthma medicines are taken using an inhaler. Inhaled asthma medications go directly to the site of inflammation and constriction in the airways instead of traveling through the bloodstream to get there. Inhaled medications are the preferred therapy for asthma. Inhaled medications only work if they get to the airways, so learn how to use your inhaler properly.

Many people do not use their inhalers properly, so the medication does not reach their airways. It is very important that you show your doctor, pharmacist, or asthma educator how you use your inhaler to make sure the medication is getting into your lungs, where you need it.

Inhalers fall into two categories:

- **Aerosol inhalers:** A pressurized metered-dose inhaler is a canister filled with asthma medication suspended in a propellant. When the canister is pushed down, a measured dose of the medication is pushed out as you breathe it in. Pressurized metered dose inhalers are commonly called "puffers."

- **Dry-powder inhalers:** Dry-powder inhalers contain a dry powder medication that is drawn into your lungs when you breathe in.

Some people prefer dry-powder inhalers to pressurized inhalers because they find it easier to coordinate breathing in medication from them. However, with some dry-powder inhalers, it's necessary to inhale more quickly to get the right dose than it is with a pressurized inhaler. You may have to experiment with a number of different devices (under your doctor's supervision) before finding the one you're most comfortable with. An asthma educator can assist you in matching you with the best device.

Some inhaler devices come with built-in counters that monitor the number of doses a person has taken and how many doses the device has left. If your inhaler doesn't have a counter, ask your doctor or an asthma educator to show you how to monitor your dose.

235

Section 16.3

How to Use Your Metered-Dose Inhaler

Excerpted from "Facts about Controlling Your Asthma," National Heart, Lung, and Blood Institute, National Institutes of Health, NIH Publication No. 97-2339, September 1997. Reviewed by David A. Cooke, MD, FACP, May 2011.

Using an inhaler seems simple, but most patients do not use it the right way. When you use your inhaler the wrong way, less medicine gets to your lungs. (Your doctor may give you other types of inhalers.)

For the next two weeks, read these steps aloud as you do them or ask someone to read them to you. Ask your doctor or nurse to check how well you are using your inhaler.

Use your inhaler in one of the three ways pictured in Figure 16.1 (A or B are best, but C can be used if you have trouble with A and B).

Steps for Using Your Inhaler

Getting ready:

1. Take off the cap and shake the inhaler.

2. Breathe out all the way.

3. Hold your inhaler the way your doctor said (see Figure 16.1).

Breathe in slowly:

4. As you start breathing in slowly through your mouth, press down on the inhaler one time. (If you use a holding chamber, first press down on the inhaler. Within five seconds, begin to breathe in slowly.)

5. Keep breathing in slowly, as deeply as you can.

Hold your breath:

6. Hold your breath as you count to ten slowly, if you can.

7. For inhaled quick-relief medicine (beta$_2$-agonists), wait about one minute between puffs. There is no need to wait between puffs for other medicines.

Clean Your Inhaler as Needed

Look at the hole where the medicine sprays out from your inhaler. If you see "powder" in or around the hole, clean the inhaler. Remove the metal canister from the L-shaped plastic mouthpiece. Rinse only the mouthpiece and cap in warm water. Let them dry overnight. In the morning, put the canister back inside. Put the cap on.

Know When to Replace Your Inhaler

For medicines you take each day (an example): Say your new canister has two hundred puffs (number of puffs is listed on canister) and you are told to take eight puffs per day. Two hundred puffs in the canister divided by eight puffs per day equals twenty-five days, so this canister will last twenty-five days. If you started using this inhaler on May 1, re-place it on or before May 25. You can write the date on your canister.

For quick-relief medicine take as needed and count each puff.

Do not put your canister in water to see if it is empty. This does not work.

A.   Hold inhaler 1 to 2 inches in front of your mouth (about the width of two fingers).

B.   Use a spacer/holding chamber. These come in many shapes and can be useful to any patient.

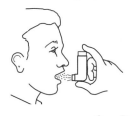

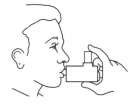

C.   Put the inhaler in your mouth. Do not use for steroids.

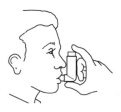

Figure 16.1. How to use your metered-dose inhaler.

Section 16.4

How to Use Your Metered-Dose Inhaler with Spacer

Excerpted from "A Patient's Guide to Aerosol Drug Delivery," © 2010 American Association for Respiratory Care (www.yourlunghealth.org). Reprinted with permission.

Steps for Correct Use of Pressured Metered-Dose Inhaler (pMDI) with Spacer/Valved Holding Chamber

When using a spacer or valved holding chamber, you should:

1. Wash and dry your hands thoroughly.

2. Warm the pMDI canister to hand or body temperature.

3. Remove the mouthpiece cover and make sure there aren't any loose parts inside the mouthpiece.

4. Shake the pMDI several times.

5. Prime the pMDI into the air if it is new or has not been used for several days.

6. Attach the pMDI to the spacer/valved holding chamber.

7. Keep the canister in an upright position.

8. Sit up straight or stand up.

9. Exhale fully.

10. Follow the instructions below based on the type of device interface being used.

   With the Mouthpiece

   - Place the mouthpiece of the spacer between your lips. Make sure that your tongue is flat under the mouthpiece and does not block the pMDI, and seal your lips around the mouthpiece.

   - Actuate the pMDI as you begin to breathe in slowly. If the device produces a "whistle," this indicates that inspiration is too rapid. (Some devices use a "whistling" sound to indicate excessively high inhalation, so hearing this "whistling" noise is a sign for you to inhale more slowly.)

- Move the mouthpiece away from your mouth and hold your breath for ten seconds or for as long as possible.

With the Mask

This is used primarily for infants, children, or those unable to use the mouthpiece:

- Place the mask completely over the nose and mouth and make sure it fits firmly against the face.
- Hold the mask in place and actuate the pMDI as the child begins to inhale slowly. If the device produces a "whistling" sound, be aware that the child is inhaling too rapidly.
- Hold the mask in place while the child takes six normal breaths (including inhalation and exhalation) and remove the mask from the child's face.

With the Collapsing Bag

- Open the bag to its full size. Press the pMDI canister immediately before inhalation.
- Keep inhaling until the bag is completely collapsed.
- Breathe in and out of the bag several times to inhale all the medication in the bag.

11. Wait fifteen to thirty seconds if another puff of medicine is needed.

12. Repeat steps above until the dosage prescribed by your doctor is reached.

13. If taking a corticosteroid, you should rinse the mouth after the last puff of medicine and spit the water out. Do not swallow it.

14. Replace the mouthpiece cover on the pMDI after each use.

General Steps to Avoid Reduced or No Dosing for pMDIs with Spacer/Valved Holding Chamber

When using pMDIs with a spacer or valved holding chamber, the following steps should be taken to avoid reduced or no dosing during the aerosol treatment. You should:

1. Assure proper fit of the pMDI to the spacer or valved holding chamber.

2. Remove cap from the pMDI boot.

3. After use, clean and reassemble the pMDI spacers and valved holding chamber according to manufacturers' instructions.

Section 16.5

Spacers

What Is a Spacer?

Spacers are excellent devices to help improve delivery of inhaled medications to the lungs, such as those used to treat asthma, cystic fibrosis, and chronic obstructive pulmonary disease (emphysema or chronic bronchitis).

A spacer is a plastic device which acts as a holding chamber for medication for the few seconds that might elapse between activating your metered dose inhaler (MDI) and breathing in the medication.

Spacers come in a variety of shapes and sizes—they may look like a clear plastic balloon or they may just look like a tube. Your doctor or pharmacist can provide advice on the type of spacer most suitable for your needs.

How Do Spacers Work?

Spacers help people with asthma to inhale their asthma medication directly into their lower airways, rather than into their throats. Spacers can either fit directly into the mouth with a mouthpiece or via a facemask. The inhaler (or "puffer") fits into the other end of the spacer. The asthma medication is then sprayed from the inhaler into one end of the spacer and breathed in, over a period of time, at the other end. The valves within spacers prevent the medication from escaping into the air, allowing you to breathe at your own pace while inhaling the medication.

Who Should Use a Spacer?

Spacers should be used by:

- adults who have poor coordination using a metered dose inhaler, as you don't have to coordinate pressing the inhaler and breathing at exactly the same time;

- children—those aged four years and under should use a small-volume spacer (with a facemask for children aged up to two years and a mouthpiece for those over two to five years), while children five years and older should use a large-volume spacer'

- people using inhaled corticosteroids (preventer medication) via an MDI, particularly at high doses, as a spacer can help minimize some of the side effects of the medication; and

- people having an acute asthma attack. Giving high doses of reliever medication via an MDI and valved spacer is an effective alternative to using a nebulizer to deliver the medication. The correct number of puffs of the MDI depends on your age; consult your doctor for specific advice and make sure that this is written into your asthma management plan.

Cleaning Your Spacer

Spacers should be washed monthly in warm water with kitchen detergent and left to drain and air dry. Do not dry your spacer with a cloth as this produces static build-up that makes the medication stick to the sides.

If you're not sure how to use your spacer, or if you suspect that you're not using it effectively, ask your doctor or pharmacist to show you how to use it correctly.

Section 16.6

How to Use Dry Powder Inhalers

How to Use a DISKUS

A DISKUS is a dry-powder inhaler that holds sixty doses. It features a built-in counter, so that you always know how many doses you have left in it.

To use your DISKUS:

1. Open your DISKUS: Hold it in the palm of your hand, put the thumb of your other hand on the thumb grip and push the thumb grip until it "clicks" into place.

2. Slide the lever away from you as far as it will go to get your medication ready.

3. Breathe out away from the device.

4. Place the mouthpiece gently in your mouth and close your lips around it.

5. Breathe in deeply until you have taken a full breath.

6. Remove the DISKUS from your mouth.

7. Hold your breath for about ten seconds, then breathe out.

8. Always check the number in the dose counter window to see how many doses are left.

If you drop your DISKUS or breathe into it after its dose has been loaded, you may cause the dose to be lost. If either of these things happens, reload the device before using it.

How to Use a Turbuhaler

A Turbuhaler is a dry-powder inhaler available in an easy-to-use format.

Some Turbuhalers feature a dose counter that shows the exact amount of medication left. If your Turbuhaler doesn't have a dose counter, then check for a red indicator in the windows on the side of the device. When you see red in the window, there are approximately twenty doses left and it's time to order a refill.

How to use a Turbuhaler:

1. Unscrew the cap and take it off. Hold the inhaler upright.

2. Twist the colored grip of your Turbuhaler as far as it will go. Then twist it all the way back. You have done it right when you hear a "click."

3. Breathe out away from the device.

4. Put the mouthpiece between your teeth and close your lips around it. Breathe in forcefully and deeply through your mouth.

5. Remove the Turbuhaler from your mouth before breathing out.

6. Always check the number in the side counter window under the mouthpiece to see how many doses are left. For the Turbuhalers that do not have a dose counter window, check the window for a red mark, which means your medication is running out. When finished, replace the cap.

If you drop your Turbuhaler or breathe into it after its dose has been loaded, you may cause the dose to be lost. If either of these things happens, reload the device before using it.

Clean your Turbuhaler as needed. To do this, first wipe the mouthpiece with a dry tissue or cloth. Never wash the mouthpiece or any other part of the Turbuhaler—if it gets wet, it won't work properly.

How to Use a Diskhaler

A Diskhaler is a dry-powder inhaler that holds small pouches (or blisters), each containing a dose of medication, on a disk. The Diskhaler punctures each blister so that its medication can be inhaled.

To use your Diskhaler:

1. Remove the cover and check that the device and mouthpiece are clean.

2. If a new medication disk is needed, pull the corners of the white cartridge out as far as it will go, then press the ridges on the sides inwards to remove the cartridge.

3. Place the medication disk with its numbers facing up on the white rotating wheel. Then slide the cartridge all the way back in.

4. Pull the cartridge all the way out, then push it all the way in until the highest number on the medication disk can be seen in the indicator window.

5. With the cartridge fully inserted, and the device kept flat, raise the lid as far as it goes, to pierce both sides of the medication blister.

6. Move the Diskhaler away from your mouth and breathe out as much as you can until no air is left in your lungs.

7. Place the mouthpiece between your teeth and lips, making sure you do not cover the air holes on the mouthpiece. Inhale as quickly and deeply as you can. Do not breathe out.

8. Move the Diskhaler away from your mouth and continue holding your breath for about ten seconds.

9. Breathe out slowly.

10. If you need another dose, pull the cartridge out all the way and then push it back in all the way. This will move the next blister into place. Repeat steps 5 through 9.

11. After you have finished using the Diskhaler, put the mouthpiece cap back on.

If you drop your Diskhaler or breathe into it after its dose has been loaded, you may cause the dose to be lost. If either of these things happens, reload the device before using it.

Your Diskhaler should always be cleaned according to its instructions and before you insert a new medication disk into it.

Chapter 17

Adverse Effects Related to the Use of Asthma Medications

Chapter Contents

Section 17.1

Don't Let Asthma Medication Side Effects Interfere with Your Asthma Control

As with all medications there are a number of asthma medication side effects that you need to be aware of. While asthma medication side effects prevent some people from actually taking their medication, asthma medications are generally well tolerated. However, knowing your asthma medication side effects is an important part of caring for your asthma. Asthma medication side effects can often be prevented, but it is equally important to know which asthma medication side effects you need to emergently seek care for and which ones you can monitor at home.

Asthma Medication Side Effects: Inhaled Corticosteroids

Asthma medication side effects for inhaled corticosteroids occur as:

- local adverse effects (in only one area of the body);
- systemic effects (throughout the body).

Inhaled Corticosteroids: Local Side Effects

While local side effects can be annoying and bothersome, they are generally not serious. More importantly, there are simple steps you can take to prevent these local side effects:

- oral candidiasis, or thrush;
- dysphonia (hoarseness);
- reflex cough and bronchospasm.

Inhaled Corticosteroids: Systemic Side Effects

While uncommon, a number of systemic effects can occur with inhaled corticosteroids. Generally, there is a higher risk with increasing doses of inhaled corticosteroids. Potential asthma medication side effects with inhaled steroids include:

- poor growth;

- decreased bone density;

- disseminated varicella infection (chickenpox that spreads to organs);

- easy bruising;

- cataracts and glaucoma;

- adrenal gland suppression.

Asthma Medication Side Effects: Short Acting Beta Agonists (SABA)

While albuterol side effects will not be experienced by most patients using albuterol and other relief medicines, being knowledgeable of common and serious albuterol side effects is an important skill.

Additionally, overusing your rescue inhaler is a sign of poor asthma control. If you are overusing your asthma inhaler, you need to speak to your physician about adjusting your asthma action plan.

Asthma Medication Side Effects: Long Acting Beta Agonists (LABA)

The side effects of LABAs are similar to those for the SABAs. However, there have been concerns regarding the possibility that LABA treatment increases severity of asthma exacerbations and risk of fatal asthma episodes.

These concerns have resulted in a black box warning from the U.S. Food and Drug Administration (FDA). Even though a LABA may decrease the frequency of asthma episodes and severity of symptoms, a LABA may make asthma episodes more severe when they occur. You should never be using a LABA alone to control your asthma. Make sure you discuss any concerns that you may have with your asthma care provider.

Asthma Medication Side Effects: Oral Steroids Like Prednisone

If you require treatment with oral steroids two or more times per year, your asthma is not well controlled and you should discuss with your asthma care provider. The longer you need oral steroids and the larger dose required to get your asthma under control puts you at greater risk for side effects. Side effects are similar to the systemic side effects noted for inhaled steroids above.

Asthma Medication Side Effects: Montelukast and Other Leukotriene Modifiers

Singulair (montelukast) and other leukotriene modifiers are generally well tolerated, but you should be aware that potential side effects include:

- stomach upset;
- headache;
- liver test abnormalities;
- skin rashes;
- Rarely, Churg-Strauss syndrome.

Additionally, Singulair (montelukast) and other leukotriene modifiers have changed their labeling to make providers and parents aware of potential mental health side effects noted with this class of drugs. It is very important to discuss any mental health side effects with your asthma care provider so the two of you can decide how to best manage these side effects.

Asthma Medication Side Effects: Cromolyn Sodium and Nedocromil

Cromolyn and nedocromil are considered alternative treatments for patients with mild persistent asthma and can be used to prevent symptoms if you know you will have an allergen exposure and use the medication beforehand.

Cromolyn sodium and nedocromil are generally well tolerated with most side effects decreasing with continued use. Make sure to tell your doctor if side effects do not resolve or become bothersome. Side effects include:

- bad taste in mouth;
- cough;
- itching or sore throat;
- headache;
- sneezing or stuffy nose.

Make sure to notify your doctor promptly if you experience:

- shortness of breath;
- wheezing.

Asthma Medication Side Effects: Xolair

Xolair, one of the immunomodulators, is given as an injection. As a result, you may experience pain or swelling at the injection site. Other common side effects include:

- viral illness;
- upper respiratory tract infections;
- sinusitis;
- headache;
- sore throat.

There are two serious potential side effects you need to be aware of and discuss with your physician:

- **Anaphylaxis:** A very small (0.2 percent) number of patients taking Xolair injections may experience this potentially life threatening condition. Symptoms of anaphylaxis may include sudden onset of asthma like symptoms such as wheezing, cough, shortness of breath, or trouble breathing; feeling dizzy or faint; hives; changes in your voice, swelling of the tongue, or difficulty swallowing. These symptoms are a medical emergency and you should seek medical care right away.

- **Cancer:** For unknown reasons, there was a small increase in risk of cancer among patients using Xolair compared to placebo in clinical trials (0.5 percent versus 0.2 percent). There was not any single predominate type of cancer noted. If this is concerning to you, be sure to discuss the risks and benefits with your doctor before starting treatment.

In Summary

All medications have risks and side effects that you and your doctor need to consider before starting a new asthma medication or if your symptoms worsen. Asthma medication side effects can be serious, but most are relatively minor or can be prevented. Be sure you know when you need to call your doctor about asthma medication side effects and when your symptoms can be monitored.

Source

National Heart, Lung, and Blood Institute. Accessed: December 8, 2009. Expert Panel Report 3 (EPR3): Guidelines for the Diagnosis and Management of Asthma

Section 17.2

Osteoporosis

"What People with Asthma Need to Know about Osteoporosis,"
National Institute of Arthritis and Musculoskeletal and Skin
Diseases, National Institutes of Health, June 2010.

What Is Asthma?

Asthma is a chronic lung disease that affects more than twenty-two million Americans, nearly six million of whom are children. Asthma is becoming more common, and African Americans are especially at risk. For people with asthma, everyday things can trigger an attack. These triggers include air pollution, allergens, exercise, infections, emotional upset, or certain foods.

Typical asthma symptoms include coughing, wheezing, tightness in the chest, difficulty breathing, rapid heart rate, and sweating. Children with asthma often complain of an itchy upper chest or develop a dry cough. These may be the only signs of an asthma attack.

Asthma itself does not pose a threat to bone health. However, certain medications used to treat asthma and some behaviors triggered by concern over the disease can have a negative impact on the skeleton.

What Is Osteoporosis?

Osteoporosis is a condition in which the bones become less dense and more likely to fracture. Fractures from osteoporosis can result in pain and disability. Osteoporosis is a major health threat for an estimated forty-four million Americans, 68 percent of whom are women.

Risk factors for developing osteoporosis include the following:

- Thinness or small frame
- Family history of the disease
- Being postmenopausal and particularly having had early menopause
- Abnormal absence of menstrual periods (amenorrhea)
- Prolonged use of certain medications, such as those used to treat lupus, asthma, thyroid deficiencies, and seizures
- Low calcium intake
- Lack of physical activity
- Smoking
- Excessive alcohol intake

Osteoporosis often can be prevented. It is known as a silent disease because, if undetected, it can progress for many years without symptoms until a fracture occurs. Osteoporosis has been called a childhood disease with consequences in old age because building healthy bones in youth helps prevent the disease and fractures later in life. However, it is never too late to adopt new habits for healthy bones.

The Connection between Asthma and Osteoporosis

People with asthma tend to be at increased risk for osteoporosis, especially in the spine, for several reasons. First, anti-inflammatory medications, known as glucocorticoids, are commonly prescribed for asthma. When taken by mouth, these medications can decrease calcium absorbed from food, increase calcium lost from the kidneys, and decrease bone formation. Doses of more than 7.5 mg (milligrams) each day can cause significant bone loss, particularly during the first year of use. Corticosteroids also interfere with the production of sex hormones in both women and men, which can contribute to bone loss, and they can cause muscle weakness, which can increase the risk of falling and related fractures.

Many people with asthma think that milk and other dairy products trigger asthma attacks, although the evidence shows that this is only likely to be true if they also have a dairy allergy. This unnecessary avoidance of calcium-rich dairy products can be especially damaging for children with asthma who need calcium to build strong bones.

Because exercise often can trigger an asthma attack, many people with asthma avoid weight-bearing physical activities that are known to strengthen bone. Those people who remain physically active often choose swimming as their first exercise of choice because it is less likely than other activities to trigger an asthma attack. Unfortunately, swimming does not have the same beneficial impact on bone health as weight-bearing exercises, which work the body against gravity. Weight-bearing exercises include walking, jogging, racquet sports, basketball, volleyball, aerobics, dancing, and weight training.

Osteoporosis Management Strategies

Strategies to prevent and treat osteoporosis in people with asthma are not significantly different from those used to treat people who do not have asthma.

Nutrition: A well-balanced diet rich in calcium and vitamin D is important for healthy bones. Good sources of calcium include low-fat dairy products; dark green, leafy vegetables; and calcium-fortified foods and beverages. Supplements can help ensure that the calcium requirement is met each day, especially in those with a proven milk allergy. The Institute of Medicine recommends a daily calcium intake of 1,000 mg each day for men and women, increasing to 1,200 mg daily for those age fifty and older.

Vitamin D plays an important role in calcium absorption and bone health. It is synthesized in the skin through exposure to sunlight. Food sources of vitamin D include egg yolks, saltwater fish, and liver. Many people obtain enough vitamin D by getting about fifteen minutes of sunlight exposure each day or from eating fortified foods. Other individuals—especially those who are older or housebound, live in northern climates, or use sunscreen—may require vitamin D supplements to achieve the recommended intake of 400 to 600 International Units (IU) each day.

Exercise: Like muscle, bone is living tissue that responds to exercise by becoming stronger. The best kind of activity for your bones is weight-bearing exercise that forces you to work against gravity. Some examples include walking, climbing stairs, weight training, and dancing. Regular exercise, such as walking, may help prevent bone loss and provide many other health benefits.

People who experience exercise-induced asthma should exercise in an environmentally controlled facility and participate in activities that fall within their limitations. They may also use medication when necessary to enable them to exercise.

Healthy lifestyle: Smoking is bad for bones, as well as the heart and lungs. Women who smoke tend to go through menopause earlier, triggering earlier bone loss. In addition, people who smoke may absorb less calcium from their diets. Alcohol also can affect bone health negatively. Those who drink heavily are more prone to bone loss and fracture because of both poor nutrition and an increased risk of falling.

Reducing exposure to asthma triggers, such as irritants and allergens, can help lessen a person's reliance on glucocorticoid medication. Avoiding people with colds and other respiratory infections and minimizing emotional stress can also be important.

Bone density test: A bone mineral density (BMD) test measures bone density at various sites of the body. This safe and painless test can detect osteoporosis before a fracture occurs and can predict one's chances of future fracture. People with asthma, particularly those receiving glucocorticoid therapy for two months or more, should talk to their doctors about whether they might be candidates for a BMD test.

Medication: Like asthma, osteoporosis is a disease with no cure. However, there are medications available to prevent and treat osteoporosis, including: bisphosphonates; estrogen agonists/antagonists (also called selective estrogen receptor modulators or SERMS); parathyroid hormone; estrogen therapy; hormone therapy; and a recently approved receptor activator of nuclear factor kappa-B ligand (RANK ligand, or RANKL) inhibitor.

Because of their effectiveness in controlling asthma with fewer side effects, inhaled glucocorticoids are preferred to oral forms of the medication. Bone loss tends to increase with increased glucocorticoid doses and prolonged use; therefore, the lowest possible dose for the shortest period of time that controls asthma symptoms is recommended.

Section 17.3

Glaucoma

Inhaled steroids are a mainstay of therapy in the treatment of asthma among adults. Yet talk of having to take "steroids" makes many people very apprehensive, because of concern about medication side effects. Inhaled steroids are important for prevention of asthmatic attacks, but are they safe? Two recent medical reports have put these questions in the forefront of our thinking about asthma. One report described a 50 percent reduction in the risk of hospitalization for asthma among patients prescribed inhaled steroids compared to others who were not taking inhaled steroids. The other report described a 40 percent increase in the risk of developing glaucoma among some persons taking inhaled steroids. Are these medications friend or foe? Where does the truth lie?

For many persons "steroids" conjure up the image of weight gain, puffy face, mood swings, and thinning bones. These are potential side effects of steroids taken in tablet form, especially when taken for many weeks to months. Steroids in tablet form act by being absorbed from the stomach, entering the bloodstream, and traveling to all parts of the body, including the bronchial tubes of the lungs. At the same time the blood carries them to the eyes, muscles, bones, skin, appetite center—to all parts of the body, where they can exert their undesirable effects.

One can avoid most of these potentially harmful side effects by inhaling the steroid medication directly into the breathing tubes. In this way the inhaled steroids are delivered directly to where they are needed, the inflamed bronchial tubes, and not to the remainder of the body. In the same way that one applies steroid creams to skin rashes without fear of side effects elsewhere in the body, so too one can apply steroid medication from inhalers to the surface of bronchial tubes without fear of generalized adverse side effects—for the most part.

Depending on how much of the inhaled steroid medication one takes—that is, depending on the strength of the medication and the number of puffs inhaled each day—some of it can be absorbed from the mouth and bronchial tubes and pass into the bloodstream. In general, at the usual doses (eight to twelve puffs or 400 to 800 micrograms/day), the amount of steroid passing into the bloodstream is trivial, especially if one uses a spacer tube and rinses one's mouth after each use. At standard doses one does not develop any side effects in the eyes, bones, muscles, and elsewhere. Consistent with this understanding, in a recent medical report of some fifty thousand persons treated by ophthalmologists in Quebec, Canada, high pressure within the eye and its consequences (glaucoma) were overall no more common among persons taking inhaled steroids than among persons not using these medications.

However, these same doctors found that persons with asthma over the age of sixty-five years who were taking large doses of inhaled steroids for at least three months had a 40 percent increased chance of developing high eye pressure or glaucoma. Among persons taking large doses of these inhaled steroids, a small amount of the medication can enter the bloodstream and be transported to the eyes. Among persons sensitive to their effects, fluid can build up within the eyes and cause injury to the nerves from the elevated pressure exerted on them.

What is considered a large dose of inhaled steroids? The authors of this report used the following criteria to define large doses: for beclomethasone (Vanceril, Beclovent), thirty-two puffs a day or more; for triamcinolone (Azmacort), sixteen puffs a day; for budesonide (Pulmicort), eight puffs a day, and for flunisolide (Aerobid), six or more puffs a day. The newer inhaled steroid, fluticasone (Flovent), was not available at the time of this study, and so what constitutes large doses of inhaled fluticasone was not considered.

Several additional studies have been performed to look for an association between inhaled steroid use and glaucoma. Some of these studies used newer inhaled steroids such as fluticasone, budesonide, and ciclesonide. These studies showed very low rates of glaucoma in patients treated with inhaled steroids, and could not clearly link treatment to eye problems.

Although the evidence suggests the risk is low, it seems reasonable to recommend that persons over the age of sixty-five who are taking large doses of inhaled steroids see an ophthalmologist for measurement of their eye pressure. This is a painless procedure that takes no more than five minutes. It is probably a good idea for all persons over the age of sixty-five years to be checked for glaucoma; now there is an especially good reason for older persons on high-dose inhaled steroids.

Before you are tempted to give up your inhaled steroid medicine for fear of complications in your eyes or elsewhere, remember that for persons taking any less than the large doses of inhaled, there is no evidence that the inhaled steroids are harmful to the eyes. And remember that your chance of having an attack of asthma severe enough to require hospitalization is reduced in half by your use of inhaled steroids. Used wisely, and in the lowest doses that are effective, these medicines are still the best long-term treatment for the majority of persons with persistent asthma.

Chapter 18

Immunotherapy and Asthma

Asthma and allergies are two quite personal conditions in the sense that they can work so differently from one person to another. Treatment plans don't come in a one-size-fits-all formula. Lifestyle choices and/or demands can make it easier or more difficult to avoid allergens. Sometimes medications that once worked have become ineffective. When medications aren't helping and you're having a hard time avoiding your allergens, it might be time to consider allergen immunotherapy, or "allergy shots."

What Is Immunotherapy?

With immunotherapy treatment, you receive increasingly higher doses of your allergens over time, gradually becoming less sensitive to them. Allergy shots have been proven effective for symptoms caused by grass, tree, and weed pollens; dust mites; cat dander; certain molds; and stinging insects.

To date, allergen immunotherapy is the only treatment that has the potential to provide long-term prevention of allergic asthma or rhinitis symptoms. Allergy shots may have a lasting effect after they are stopped, whereas medications do not.

"Immunotherapy," Reprinted with permission from the Asthma and Allergy Foundation of America, www.aafa.org, © 2005. All rights reserved. Reviewed by David A. Cooke, M.D., FACP, May 2011.

Who Is Eligible?

To help determine if you will be a good candidate for allergy shots, your physician will look at two key factors: how long you experience allergy symptoms each year and how well other treatments are controlling them. People with perennial or prolonged allergies are generally the best match, as well as those needing multiple medications for their symptoms. A switch to allergy shots is usually not cost-effective for patients whose seasons last only a few months and who are achieving good control with cromolyn sodium inhalers, topical corticosteroids, or nonsedating antihistamines.

Additional considerations include your age and health. Patients into their sixties can be good candidates for treatment. However, the younger the patient, not only the better the chances for relief, but also the more years of potential benefit. Your body must also be able to respond to epinephrine, which would be used in the rare event that you should have a severe reaction from the injections. Arrhythmia or other heart problems would make you ineligible in this case.

How Does the Process Work?

Once your doctor has verified that immunotherapy is a good option for you, he or she will conduct tests that will determine what allergens should be in your allergy extract. Skin testing is one of the most common, accurate, and inexpensive ways to do this.

In prick/scratch testing, a small drop of a possible allergen is placed on the skin, followed by lightly pricking or scratching through the drop with a needle. In intradermal (under the skin) testing, a very small amount of allergen is injected into the outer layer of skin. With either test, if you are allergic to the substance, you will develop redness, swelling, and itching at the test site within twenty minutes. You may also see a raised, round area that looks like a hive. Usually, the larger the area, or wheal, the more sensitive you are to the allergen. Most people are tested for about five to twenty-five allergens at a time, depending on whether sensitivity is being tested for indoor allergens only, or for both indoor and outdoor allergens.

After allergen identification comes the actual treatment. You'll begin with shots once or twice a week, until you start to feel relief (this process usually takes four to six months). Monthly maintenance doses are then given to help keep your "allergen resistance level" steady. You can expect your symptoms to be reduced after your first year of immunotherapy. If not, the use of allergy shots for your condition should be reconsidered. After you've been taking allergy shots for three to five years, it's time to stop for a reevaluation of treatment and symptoms. If the result is a return of symptoms, another course of therapy may be recommended, as a gradual relapse has been known to occur in some patients.

A Quicker Alternative

Because of time, cost, and convenience issues, rush immunotherapy has reemerged as a viable option to conventional allergy shots. First suggested sixty-five years ago by British physician John Freeman, this accelerated version of the traditional course of shots brings patients to maintenance dosing levels within several weeks instead of months.

A typical rush regimen schedules four daily injections at one-hour intervals on five consecutive days. Maintenance doses are reached in five to ten days. After maintenance is achieved, injections move to a weekly, then biweekly, and finally, a monthly schedule.

In one recent study, forty-four patients, ages two to fifty, successfully achieved full maintenance dosing in one day. Diagnosed with a variety of conditions including asthma, allergic rhinoconjunctivitis, and chronic sinusitis, all were able to complete the therapy and showed no signs of blood pressure changes. Peak flow meter readings also remained stable. Participants had been pre-medicated with prednisone and various antihistamines for two days prior to the study as well as on the morning it began. Two patients developed and were treated for generalized itching.

Chapter 19

Alternative and Complementary Asthma Therapies

Chapter Contents

Section 19.1

Alternative and Complementary Therapies for Treating Asthma: How Effective Are They?

"Complementary or Alternative Asthma Treatments,"
reprinted with permission from www.getasthmahelp.org, the
website of the Asthma Initiative of Michigan, © 2010.

There is no good reason to take a chance on risky alternative medicines when proven medical treatment is available that can keep you symptom-free.

The only proven way to control asthma is by using prescription medications and avoiding triggers. Alternative treatments for asthma usually mean treatments that do not use drugs prescribed by doctors. The Expert Panel Report 3 (2007) does not recommend any other kind of treatment for asthma, based on a thorough review of scientific studies. However, surveys show that many people with chronic diseases, including asthma, are using treatments other than prescription drugs and trigger avoidance to try to control their asthma.

Anyone thinking about trying an alternative treatment should talk it over with his or her doctor first. These treatments are not only unproven, but can also be harmful. It is important to keep using treatments as prescribed unless your doctor either tells you to stop taking the medication or tells you to change your current prescribed dose. Using an alternative treatment may worsen your asthma symptoms and might even lead to other health problems. It is possible that some treatments, like relaxation techniques, could be used complementary (in addition) to your prescribed medication. Your doctor may tell you that it is okay to practice this kind of treatment.

The following statements represent the opinions of the Expert Panel (2007) regarding common complementary and alternative medications (CAMs) used in the treatment of asthma (EPR-3, p. 240).

Acupuncture

The Expert Panel does not recommend the use of acupuncture for the treatment of asthma.

Acupuncture involves the insertion of thin needles along acupuncture points or acupoints on the body. (Acupressure is a different way of stimulating the same acupoints.) Two Cochrane reviews (Linde et al. 2000; McCarney et al. 2004) of randomized trials with hundreds of participants using real acupuncture and sham acupuncture to treat asthma or asthma-like symptoms found no clinical improvement for acupuncture compared to sham acupuncture. Both reviews stated that there is not enough evidence to make recommendations about the value of acupuncture in asthma treatment. Additional studies published between 1970 and 2000, comparing real acupuncture with sham acupuncture, found no evidence of acupuncture reducing asthma symptoms (Martin et al. 2002).

In addition, people can become very sick after acupuncture treatment. These people usually became sick because of infected needles or puncture injuries.

Chiropractic Therapy

The Expert Panel concludes that there is not enough evidence to recommend the use of chiropractic or related techniques in the treatment of asthma.

Chiropractic therapy and other forms of spinal or bodily manipulation or massage have been reported to benefit some patients who have asthma. However, systematic reviews of chiropractic techniques in asthma (Balon and Mior 2004) and related therapies, such as the Alexander technique (Dennis 2000), found few randomized, controlled studies (studies that use scientific methods to prove something works or doesn't work). Those studies, where available, showed mixed results, with perhaps some benefit in symptoms or health-related quality-of-life measures but no absolute improvement on more objective measures of asthma outcomes (such as improved spirometry tests).

Homeopathy and Herbal Medicine

The Expert Panel concludes that there is not enough evidence to support the value of homeopathy or herbal products for the treatment of asthma, and that more scientific studies are needed. Furthermore, because herbal products are not made in a uniform way by all companies, one must be aware that some products may have harmful ingredients, and that some may interact with other medications that the patient may be taking.

Homeopathy deals with the use of diluted substances, which cause symptoms when used at full strength. A review of homeopathy studies showed that they were of uneven quality and used different homeopathic treatments, which made it hard to reliably assess the possible role of homeopathy in asthma (McCarney et al. 2004). A variety of herbal products have been used alone and as additional therapy for asthma with positive results in small trials that have not been copied (Gupta et al. 1998; Khayyal et al. 2003; Lee et al. 2004; Urata et al. 2002). The National Center for Complementary and Alternative Medicine of the National Institutes of Health encourages the development of well-designed studies to find the role of herbal products.

Breathing Techniques

The Expert Panel concludes there is not enough evidence to suggest that breathing techniques have clinical benefit for patients who have asthma.

Scientific studies have been done with breathing exercises (Holloway and Ram 2004), inspiratory (inhale) muscle training (Ram et al. 2003; Weiner et al. 2002), and Buteyko breathing (Cooper et al. 2003) (raising blood carbon dioxide partial pressure [PCO_2] through hypoventilation). Seven studies on breathing exercises (Holloway and Ram 2004) showed that treatment interventions and outcome measurements varied greatly. So, although there was a suggestion of improvement in things like quick-relief inhaler use, quality of life, and flare-ups in persons who have asthma, no reliable conclusions about the use of breathing exercises for treatment of asthma in clinical practice could be found (Holloway and Ram 2004).

Inspiratory muscle training studies have also been scientifically reviewed (Ram et al. 2003), and in three studies in which the maximum inspiratory pressure (PImax) was reported, it was significantly improved compared to controls (those who did not do the training). In another study of breathing techniques, outcomes suggests that, in mild persistent asthma, using the techniques before using a quick-relief inhaler might curb overuse of the quick-relief inhaler, and that the process of practicing breathing techniques may be more important than the type of breathing technique used (Slader et al. 2006). Larger studies are needed to confirm study findings.

Relaxation Techniques

The Expert Panel concludes that, despite some encouraging data from small studies, more positive data from randomized, controlled studies is needed before relaxation techniques can be recommended in the treatment of asthma.

Recent controlled studies have been done to find whether relaxation techniques, including biofeedback and hypnotherapy, may be helpful in asthma. Early data suggest that relaxation techniques may help improve not only symptoms (which in studies appeared to improve generally) but also lung function (Lehrer et al. 2004; Loew et al. 2001). Due to the smallness of the study and other concerns, these studies would need more confirmation.

A systematic review of scientific studies of relaxation techniques (Huntley et al. 2002) stated that there was a lack of data from well-done studies of relaxation therapies to recommend them in the treatment of asthma. This review did find some support, however, for muscle relaxation techniques in particular, which may lead to improvements in lung function.

Yoga

There are not enough well-controlled studies on the effects of yoga on asthma.

A recent, well-controlled pilot study of one type of yoga (Iyengar) showed no major results for health-related quality-of-life measures (Sabina et al. 2005).

Section 19.2

Magnesium Supplements for the Treatment of Asthma

"Magnesium Supplements May Benefit People with Asthma,"
National Center for Complementary and Alternative Medicine,
National Institutes of Health, April 17, 2011.

Some previous studies have reported associations between low magnesium consumption and the development of asthma. Now, recent research supported by the National Center for Complementary and Alternative Medicine (NCCAM) and published in the *Journal of Asthma* provides additional evidence that adults with mild to moderate asthma may benefit from taking magnesium supplements.

Researchers from Bastyr University in Kenmore, Washington, and the University of California, Davis, enrolled fifty-two men and women aged twenty-one to fifty-five with mild to moderate asthma. The participants consumed either 340 mg of magnesium citrate or placebo daily for 6.5 months. The researchers examined clinical asthma symptoms and control using tests to measure lung responsiveness and pulmonary function, inflammation markers, and magnesium levels at the beginning of the study and every month thereafter.

The researchers found that those who took magnesium experienced significant improvement in lung activity and the ability to move air in and out of their lungs. Those taking magnesium also reported other improvements in asthma control and quality of life compared with people who received placebo. There were no significant changes for objective measures of forced expiratory volume in one second (the volume of air that can be exhaled in one second after taking a deep breath) or inflammation and magnesium levels in either group.

During the study the researchers indicated that members of both groups had similar levels of magnesium in serum or within red blood cells. Participants in both groups also had similar levels of C-reactive protein (a marker of inflammation) throughout the study. Airway inflammation is an important component of asthma.

The researchers noted that this study adds to the body of research that shows subjective and objective benefits of magnesium supplements in people with mild to moderate asthma.

Reference

Kazaks AG, Uriu-Adams JY, Albertson TE, et al. Effect of oral magnesium supplementation on measures of airway resistance and subjective assessment of asthma control and quality of life in men and women with mild to moderate asthma: a randomized placebo controlled trial. *Journal of Asthma*. 2010;47(1):83–92.

Section 19.3

Traditional Chinese Herbs May Benefit People with Asthma

Reprinted from National Center for Complementary and Alternative Medicine, National Institutes of Health, April 17, 2011.

Asthma affects millions of adults and children in the United States. Its increasing prevalence, the absence of curative treatments, and concerns about side effects from long-term use of asthma drugs have prompted interest in complementary and alternative therapies such as traditional Chinese medicine (TCM) herbs.

In a recent article, National Center for Complementary and Alternative Medicine (NCCAM)–supported scientists from the Mount Sinai School of Medicine reviewed research evidence on TCM herbs for asthma, focusing on studies reported since 2005:

- Preliminary clinical trials of formulas containing *Radix glycyrrhizae* in combination with various other TCM herbs have had positive results. One study compared an herbal formula called ASHMI (anti-asthma herbal medicine intervention) with the drug prednisone in adults; three others looked at herbal formulas as complementary therapies in children. All of the trials reported improvement in lung function with the herbal formulas and found them to be safe and well tolerated. Most of the trials showed significant improvements in asthma symptom scores, although one did not.

- A three-year follow-up of fourteen patients with asthma taking an extract of *Sophora flavescens* Ait (a component of ASHMI) reported positive clinical results and no side effects.

- Laboratory findings on TCM herbal remedies suggest several possible mechanisms of action against asthma, including an anti-inflammatory effect, inhibition of smooth-muscle contraction in the airway, and modulation of immune system responses. The authors noted that clinical trials are under way for ASHMI. They also summarize research on a TCM formula being developed to combat peanut allergy.

Reference

Li X-M, Brown LV. Efficacy and mechanisms of action of traditional Chinese medicines for treating asthma and allergy. *Journal of Allergy and Clinical Immunology*. 2009;123(2):297–306.

Chapter 20

New Developments in Asthma Treatment

Chapter Contents

Section 20.1

Beta Blockers as Asthma Treatment

Just when the Food and Drug Administration (FDA) is reconsidering the use of stimulants to treat asthma, a new research study offers further evidence to support a University of Houston professor's theory that an opposite approach to asthma treatment may be in order.

Richard A. Bond, professor of pharmacology at the University of Houston College of Pharmacy (UHCOP), has been investigating whether beta-2 adrenoreceptor antagonist drugs (or beta blockers) ultimately might be a safer, more effective strategy for long-term asthma management than the currently used beta-2 adrenoreceptor agonists (or stimulants).

The beta-2 adrenoreceptor is a receptor found in many cells, including the smooth muscle lining the airways, and has long been a target for asthma drugs. However, a recent study shows the absence of asthma-like symptoms in a mouse model that lacks the key gene that produces the receptor. This lends further evidence to Bond's theory that questions whether the pharmaceutical industry should be working to block or inhibit the receptor instead of the current approach of chronically stimulating it to reduce asthma symptoms.

The study, "Beta2-Adrenoreceptor Signaling Is Required for the Development of an Asthma Phenotype in a Murine Model," is in the January 26, 2009, online issue of the journal *Proceedings of the National Academy of Sciences (PNAS)*, one of the world's most-cited multidisciplinary scientific serials. A follow-up commentary by an independent scientist in the field also was published in the print issue of *PNAS* in February 2009.

The timely release of this study comes on the heels of the FDA considering a renewed look at the use of long-acting beta agonist drugs (LABAs)—at least those used alone, without a steroidal component—for the management of asthma symptoms. In an FDA report released in December 2009, an analysis of more than one hundred trials on four drugs (two LABAs alone and two LABA/corticosteroid combinations) found an increased risk of hospitalization and asthma-related deaths with the LABA-only therapy. During the same month, an FDA advisory panel urged the FDA to ban the LABA-only drugs and strengthen warnings on the combination drugs.

Bond and his colleagues propose an alternative to stimulants, using antagonists (or beta blockers) instead. This approach, termed paradoxical pharmacology, suggests patients may be treated with medication that initially worsens their symptoms before eventually improving their overall health.

Beta-blockers currently are contraindicated for asthma because they typically trigger bronchoconstriction, decreasing the flow of air to the lungs. Bond has suggested, however, that although beta-blockers would not replace the need for emergency inhalers for acute episodes, the negative effects associated with beta-blockers eventually taper off to provide long-term relief from asthma symptoms. In addition, several studies have shown chronic use of the beta-2 agonists (or stimulants) can negatively affect asthma control and airway hyperresponsiveness by desensitizing the beta-2 adrenoreceptor through regular stimulation.

In this latest study, the research team was unable to trigger the development of asthma-like symptoms in a mouse model in which the beta-2 adrenoreceptor gene had been removed as compared to the mouse model with the intact receptor gene.

"The study indicates that, with regard to developing asthma-like features, the mouse is better off without the beta-2 adrenoreceptor at all," Bond said. "It means that whether we block receptor signaling pharmacologically by using beta blockers or genetically by 'removing' the receptor, we get the same answer. The research shows that blocking or inhibiting the receptor with antagonists, instead of stimulating it with agonists, reduces the asthma-like features of the mouse model."

Bond's co-authors come from a multi-institutional research team that include current University of Houston (UH) pharmacology graduate student Long P. Nguyen; UH pharmacology Ph.D. graduate Rui Lin; former UH post-doc fellow Sergio Parra; UH biology graduate student Ozozoma Omoluabi; Baylor College of Medicine's Dr. Nicola A. Hanania; M.D. Anderson Cancer Center's Michael J. Tuvim and Dr. Burton F. Dickey; and fellow UH College of Pharmacology faculty researcher Brian J. Knoll.

With support from the Strategic Program for Asthma Research of the American Asthma Foundation, a second human clinical trial based on Bond's research is under way using the beta-blocker drug nadolol in patients with mild asthma. In the first clinical trial, sponsored by

San Francisco-based Inverseon Inc., eight of ten patients had less airway hyperresponsiveness on beta-blocker therapy at the end of the trial, although some did experience an initial negative response.

Commenting on the results of the first clinical trial, two United Kingdom researchers wrote in the January 10, 2009, issue of the British journal *The Lancet* that the use of beta-blocker therapy for asthma warrants serious, but careful, consideration and further investigation, including the use of specific alternative types of beta blockers.

To those ends, Inverseon, of which Bond is scientific founder, has filed U.S. patent applications for using beta-blockers to treat airway disease. Dr. William Garner, chairman of Inverseon, said the company recently received a notice of allowance—one of several procedural steps on the path to patent approval—from the U.S. Patent Office.

"The comment in *The Lancet* on Inverseon's human asthma study, combined with the notice of allowance from the U.S. Patent Office, represents important external validation of Inverseon's approach to asthma," Garner said. "We believe that our oral therapy has the potential to be a significant product for the chronic treatment of asthma."

Section 20.2

Bronchial Thermoplasty

On April 27, 2010, the U.S. Food and Drug Administration (FDA) approved the first medical device that uses heat, produced by radio-frequency energy, to treat severe asthma. The Alair Bronchial Thermoplasty System is intended for patients eighteen and older whose severe and persistent asthma is not well controlled with inhaled corticosteroids and long-acting beta-agonist medications.

The FDA based its approval on data from a clinical trial of 297 patients. The trial showed a reduction of severe asthma attacks after treatment. The University of Chicago Medical Center was one of about thirty centers around the world, and the only one in Illinois, that participated in the Asthma Interventional Research 2 (AIR2) clinical trial.

"The approval of the Alair system provides adult patients suffering from severe and persistent asthma with an additional treatment option for a disease that is often difficult to manage," said Jeffrey Shuren, MD, JD, director of the FDA's Center for Devices and Radiological Health.

The FDA is requiring a five-year post-approval study of the device to study its long-term safety and effectiveness. The device manufacturer, Asthmatx, will follow many of the patients who participated in the initial trial and enroll three hundred new patients at several medical centers across the United States.

The study found that this treatment, known as "bronchial thermoplasty," improved asthma-specific quality of life when assessed at six, nine, and twelve months after therapy. Although 6 percent more treated patients than controls were hospitalized for complications soon after treatment, the treated group over the first year had 32 percent fewer severe asthma exacerbations, an 84 percent decrease in emergency room visits, and 66 percent fewer days missed from work.

Although the Alair system is designed to reduce severe asthma attacks on a long-term basis, there is a risk of asthma attacks during the course of the treatment. Possible side effects during this period may also include wheezing, chest tightness or pain, partially collapsed lung, coughing up blood, anxiety, headaches, and nausea.

The short-term risks, however, were "outweighed by the benefits that persist for at least a year," said pulmonologist Kyle Hogarth, MD, assistant professor of medicine at the University of Chicago and a member of the AIR2 study group.

Bronchial thermoplasty is designed to prevent the airway constriction that is a hallmark of asthma by eliminating some of the smooth muscle that surrounds the breathing passages. When irritated or inflamed, this airway smooth muscle contracts, narrowing the breathing passages. This causes wheezing and reduced breathing capacity that can be severe and even life threatening.

Prior to the AIR2 trial, fewer than one hundred patients have ever been treated with bronchial thermoplasty, and none in the United States. In a Canadian trial involving sixteen asthma patients, the procedure improved average air-flow rates in and out of the lungs, even when tested two years after treatment. About 75 percent of those treated reported that they were "less limited" in their daily activities one to three years after therapy.

"This is an entirely novel and quite exciting approach to treating asthma, unlike anything else available," said pulmonologist Imre Noth, MD, associate professor of medicine and co-director of the study at the University of Chicago.

In bronchial thermoplasty, physicians insert a thin, flexible tube through the nose or mouth, down the throat, and into the major airways of the lungs. Then they pass a narrow catheter, with a small expandable heat source at the tip, through that tube.

Once the catheter is in position it is expanded to hold it snugly in place and heated, using radiofrequency energy, to about 150 degrees Fahrenheit—a little cooler than a cup of hot coffee—for ten seconds. This kills about half of the smooth muscle cells that line that segment of the airway. Then the catheter is slightly repositioned and reheated.

This routine is repeated about thirty times, until all the accessible airways from one lobe of the lung have been treated, a process that takes about thirty to forty-five minutes.

Patients in this study were given three separate thermoplasty procedures, with at least three weeks between sessions. Each procedure treated the small- to medium-size airways, those at least 3 mm in diameter, in a different part of the lung.

The smooth muscle that lines the human airway "is a lot like the appendix, it serves no known purpose," Noth said, "other than to cause serious medical problems." There is no disease or deficit caused by the loss of airway smooth muscle.

In people with asthma, however, this vestigial tissue can become hypersensitive, responding vigorously to all sorts of stimuli, gaining size and strength over time and contracting when irritated. It is these contractions that narrow the airway and restrict breathing for patients with asthma.

Although there are many different triggers, an acute asthma attack is always characterized by contraction of the smooth muscle in the airway wall. Fortunately, smooth muscle is uniquely heat sensitive. It can be eliminated without lasting damage to the epithelial cell layers that line the inner surface of the airways. After thermoplasty, epithelial regrowth is quick and complete. The smooth muscle at the treatment site is replaced by loose connective tissue.

According to asthma specialist Alan Leff, MD, professor of medicine at the University of Chicago, who worked as a paid consultant to Asthmatx on development of this instrument over an eight-year period: "The compelling use of this procedure is for patients who are inadequately controlled on current drug therapy. But if this therapy lives up to its early promise, bronchial thermoplasty may eventually have a very broad application."

The AIR2 clinical trial enrolled nearly three hundred patients with persistent asthma. Participants were nonsmokers, between eighteen and sixty-five years of age, who were willing to commit to fourteen clinic visits over a period of fourteen months, with annual follow-up visits for the next four years.

Patients kept a daily diary of symptoms, medication use, and morning and evening expiratory flow rates. They filled out questionnaires and went through a series of medical tests, including lung function tests, x-rays, computed tomography (CT) scan, heart tests, and three separate bronchoscopic procedures.

Only two out of three participants were treated with bronchial thermoplasty. The other third, selected at random, received "sham" treatments—bronchoscopies, but without heat treatment of the airways. The patients and the study's data collectors did not know who received thermoplasty or who received only the sham treatment.

The long-term risks associated with thermoplasty are not yet fully known. Patients in the AIR2 trial will be followed for five years.

The Alair system is not for use in asthma patients with a pacemaker, internal defibrillator, or other implantable electronic device. Patients with known sensitivities to lidocaine, atropine, or benzodiazepines should not use the device. Alair has not been studied for success in retreatment of the same area of the lung. Currently, patients should not be retreated with the Alair system in the same area of the lung.

Asthma patients considering the Alair system should not be treated while the following conditions are present: an active respiratory infection, coagulopathy (bleeding disorder), asthma exacerbations, or if they have had changes to their corticosteroid regimen fourteen days before the proposed treatment.

The study was sponsored by Asthmatx, Inc., of Sunnyvale, California, which makes the treatment device.

Section 20.3

Folic Acid for the Treatment of Asthma

"Folic Acid May Help Treat Allergies, Asthma," April 30, 2009
© Johns Hopkins Children's Center (www.hopkinschildrens.org).
Reprinted with permission.

Folic acid, or vitamin B9, essential for red blood cell health and long known to reduce the risk of spinal birth defects, may also suppress allergic reactions and lessen the severity of allergy and asthma symptoms, according to new research from the Johns Hopkins Children's Center.

In what is believed to be the first study in humans examining the link between blood levels of folate—the naturally occurring form of folic acid—and allergies, the scientists say results add to mounting evidence that folate can help regulate inflammation. Recent studies, including research from Johns Hopkins, have found a link between folate levels and inflammation-mediated diseases, including heart disease. A report on the Johns Hopkins Children's findings appears online ahead of print in the *Journal of Allergy & Clinical Immunology*.

Cautioning that it's far too soon to recommend folic acid supplements to prevent or treat people with asthma and allergies, the researchers emphasize that more research needs to be done to confirm their results, and to establish safe doses and risks.

Reviewing the medical records of more than eight thousand people ages two to eighty-five, the investigators tracked the effect of folate levels on respiratory and allergic symptoms and on levels of immunoglobulin

E (IgE) antibodies, immune system markers that rise in response to an allergen. People with higher blood levels of folate had fewer IgE antibodies, fewer reported allergies, less wheezing, and lower likelihood of asthma, researchers report.

"Our findings are a clear indication that folic acid may indeed help regulate immune response to allergens, and may reduce allergy and asthma symptoms," says lead investigator Elizabeth Matsui, M.D., M.H.S., pediatric allergist at Johns Hopkins Children's. "But we still need to figure out the exact mechanism behind it, and to do so we need studies that follow people receiving treatment with folic acid, before we even consider supplementation with folic acid to treat or prevent allergies and asthma."

The current recommendation for daily dietary intake of folic acid is 400 micrograms for healthy men and nonpregnant women. Many cereals and grain products are already fortified with folate, and folate is found naturally in green, leafy vegetables, beans, and nuts.

Other findings of the study:

- People with the lowest folate levels (below 8 nanograms [ng] per milliliter [ml]) had 40 percent higher risk of wheezing than people with the highest folate levels (above 18 ng/ml).

- People with the lowest folate levels had a 30 percent higher risk than those with the highest folate levels of having elevated IgE antibodies, markers of allergy predisposition.

- Those with the lowest folate levels had 31 percent higher risk of atopy (allergic symptoms) than people with the highest folate levels.

- Those with the lowest folate levels had 16 percent higher risk of having asthma than people with the highest folate levels.

Blacks and Hispanics had lower blood folate levels—12 and 12.5 nanograms per milliliter, respectively—than whites (15 ng/ml), but the differences were not due to income and socioeconomic status.

The Johns Hopkins team is planning a study comparing the effects of folic acid and placebo in people with allergies and asthma.

Asthma affects more than 7 percent of adults and children in the United States, and is the most common chronic condition among children, according to the Centers for Disease Control and Prevention (CDC). Environmental allergies are estimated to affect twenty-five million Americans, according to the CDC.

Co-investigator on the study: William Matsui, M.D, of the Johns Hopkins Kimmel Cancer Center.

The research was funded by the National Institutes of Health.

Section 20.4

Tiotropium Bromide Possible Alternate Therapy for Asthma

Excerpted from "Possible Alternate Therapy for Adults with Poorly Controlled Asthma," NIH News, National Institute of Health, September 19, 2010.

A drug commonly used for the treatment of chronic obstructive pulmonary disease (COPD) successfully treats adults whose asthma is not well controlled on low doses of inhaled corticosteroids, reported researchers supported by the National Heart, Lung, and Blood Institute (NHLBI), part of the National Institutes of Health.

"This study's results show that tiotropium bromide might provide an alternative to other asthma treatments, expanding options available to patients for controlling their asthma," said NHLBI Acting Director Susan B. Shurin, M.D. "The goal in managing asthma is to prevent symptoms so patients can pursue activities to the fullest."

According to the study, adding tiotropium bromide to low doses of inhaled corticosteroids is more effective at controlling asthma than doubling inhaled corticosteroids alone, and as effective as adding the long-acting beta agonist salmeterol. The results were published online on September 19, 2010 in the *New England Journal of Medicine* and presented at the Annual Congress of the European Respiratory Society in Barcelona, Spain.

Increasing inhaled corticosteroids or supplementing them with long-acting beta agonists like salmeterol are the two preferred treatment options available for adults whose asthma is poorly controlled on low doses of inhaled corticosteroids. However, higher doses of corticosteroids do not improve symptoms for all patients and can have significant side effects, while long-acting beta agonists have come under scrutiny for their risk of worsening asthma symptoms that could result in hospitalization and, rarely, death.

"Tiotropium relaxes smooth muscle in the airways through a different mechanism than beta agonists, and thus may help people who do not respond well to currently recommended treatments," said study lead Stephen Peters, M.D., Ph.D., of Wake Forest University Baptist Medical Center, Winston-Salem, North Carolina. "Further analysis of the study data will help us better understand which patients respond best to tiotropium. Then we will need to conduct longer-term studies to establish its safety for asthma patients and to determine its effect on the frequency and severity of asthma exacerbations."

Conducted by the NHLBI's Asthma Clinical Research Network, the study compared three treatment methods: doubling the dose of inhaled corticosteroids alone, supplementing a low dose of inhaled corticosteroids with a long-acting beta agonist (salmeterol), and supplementing a low dose of inhaled corticosteroids with a long-acting anticholinergic drug (tiotropium bromide). Anticholinergics block a part of the autonomic nervous system that can cause airway muscles to contract. The study followed 210 adults whose asthma was not well controlled on low doses of inhaled corticosteroids alone. Participants received each treatment for fourteen weeks with two-week breaks in between, for a total of forty-eight weeks.

Tiotropium bromide was shown to be effective using several asthma control measurements, including patients' day-to-day lung function as well as the number of days in which they had no asthma symptoms and did not need to use their albuterol rescue inhalers. When patients began the trial, their average number of such "asthma control days" was seventy-seven per year (extrapolated from the treatment period). Doubling corticosteroids gave patients another nineteen symptom-free days on average, while adding tiotropium to low-dose corticosteroids gave them another forty-eight.

"Much research over the last century has explored the role of cholinergic mechanisms [which constrict the airways] and anticholinergic therapies in asthma. However, this is the first study to explore adding an anticholinergic inhaler to low-dose inhaled corticosteroids," said James Kiley, Ph.D., director of the NHLBI's Division of Lung Diseases. "The Asthma Clinical Research Network is designed to address exactly these kinds of practical and important management questions, with the ultimate goal of helping asthma patients."

Chapter 21

Ongoing Asthma-Related Clinical Trials

Clinical trials are research studies. They may be used to answer questions about new ways of treating or preventing asthma attacks. Clinical trials may also be used to answer other questions about caring for people with asthma. Questions that a clinical trial may answer include:

- Does a drug prevent or treat asthma?

- Is a new test helpful in monitoring people with asthma?

- Does a drug cause problems when it is taken over a long period of time?

Clinical trials are run by doctors and nurses who use a set of rules called a protocol. The protocol explains exactly how the trial will be run and who will enroll. To be in an asthma clinical trial:

- You must have asthma or be at risk for it.

- You must be able to take the treatment that is being studied, if treatment is part of the study.

- You must be able to follow the study rules.

Before you enter the study, the medical team will make sure that you can take part. They may ask you questions about your health, give you a physical exam, and draw some blood or perform other medical tests.

"Clinical Trials," reprinted with permission from www.getasthmahelp.org, the website of the Asthma Initiative of Michigan, © 2010.

There are laws that protect the rights of people in clinical trials. One of these laws requires study doctors and nurses to enroll patients only after they have given informed consent. This means that the study doctors and nurses must tell you everything that would affect whether or not you would want to be in the trial. Also, before you enter the trial, they must have your agreement in writing that you have been given this information and that you are willing to take part in the study.

After you enter the trial, you will need to attend regularly scheduled study visits. If you are taking a drug as part of the study, the doctor or nurse will check you for side effects and signs of whether the drug is working. Studies that do not involve drugs also require regular visits. Some studies can last several years.

If you decide that you no longer want to take a study treatment or take part in other study activities, you can stop at any time. Just be sure that your doctor knows about your decision. If a study treatment is not working for you or if it causes harmful side effects, your doctor will stop your treatment. If you stop a study treatment or taking part in other study activities, you will still be in the study, and you will be asked to keep attending your scheduled visits until the study ends. Of course, you are free to withdraw from the study at any time. If you get sick from taking a study drug, the people running the trial will make sure that you are able to get treatment if you need it.

If you are thinking about taking part in a clinical trial, you should not hesitate to ask your doctor or nurse questions. Here are some examples of questions you may want to ask:

- What are the side effects of the study drug?
- Are there any drugs, food, etc., that I should not take while I am taking the study drug?
- Has the study drug been used before?
- Will a placebo be used in the study?
- What other treatment choices do I have?
- How long will the study last?
- Will I be given travel money for this study?
- How will my part in the study be kept secret?
- Who will provide my medical care after the study is over?
- Who do I call if I have more questions?

Part Four

Living with Asthma

Chapter 22

Working with Your Doctor

Chapter Contents

Section 22.1

Choosing an Asthma Doctor

Reprinted with permission from the Asthma and Allergy
Foundation of America, www.aafa.org, © 2005. All rights reserved.
Reviewed by David A. Cooke, M.D., FACP, May 2011.

Pediatricians, general practitioners, internists, allergists, and pulmonologists can all treat asthma and allergies.

Allergists or immunologists are internists and pediatricians who have additional training in the immune system and special skills in evaluating and treating asthma and allergies.

They become board certified when they pass an examination in the specialty area of allergy and immunology. Because allergists tend to see more allergic and asthmatic people than other kinds of doctors, they are more experienced in treating them.

This is especially important because about 90 percent of children and 50 percent of adults with asthma have allergies that trigger asthma symptoms. Identifying and learning to control these allergies can be the key to better asthma control.

Your primary care physician may refer you to an allergist to test you for allergies and to get your asthma under better control. Once your asthma and allergies are better controlled, you can expect to visit your allergist less often as he or she works with your primary care physician to keep your asthma in check.

What can I expect from my asthma and allergy treatment?

If you are carefully following your doctor's instructions and you are still experiencing the following problems, you may need to seek a second opinion.

With proper medical treatment, your asthma and allergy symptoms should not:

- interfere with daily activities;

- wake you up at night;

- cause you to miss school or work;

- cause you to wheeze during strenuous physical activities;

- send you to the emergency room.

How can I find a professionally trained allergist?

You can start by looking in the white pages of your phone book for your local medical society. They are usually listed as (city name) Medical Society.

You can also look in the Yellow Pages of your phone book under Physicians. The physicians will be listed under their specialty area, such as "Allergy & Immunology." Choose an allergist that is "board certified."

Section 22.2

Your Asthma Healthcare Team

"Your Healthcare Team," reprinted with permission from the Asthma Society of Canada, © 2011. All rights reserved. For additional information, please visit http://www.asthma.ca.

Asthma is a variable condition. In other words, it can vary over time, under different circumstances, and for different individuals. Because of this, your doctor will create a customized treatment plan that fits your particular needs, lifestyle, and triggers, as well as the frequency and intensity of your symptoms.

This plan may include referrals to other healthcare professionals—individuals who can help you with specific aspects of asthma treatment and management.

Family Doctor

Your family doctor is an essential part of your healthcare team. He or she is familiar not just with how asthma affects you, but also with your medical history and overall state of health.

Under certain circumstances, your doctor may refer you to a specialist. If, for example, your asthma is associated with allergies, you might be referred to an allergist. If you need help learning how to manage your asthma, you may be referred to an asthma educator. If you have difficulty managing asthma, you may be referred to a respirologist.

Whatever course of action of your doctor decides on, he or she will monitor the outcomes of your referrals. That way, you and your doctor can keep "the big picture" in mind while determining how well all the elements of your asthma management are working.

Certified Asthma Educator

A certified asthma educator (CAE) is a healthcare professional, usually a respiratory therapist, nurse, or pharmacist, who has completed a special asthma education program that includes written exams.

If you are unable to locate a CAE in your community, call your local hospital and ask to speak with a respiratory therapist. He or she will watch your inhaler technique and give you tips on how to best manage your asthma.

You can find CAEs in doctors' offices, hospitals, clinics, pharmacies, and pharmaceutical companies. Their training allows them to create personalized education and lifestyle-modification programs for individuals with asthma.

Registered Respiratory Therapist (RRT) or Registered Respiratory Care Practitioner (RRCP)

A registered respiratory therapist (RRT/RRCP) has been specially trained to treat people who have problems breathing. If an asthma episode requires you to go to a hospital, an RRT/RRCP may be among the team of professionals helping you there. He or she can assist in stabilizing a person who's having an asthma attack, administer inhaled medications, and conduct lung-function tests. RRT/RRCPs also provide training and education to people with asthma.

Respiratory Nurse

A respiratory nurse is a nurse who has undergone additional training in pulmonary (lung) health. Respiratory nurses can be found in doctors' offices, hospitals, clinics, and health departments, assist in the treatment of people with asthma, and also provide training and education.

Pharmacist

A pharmacist is a great source of information and education for anyone. If you have concerns about medication you've been prescribed, your local pharmacist is generally easier to reach than your family doctor, and is always happy to answer questions. He or she can also demonstrate the correct techniques for using inhaler medicines and check your own techniques to make sure you're taking them correctly.

Respirologist

A respirologist is a medical doctor who specializes in the study of lung diseases and related conditions such as asthma and chronic obstructive lung disease.

Allergist

An allergist is a medical doctor who has specialized in the study of allergies and the conditions associated with them, including asthma.

If you have been referred to an allergist, he or she will probably administer a series of tests to determine exactly what substances or conditions you're allergic to. Once those allergens have been identified, your allergist can recommend specific treatments for your symptoms, and advise you on how best to avoid allergens in your day-to-day life.

Section 22.3

How to Work with Your Healthcare Professional

"Working with Your Health Care Professional," reprinted with
permission from www.getasthmahelp.org, the website of the
Asthma Initiative of Michigan, © 2010.

You do not need to accept having asthma symptoms as being normal.
If you are having asthma symptoms, you and your doctor or asthma
educator can work together to find ways to improve your health. But
how do you make sure that you are getting the best care? Follow these
tips to get the most out of your doctor or asthma educator visits.

Learn

Find out what triggers your asthma and what you need to do to stay
healthy. In fact, everyone in your family needs to know what triggers
your asthma and what they can do if you need help. Learn all you can
about the medications you take. Know what to do for asthma attacks.

What You Should Expect from Your Asthma Management Program

Think about the goals you have for your breathing health. Below
is a list of what some of those goals could be:

- Have an Asthma Action Plan
- No symptoms or minor symptoms of asthma, such as wheezing, coughing, shortness of breath, or chest tightness
- Sleeping through the night without asthma symptoms
- No time off from school or work due to asthma
- Full participation in physical activities
- No emergency room visits or stays in the hospital
- Few or no side effects from asthma medications

Ask Questions

Make a list of all of the goals that are not being met, and ask questions about how you can improve.

Between visits to your healthcare professional, write down all of your questions so that you can bring up all of your concerns at the next visit.

Give Information

Tell your doctor or asthma educator what your symptoms have been since your last visit. Be honest and as detailed as possible. Provide peak flow meter readings, if you have them. Talk about how and when you take your medicines. Talk about problems or concerns you have about your medicines. Use the checklist of treatment goals (above) to talk about how all of your goals can be met.

State What You Expect at Each Visit

Tell your doctor or asthma educator what you want from the visit. You may simply want some questions answered, or maybe you might want to go over your current medications to see if you need a change. You may want to review and update your Asthma Action Plan. Try to be positive—this will help both you and your healthcare professional keep an open mind and improve how you relate to each other.

Follow Directions

Make an Asthma Action Plan with your healthcare professional and demonstrate back what the doctor wants you to do. This helps you to be sure that you know what you are supposed to do. Don't agree to do something that you do not plan to do. Unless your doctor is told that a treatment plan is hard for you, he or she will not know to make changes. If you are confused, ask the doctor to say the information in another way. Take your medicine as your doctor tells you.

Know When to See Your Doctor or Asthma Educator

You should see your doctor at least twice a year for your asthma, even if you are feeling good. These visits will help both of you to keep track of your asthma and make changes in your Asthma Action Plan as needed. Ask your doctor or asthma educator for guidelines about when you need to call or come in between these regular visits. Here is a sample set of guidelines the doctor may want you to follow.

You should follow your Asthma Action Plan and see the doctor as soon as possible if:

- your asthma symptoms seem worse than usual or happen more often;

- you are taking your medicine more often to relieve the symptoms of asthma;

- a medicine does not seem to be working, or is making you feel worse.

You should get help right away if:

- your asthma keeps getting worse even after taking your medicine and following your action plan;

- your peak flow reading falls into the red zone;

- your lips or fingernails turn blue;

- your breathing is rapid and you can talk only in single words.

Keep Your Doctor's Visit

Have a way to remind yourself to keep your doctor's visit. Put a note on the refrigerator, your dresser, or some other place. If you cannot keep your visit, call and change it. With time, you and your doctor will find the treatment that works best for you. Remember asthma symptoms can change over time. It's important to see your doctor or asthma educator at least twice every year for your routine asthma care (this doesn't include visits to the doctor when your asthma is not in control).

Section 22.4

What to Ask the Doctor

Excerpted from "Asthma: What to Ask the Doctor—Adult,"
© 2011 A.D.A.M., Inc. Reprinted with permission.

Asthma is a problem with the airways that bring oxygen to your lungs. A person with asthma may not feel symptoms all the time. But when an asthma attack happens, it becomes hard for air to pass through your airways. The symptoms are coughing, wheezing, chest tightness, or shortness of breath.

Below are some questions you may want to ask your doctor or nurse to help you take care of your asthma.

- Am I taking my asthma medicines the right way?

  - What drugs should I be taking every day (called controller drugs)? What should I do if I miss a day?

  - Which drugs should I take when I am short of breath (called rescue drugs)? Is it okay to use these rescue drugs every day?

  - What are the side effects of my medicines? For what side effects should I call the doctor?

  - How will I know when my inhalers are getting empty? Am I using my inhaler the right way? Should I be using a spacer?

- What are some signs that my asthma is getting worse and that I need to call the doctor? What should I do when I feel short of breath?

- What shots or vaccinations do I need?

- What will make my asthma worse?

  - How can I prevent getting a lung infection?

  - How can I get help quitting smoking?

  - How do I find out when smog or pollution is worse?

- What sort of changes should I make around my home?
  - Can I have a pet? In the house or outside? How about in the bedroom?
  - Is it okay for me to clean and vacuum in the house?
  - Is it okay to have carpets in the house?
  - What type of furniture is best to have?
  - How do I get rid of dust and mold in the house? Do I need to cover my bed or pillows?
  - How do I know if I have cockroaches in my home? How do I get rid of them?
  - Can I have a fire in my fireplace or wood-burning stove?
- What sort of changes do I need to make at work?
- What exercises are better for me to do?
  - Are there times when I should avoid being outside and exercising?
  - Are there things that I can do before I start exercising?
- Do I need tests or treatments for allergies? What should I do when I know I'm going to be around something that triggers my asthma?
- What type of arrangements do I need to make when I am planning to travel?
  - What drugs should I bring? How do I get refills?
  - Whom should I call if my asthma gets worse?

Chapter 23

How to Monitor Your Asthma

Chapter Contents

Section 23.1

Monitoring Your Symptoms

"Monitoring Symptoms," Reprinted with permission © 2011 American Lung Association. For more information about the American Lung Association or to support the work it does, call 800-LUNG-USA (800-586-4872) or log on to www.LungUSA.org.

Monitoring your symptoms is an important step in controlling your asthma. There are four key symptoms that you should monitor to help you keep your asthma under control:

- **Daytime symptoms:** How often do you have asthma symptoms during the day, such as: coughing, wheezing, chest tightness, or shortness of breath?

- **Nighttime symptoms:** Do you wake up at night with asthma symptoms, such as: coughing, wheezing, chest tightness, or shortness of breath?

- **Rescue inhaler use:** How often do you use your rescue inhaler to relieve asthma symptoms?

- **Activity level:** Do you have difficulty performing normal activities, such as: walking, climbing stairs, daily chores, or playing with the kids?

Keep a journal or diary to help you monitor your symptoms. A symptoms journal or diary can be an important communication tool to share with you healthcare provider about your asthma. Also, it can help you determine if your asthma is getting worse.

Tracking asthma symptoms is an important component to any asthma action plan.

Section 23.2

Peak Flow Monitoring

"Measuring Your Peak Flow Rate," Reprinted with permission © 2011 American Lung Association. For more information about the American Lung Association or to support the work it does, call 800-LUNG-USA (800-586-4872) or log on to www.LungUSA.org.

A peak flow meter is a portable, inexpensive, hand-held device used to measure how air flows from your lungs in one "fast blast." In other words, the meter measures your ability to push air out of your lungs.

Peak flow meters may be provided in two ranges to measure the air pushed out of your lungs. A low-range peak flow meter is for small children, and a standard-range peak flow meter is for older children, teenagers, and adults. An adult has much larger airways than a child and needs the larger range.

There are several types of peak flow meters available. Talk to your healthcare provider or pharmacist about which type to use.

Who Can Benefit from Using a Peak Flow Meter?

Many healthcare providers believe that people who have asthma can benefit from the use of a peak flow meter. If you need to adjust your daily medication for asthma, a peak flow meter can be an important part of your asthma management plan.

Patients age five and older are usually able to use a peak flow meter to help manage their asthma. In addition, some people with chronic bronchitis and emphysema may also benefit from the use of a peak flow meter.

Not all healthcare providers use peak flow meters in their management of children and adults with asthma. Many healthcare providers believe a peak flow meter may be of most help for people with moderate and severe asthma. If your asthma is mild or you do not use daily medication, a peak flow meter may not be useful for asthma management.

Why Should I Measure My Peak Flow Rate?

Your peak flow rates can show you if your asthma is getting worse, even before you feel symptoms. In addition, measurements with a peak flow meter can help your healthcare provider make decisions about your treatment and adjust your medicines as necessary.

A peak flow meter can be used as a signal of when your asthma is getting worse. Asthma sometimes changes gradually. Your peak flow may show changes before you feel them. Peak flow readings can show you when to start following the steps on your asthma action plan that you developed with your healthcare provider. It can help you determine the severity of the episode, decide when to use your rescue medicine, and decide when to seek emergency care.

A peak flow meter may help you and your healthcare provider identify causes of your asthma at work, home, or play. It may help parents to determine what might be triggering their child's asthma.

How Do You Use a Peak Flow Meter?

Step 1: Before each use, make sure the sliding marker or arrow on the peak flow meter is at the bottom of the numbered scale (zero or the lowest number on the scale).

Step 2: Stand up straight. Remove gum or any food from your mouth. Take a deep breath (as deep as you can). Put the mouthpiece of the peak flow meter into your mouth. Close your lips tightly around the mouthpiece. Be sure to keep your tongue away from the mouthpiece. In one breath, blow out as hard and as quickly as possible. Blow a "fast hard blast" rather than "slowly blowing" until you have emptied out nearly all of the air from your lungs.

Step 3: The force of the air coming out of your lungs causes the marker to move along the numbered scale. Note the number on a piece of paper.

Step 4: Repeat the entire routine three times. (You know you have done the routine correctly when the numbers from all three tries are very close together.)

Step 5: Record the highest of the three ratings. Do not calculate an average. This is very important. You can't breathe out too much when using your peak flow meter but you can breathe out too little. Record your highest reading.

Step 6: Measure your peak flow rate close to the same time each day. You and your healthcare provider can determine the best times. One suggestion is to measure your peak flow rate twice daily between 7 and 9 a.m. and between 6 and 8 p.m. You may want to measure your peak flow rate before or after using your medicine. Some people measure peak flow both before and after taking medication. Try to do it the same way each time.

Step 7: Keep a chart of your peak flow rates. Discuss the readings with your healthcare provider.

How Do I Chart My Peak Flow Rates?

Chart the *highest* of the three readings. This is called "your personal best." The chart could include the date at the top of the page with a.m. and p.m. listed. The left margin could list a scale, starting with zero (0) liters per minute (L/min) at the bottom of the page and ending with 600 L/min at the top.

You could leave room at the bottom of the page for notes to describe how you are feeling or to list any other thoughts you may have.

What Is a "Normal" Peak Flow Rate?

A "normal" peak flow rate is based on a person's age, height, sex, and race. A standardized "normal" may be obtained from a chart comparing the patient with a population without breathing problems.

A patient can figure out what is normal for them, based on their own peak flow rate. Therefore, it is important for you and your healthcare provider to discuss what is considered "normal" for you.

Once you have learned your usual and expected peak flow rate, you will be able to better recognize changes or trends in your asthma.

How Can I Determine a "Normal" Peak Flow Rate for Me?

Three zones of measurement are commonly used to interpret peak flow rates. It is easy to relate the three zones to the traffic light colors: green, yellow, and red. In general, a normal peak flow rate can vary as much as 20 percent.

Be aware of the following general guidelines. Keep in mind that recognizing changes from "normal" is important. Your healthcare provider may suggest other zones to follow.

Green zone: Eighty to 100 percent of your usual or "normal" peak flow rate signals all clear. A reading in this zone means that your asthma is under reasonably good control. It would be advisable to continue your prescribed program of management.

Yellow zone: Fifty to 80 percent of your usual or "normal" peak flow rate signals caution. It is a time for decisions. Your airways are narrowing and may require extra treatment. Your symptoms can get better or worse depending on what you do, or how and when you use your prescribed medication. You and your healthcare provider should have a plan for yellow zone readings.

Red zone: Less than 50 percent of your usual or "normal" peak flow rate signals a medical alert. Immediate decisions and actions need to be taken. Severe airway narrowing may be occurring. Take your rescue medications right away. Contact your healthcare provider now and follow the plan he has given you for red zone readings.

Some healthcare providers may suggest zones with a smaller range, such as 90 to 100 percent. Always follow your healthcare provider's suggestions about your peak flow rate.

Asthma Action Plan Based on Peak Flow Readings

It is important to know your peak flow reading, but it is even more important to know what you will do based upon that reading. Work with your healthcare provider to develop an asthma action plan that follows your green-yellow-red zone guidelines.

Record the peak flow readings that your healthcare provider recommends for your green zone, yellow zone, and red zone. Then work out with your healthcare provider what you plan to do when your peak flow falls in each of those zones.

When Should I Use My Peak Flow Meter?

Use of the peak flow meter depends on a number of things. Its use should be discussed with your healthcare provider.

If your asthma is well controlled and you know the "normal" rate for you, you may decide to measure your peak flow rate only when you sense that your asthma is getting worse. More severe asthma may require several measurements daily.

Don't forget that your peak flow meter needs care and cleaning. Dirt collected in the meter may make your peak flow measurements inaccurate. If you have a cold or other respiratory infection, germs or mucus may also collect in the meter.

Proper cleaning with mild detergent in hot water will keep your peak flow meter working accurately and may keep you healthier.

Section 23.3

Keeping a Daily Asthma Diary

By monitoring symptoms and practicing self-management, people who have asthma can control their asthma symptoms. An important part of learning to control asthma is keeping a daily asthma diary. The asthma diary is used to:

- record daily peak expiratory flow (PEF) readings and asthma symptoms;

- compare PEF readings and symptoms with asthma zones; and

- keep track of how often rescue medications are used.

Recording this information will help you become aware of early signs of asthma episodes. Your doctor will also use this diary to evaluate how well your or your child's treatment plan is working.

How to Keep a Daily Asthma Diary

First, record your peak flows in the appropriate asthma zone so that you can refer to them easily.

Green zone: Asthma is well controlled. There are no asthma symptoms. You (or your child) can complete regular activities and sleep without coughing, wheezing, or difficulty breathing. PEF is 80 to 100 percent of personal best.

My green zone is _____ to _____.

Yellow zone: A flare-up, or asthma is poorly controlled. Cough, wheeze, shortness of breath, or chest tightness may be present. PEF is 50 to 80 percent of personal best.

My yellow zone is _____ to _____.

Red zone: A severe flare-up or medical emergency. Symptoms are: frequent cough, severe shortness of breath, trouble talking, rapid breathing, wheezing, and difficulty sleeping. Start emergency asthma medication immediately and call your asthma care provider. If there is no change after starting the medication, go to the emergency room.

My red zone is _____.

To complete the diary:

- Fill in the date each day.

- Fill in your or your child's PEF reading using the peak flow meter. Measure PEF before taking asthma medications.

- Compare your PEF readings to the asthma zones listed above. Follow instructions on the asthma action plan.

- Fill in the amount of rescue medication (metered dose inhaler [MDI], dry powder inhaler [DPI], or nebulizer) used over the past twenty-four hours.

- Rate any asthma symptoms you or your child had during the day.

- Remember to take your asthma daily diary with you to appointments with your doctor or healthcare provider so they can review it with you.

Date	PEF Readings AM	PEF Readings PM	No. of Puffs of Rescue MDI/DPI	Cough	Wheeze	Shortness of Breath	Chest Tightness

Form 23.1. Asthma Diary. For cough, none = 0; occasional = 1; frequent = 2; continuous = 3. For wheeze, shortness of breath, and chest tightness, none = 0; some = 1; medium = 2; severe = 3.

Chapter 24

Asthma Action Plan

If you have asthma, it is recommended that you have a plan developed between you and your healthcare provider that gives specific instructions for early treatment of asthma symptoms. An asthma action plan is a written, individualized worksheet that shows you the steps to take to prevent your asthma from getting worse. It also provides guidance on when to call your healthcare provider or when to go to the emergency room right away.

General Information

You asthma action plan should include:

- your name;

- emergency contact information;

- contact information for your healthcare provider;

- your asthma severity classification;

- a list of triggers that may cause an asthma attack.

Asthma Zones

An asthma action plan is divided into three zones (green, yellow, and red). The green zone is where you want to be on a daily basis. In this zone, you have no asthma symptoms and you feel good. Continue to take your long-term control medicine(s) even if you're feeling well. The yellow zone means that you are experiencing symptoms. This is where you should slow down and follow the steps including the use of your quick-relief medicine to keep your asthma from getting worse. And, the red zone means you are experiencing severe asthma symptoms or an asthma flare-up. Follow the steps of your asthma action plan and get immediate medical treatment if your symptoms do not improve.

You should work with your healthcare provider to determine your zones. Your asthma action plan can be based on peak flow rate or asthma symptoms.

Peak flow rate: Peak flow monitoring is recommended for people with moderate to severe asthma. Your peak flow rate can show if your asthma is getting worse, even before you feel symptoms. Your peak flow rate is measured with a peak flow meter. To use your peak flow rate to determine the zones on your asthma action plan, first, you will need to spend some time determining your personal best. Your personal best is the highest peak flow number you achieve in a two- to three-week period. Your healthcare provider will use your personal best peak flow rate to calculate the zones in your asthma action plan.

Symptoms: Another way to monitor your asthma control is to track your symptoms. Common asthma symptoms that indicate there is a problem include:

- daytime symptoms (cough, wheeze, or chest tightness);
- problems with activity level (working, exercising, or playing);
- nighttime symptoms.

Medicines

Your asthma action plan will include your medicines and instructions for what to do when you are feeling well, what to do when you have asthma symptoms, and what to do when your asthma symptoms are getting worse. It should include the names of your medicines, how much to take, and when to take it. The dose and frequency may change depending on your asthma zone.

Asthma Action Plan

Asthma Action Plan

✚ **AMERICAN LUNG ASSOCIATION.**

General Information:

- Name _____
- Emergency contact _____ Phone numbers _____
- Physician/healthcare provider _____ Phone numbers _____
- Physician signature _____ Date _____

Severity Classification	Triggers	Exercise
○ Intermittent ○ Moderate Persistent ○ Mild Persistent ○ Severe Persistent	○ Colds ○ Smoke ○ Weather ○ Exercise ○ Dust ○ Air Pollution ○ Animals ○ Food ○ Other _____	1. Premedication (how much and when) _____ _____ 2. Exercise modifications _____ _____

Green Zone: Doing Well | **Peak Flow Meter Personal Best =** _____

Symptoms

- Breathing is good
- No cough or wheeze
- Can work and play
- Sleeps well at night

Peak Flow Meter

More than 80% of personal best or _____

Control Medications:

Medicine	How Much to Take	When to Take It
_____	_____	_____
_____	_____	_____
_____	_____	_____

Yellow Zone: Getting Worse

Contact physician if using quick relief more than 2 times per week.

Symptoms

- Some problems breathing
- Cough, wheeze, or chest tight
- Problems working or playing
- Wake at night

Peak Flow Meter

Between 50% and 80% of personal best or _____ to _____

Continue control medicines and add:

Medicine	How Much to Take	When to Take It
_____	_____	_____
_____	_____	_____

IF your symptoms (and peak flow, if used) return to Green Zone after one hour of the quick-relief treatment, THEN

- ○ Take quick-relief medication every 4 hours for 1 to 2 days.
- ○ Change your long-term control medicine by _____
- ○ Contact your physician for follow-up care.

IF your symptoms (and peak flow, if used) DO NOT return to Green Zone after one hour of the quick-relief treatment, THEN

- ○ Take quick-relief treatment again.
- ○ Change your long-term control medicine by _____
- ○ Call your physician/Healthcare provider within _____ hour(s) of modifying your medication routine.

Red Zone: Medical Alert

Ambulance/Emergency Phone Number: _____

Symptoms

- Lots of problems breathing
- Cannot work or play
- Getting worse instead of better
- Medicine is not helping

Peak Flow Meter

Less than 50% of personal best or _____ to _____

Continue control medicines and add:

Medicine	How Much to Take	When to Take It
_____	_____	_____
_____	_____	_____
_____	_____	_____

Go to the hospital or call for an ambulance if:

- ○ Still in the red zone after 15 minutes.
- ○ You have not been able to reach your physician/healthcare provider for help.
- ○ _____

Call an ambulance immediately if the following danger signs are present:

- ○ Trouble walking/talking due to shortness of breath.
- ○ Lips or fingernails are blue.

Rev_July_2008

Figure 24.1. *Asthma Action Plan*

What to Do in an Emergency

The Red Zone of your asthma action plan tells you the steps you need to take in an emergency situation. This portion of your plan should include: emergency telephone numbers for the doctor, emergency department, rapid transportation, and family/friends for support.

Long-Term Control Medicines/Quick-Relief Medicines: What You Need to Know

Long-term control medicines (also called controller, maintenance, or anti-inflammatory medicines) help prevent asthma symptoms by controlling the swelling in your lungs and decreasing mucus production. These medicines work slowly but help control your asthma for hours. They must be taken regularly (even when you don't have asthma symptoms) in order to work.

Quick-relief medicines (also called rescue medicines) relieve or stop asthma symptoms once they have started. They are inhaled and work quickly to relax the muscles that tighten around your airways. When the muscles relax, your airways open up and you breathe easier. Quick-relief medicines can be used before you exercise to avoid asthma symptoms.

Chapter 25

Minimizing Indoor Asthma Triggers

Chapter Contents

Section 25.1

What Are Indoor Asthma Triggers?

Excerpted from "Indoor Environmental Asthma Triggers,"
U.S. Environmental Protection Agency, October 5, 2010.

Americans spend up to 90 percent of their time indoors. Therefore, indoor allergens and irritants can play a significant role in triggering asthma attacks. It is important to recognize potential asthma triggers in the indoor environment and reduce your exposure to those triggers. You may not be affected by all of the triggers listed here. Your doctor can help you to determine which triggers affect your asthma and develop a specific plan to reduce your triggers.

Indoor environmental asthma triggers:

- Secondhand smoke
- Dust Mites
- Molds
- Cockroaches and pests
- Pets
- Nitrogen dioxide
- Outdoor air

When you and your doctor make the plan, be sure to include the following:

- You or your child's asthma triggers
- Instructions for asthma medicines
- What to do if you or your child has an asthma attack
- When to call your doctor
- Emergency telephone numbers

Some of the most common indoor asthma triggers include secondhand smoke, dust mites, mold, cockroaches and other pests, household pets, and combustion byproducts.

Secondhand Smoke

Secondhand smoke is a mixture of smoke from the burning end of a cigarette, pipe, or cigar and the smoke exhaled by the smoker that is often found in homes and cars where smoking is allowed.

Dust Mites

Dust mites are too small to be seen, but can be found in almost every home in mattresses and bedding materials, carpets, upholstered furniture, stuffed toys, and curtains.

Mold

Mold can grow indoors when mold spores land on wet or damp surfaces. In the home, mold is most commonly found in the bathroom, kitchen, and basement.

Cockroaches and Other Pests

Cockroach body parts, secretions, and droppings, and the urine, droppings, and saliva of pests, such as rodents, are often found in areas where food and water are present.

Warm-Blooded Pets (Such as Cats and Dogs)

Pets' skin flakes, urine, and saliva can be found in homes where pets are allowed inside.

Nitrogen Dioxide

Nitrogen Dioxide is a reddish-brown, irritating odor gas that can be a byproduct of indoor fuel-burning appliances, such as gas stoves, gas or oil furnaces, fireplaces, wood stoves, and unvented kerosene or gas space heaters.

Section 25.2

Dealing with Cockroaches and Other Pests

For many people the mere mention of the word "cockroach" makes one's hair stand on edge. We associate these small insects with indoor dirt and decay, and we know how hard it can be to rid one's home of an infestation of roaches once they settle in. But roaches are a fact of modern urban and suburban life. For some of us, exposure to roaches is an important cause of our asthma. For all of us, an important lesson can be learned from understanding the emerging information about the relationship between cockroach exposure and asthma.

Some people are born with the tendency to make allergic responses. Others seem to acquire the tendency along the way as they grow older. Most people with asthma have the tendency to make allergic responses in their bronchial tubes to certain things that we breath in.

This predisposition to make allergic reactions is only half the story in asthma. The other half involves exposure to those things that can elicit an allergic reaction. Certain things that we breathe in stimulate allergic responses; other things do not. Cat dander and ragweed pollen provoke allergic reactions in many people. Automobile exhaust and fog do not. To cause an allergic reaction, what we breathe needs to be of the right size and shape and composed of materials recognized by our allergic immune system.

Here's where the unloved cockroach fits into the story. It turns out that excrement and debris from decomposing cockroach bodies are of just the right size to be lifted into the air, breathed onto the bronchial tubes, and recognized by the immune system—in certain people—as a signal to make an allergic reaction. As you know, the allergic reaction in the bronchial tubes is asthma.

Recently, a major, federally funded research project looked for allergy-producing substances in the homes of several hundred children with asthma living in several major cities across the United States. Specifically, they measured the amount of cat, dust mite, and cockroach allergen in the bedrooms of these children aged four to nine years. The results were quite striking.

The most important allergen in these inner-city homes came from cockroaches. And the worst asthma was found in those children who had both the allergic tendency to make reactions to cockroach allergens and exposure to high concentrations of those cockroach allergens in their homes. Children in heavily cockroach-infested homes who did not have an allergic sensitivity to cockroaches were not as likely to have severe asthma. Similarly, children who had the tendency for allergic reactions to cockroach parts but lived in homes with a low burden of cockroach allergens were also less likely to have severe asthma. It was the combination of both the allergic tendency and the allergen exposure that put the children at the greatest risk for troublesome asthma.

The lesson to be learned here is greater than just the following: If you happen to be a person whose immune system makes allergic reactions to cockroach debris, keep your home free of cockroaches. You could just as easily substitute cats or dogs or dust mites or pollens for cockroaches in the above equation. For example, if you are a person whose immune systems happens to make allergic reactions to cat dander, having heavy exposures to cat allergens will put you at increased risk for severe asthma. It appears that any allergic predisposition combined with heavy allergic exposure to those specific things to which one is sensitive fuels the fire of bronchial inflammation that we recognize as asthma.

The lesson that we learn from the study of cockroaches in asthma is this. If your asthma is difficult to control, make an effort to determine what your allergic tendencies are. If you find that you have allergic sensitivities to things in your home or workplace, make every effort to reduce your exposure to those allergens. Although we cannot yet change our allergic tendencies, we can protect ourselves from breathing in large amounts of the substances to which we are allergic. By doing so, we can make our asthma better without taking a single prescription to be filled at the pharmacy.

Section 25.3

Minimizing Dust Mites

A common asthma trigger is the house dust mite, which has adapted to live by the tens of thousands in the dust of our houses, generally in bedding, mattresses, cushions, and soft furnishings.

What Is a House Dust Mite?

House dust mites are tiny creatures, usually not visible to the human eye—they measure about one-third of a millimeter in length. They are relatives of spiders and ticks. The house dust mite survives by eating the many dead skin cells that each of us sheds every day, along with pollen grains, insect scales, dead mites, and even their own droppings.

Our dead skin cells are a main component of household dust. If dust builds up in areas of the house where the air is a bit damp (humid), this dust is likely to contain dust mites, as they not only need food to survive, but also moist air.

High numbers of dead skin cells are shed in the bedroom, accumulating in mattresses and pillows as we sleep, making the bedroom a favored haunt of the house dust mite.

How Do House Dust Mites Affect My Asthma?

Dust mite droppings can become airborne and are so small that they can flow deep into your airways each time you take a breath. These inhaled droppings, rather than the mite itself, can then cause asthma in sensitive people by means of an allergic reaction, leading to the typical asthma symptoms of wheeze, tightness in the chest, coughing, and difficulty breathing.

Dust mite droppings are sometimes called dust mite "allergen" due to this ability to trigger an allergic reaction in some people. Often dust mite allergy also causes inflammation in the nose, called perennial (meaning persistent or year-round) allergic rhinitis, which results in sneezing, a blocked and stuffy nose, or a runny nose.

Although the greatest number of dust mites is found in the bedroom, their droppings can become airborne when dust is disturbed—as occurs when people move within the house—and spread, making any part of the house a source of this allergen for someone who has a house dust mite allergy.

How to Find Out If You Are Allergic to Dust Mite Droppings

Although many people with asthma will be sensitive to the allergen in house dust mite droppings, your doctor may suggest that you have skin-prick tests or blood tests called RASTs (radioallergosorbent tests) to confirm whether or not you have this allergy. Having your symptoms improve when you go on holiday, or stay somewhere other than your house, may also indicate to your doctor that dust mites or another trigger in your home may be causing problems with your asthma.

Is It Worth Trying to Avoid House Dust Mite Allergen If You Have Asthma?

There is not yet any solid evidence that reducing your exposure to house dust mites can effectively control your asthma.

Nevertheless, some people with asthma do find that their symptoms benefit from avoiding house dust mites. If you are thinking of trying these approaches, which can be inconvenient and expensive, first see your doctor to confirm the diagnosis.

How to Avoid High Levels of Dust Mites in Your House

Natural climate patterns can favor the buildup of dust mites in houses, and some areas are more favorable for dust mites than others.

In the past, chemicals were thought to be the best way to control dust mites, however, it is now believed that measures that make your house a less favorable habitat for dust mites are a better approach.

Most advice for controlling dust mites centers around:

- improving ventilation in your house to avoid the buildup of moist air;

- selecting flooring and furniture that is easy to clean and does not encourage the accumulation of dust and dead skin cells; and

- using household cleaning methods that are effective in removing or killing dust mites, for example, using a damp or electrostatic duster and mop.

If you live in a humid area, eliminating dust mites completely is difficult, but you can aim to reduce their numbers significantly. Following are some examples of how to do this.

Things You Can Do to Keep Dust Mite Levels Low in Your House

- Enclose mattresses, duvets, and pillows in dust-proof covers. These covers must be washed every two months.

- Wash bedclothes in hot water (more than 55 degrees C) once a week. If you can't wash in hot water, use a commercial product formulated to kill dust mites in cold water.

- Air pillows and bedding in sunlight for a few hours each week.

- Clean noncarpeted floors with a wet or electrostatic mop rather than using a vacuum cleaner.

- Clean carpets weekly with a vacuum cleaner that has a suitable filter such as a HEPA (high efficiency particulate air) filter. However, even this type of filter briefly increases the amount of house dust mite allergen in the air after vacuuming. It's therefore best if the allergic person does not vacuum and does not enter the room for twenty minutes after it has been vacuumed by someone else.

- Get a ducted vacuum cleaner, if practical and affordable, with an exhaust pipe opening to the outside of the house.

- Dust surfaces with a damp or electrostatic cloth two to three times weekly.

- Remove fluffy, stuffed toys from your child's bedroom. Although putting this type of toy in the freezer overnight once a fortnight can kill mites contained in the toy, this does not remove the allergen. Washing these toys in hot water once a week is the best approach.

- Remove soft, upholstered furniture from the bedroom.

- Select furniture that is upholstered in vinyl or leather rather than cloth.

- Ensure good ventilation throughout your house to avoid moist air buildup, which occurs with cooking, bathing, showering, and, more simply, as a result of people breathing inside the house.

For further information on dust mite control measures, speak to your doctor or contact your local asthma or allergy association.

Section 25.4

Preventing and Eradicating Mold

"Molds," U.S. Environmental Protection Agency, October 5, 2010.

What Are Molds?

Molds are microscopic fungi that live on plant and animal matter. Molds can be found almost anywhere; they grow on virtually any substance when moisture is present.

Molds produce tiny spores to reproduce, just as plants produce seeds. Mold spores waft through the indoor and outdoor air continually. When mold spores land on a damp spot indoors, they may begin growing and digesting whatever they are growing on in order to survive. Some molds can grow on wood, paper, carpet, foods, and even dynamite.

There is no practical way to eliminate all molds indoors; the way to control indoor mold growth is to control moisture. If you think you have a mold problem and can see mold growth, you do not need environmental testing to determine what kind of mold you have. Instead, simply clean the mold from the surface it's growing on and dry the surface thoroughly.

How Does Mold Affect Asthma?

For people sensitive to molds, inhaling mold spores can cause an asthma attack.

Actions You Can Take

If mold is a problem in your home, you need to clean up the mold and eliminate sources of moisture:

- Wash mold off hard surfaces and dry completely. Absorbent materials, such as ceiling tiles and carpet, may have to be replaced if they are contaminated with mold.

- Fix leaky plumbing or other sources of water.

- Keep drip pans in your air conditioner, refrigerator, and dehumidifier clean and dry.

- Use exhaust fans or open windows in kitchens and bathrooms when showering, cooking, or using the dishwasher.

- Vent clothes dryers to the outside.

Maintain low indoor humidity, ideally between 30 and 50 percent relative humidity. Humidity levels can be measured by hygrometers, which are available at local hardware stores.

Section 25.5

Dealing with Nitrogen Dioxide

"Nitrogen Dioxide (NO$_2$), "U.S. Environmental Protection Agency, October 5, 2010.

What Is Nitrogen Dioxide?

Nitrogen dioxide (NO$_2$) can be a byproduct of fuel-burning appliances, such as gas stoves, gas or oil furnaces, fireplaces, wood stoves, and unvented kerosene or gas space heaters. NO$_2$ is an odorless gas that can irritate your eyes, nose, and throat and cause shortness of breath. In people with asthma, exposure to low levels of NO$_2$ may cause increased bronchial reactivity and make young children more susceptible to respiratory infections. Long-term exposure to high levels of NO$_2$ can lead to chronic bronchitis.

Actions You Can Take

- Properly ventilate a room where a fuel-burning appliance is used and use appliances that vent to the outside whenever possible.

- Do not idle the car inside your garage.

- Have the entire heating system—including furnace, flues, and chimneys—professionally inspected and cleaned annually.

- Always open the flue on your fireplace before building a fire to ensure that smoke escapes through the chimney.

- Make sure the doors are tight fitting on your wood-burning stove and follow the manufacturer's directions for starting, stoking, and putting out the fire.

- Follow the manufacturer's directions for proper fuel use on un-vented kerosene or gas space heaters and keep the heater prop-erly adjusted. Open a window slightly or use an exhaust fan in the room while using the heater.

- Install and use an exhaust fan over a gas stove and vent it outdoors.

Section 25.6

Managing Pets When You Have Asthma

"Pets," U.S. Environmental Protection Agency, October 5, 2010.

About Pets and Asthma

Your pet's dead skin flakes, urine, feces, saliva, and hair can trig-ger asthma. Dogs, cats, rodents (including hamsters and guinea pigs), and other mammals can trigger asthma in individuals with an allergic reaction to animal dander. Proteins in the dander, urine, or saliva of warm-blooded animals (e.g., cats, dogs, mice, rats, gerbils, birds, etc.) have been reported to sensitize individuals and cause allergic reac-tions or trigger asthma episodes in individuals sensitive to animal allergens.

The most effective method to control animal allergens in the home is to not allow animals in the home. If you remove an animal from the home, it is important to clean the home (including floors and walls, but especially carpets and upholstered furniture) thoroughly.

Pet allergen levels are reported to stay in the home for several months after the pet is removed, even with cleaning. Isolation methods to reduce animal allergen in the home have also been suggested by reputable health authorities (e.g., keeping the animal in only one area of the home, keeping the animal outside, or ensuring that people with allergies or asthma stay away from the animal) but the effectiveness of these methods has not been determined. Several reports in the literature indicate that animal allergen is carried in the air and by residents of the home on their clothing to all parts of the home, even when the animal is isolated. In fact, animal allergen is often detected in locations where no animals were housed.

Often, people sensitive to animal allergens are advised to wash their pets regularly. Recent research indicates that washing pets may only provide temporary reductions in allergen levels. There is no evidence that this short-term reduction is effective in reducing symptoms, and it has been suggested that during the washing of the animal the sensitive individual may be initially exposed to higher levels of allergens.

Thus, the most effective method to control exposure to animal allergens is to keep your home pet free. However, some individuals may find isolation measures to be sufficiently effective. Isolation measures that have been suggested include keeping pets out of the sleeping areas, keeping pets away from upholstered furniture, carpets, and stuffed toys, keeping the pet outdoors as much as possible, and isolating sensitive individuals from the pet as much as possible.

Actions You Can Take

- If pets are one of your asthma triggers, strongly consider finding a new home for your pets.

- Keep pets out of the bedroom and other sleeping areas at all times and keep the door closed.

- Keep pets away from fabric-covered furniture, carpets, and stuffed toys.

- Vacuum carpets, rugs, and furniture two or more times per week.

Section 25.7

Dealing with Tobacco Smoke

Reprinted from "Secondhand Smoke," U.S. Environmental Protection Agency, October 5, 2010, and "Five Keys for Quitting Smoking," Centers for Disease Control and Prevention, January 26, 2011.

Secondhand Smoke

What Is Secondhand Smoke?

Secondhand smoke, also known as environmental tobacco smoke (ETS), consists of exhaled smoke from smokers and side stream smoke from the burning end of a cigarette, cigar, or pipe. Secondhand smoke contains more than four thousand substances, including several compounds that are known carcinogens.

How Does Secondhand Smoke Affect Asthma?

Secondhand smoke can trigger asthma episodes and increase the severity of attacks. Secondhand smoke is also a risk factor for new cases of asthma in preschool-aged children who have not already exhibited asthma symptoms. Scientists believe that secondhand smoke irritates the chronically inflamed bronchial passages of people with asthma. Secondhand smoke is linked to other health problems, including lung cancer, ear infections, and other chronic respiratory illnesses, such as bronchitis and pneumonia.

Many of the health effects of secondhand smoke, including asthma, are most clearly seen in children because children are most vulnerable to its effects. Most likely, children's developing bodies make them more susceptible to secondhand smoke's effects and, due to their small size, they breathe more rapidly than adults, thereby taking in more secondhand smoke. Children receiving high doses of secondhand smoke, such as those with smoking mothers, run the greatest relative risk of experiencing damaging health effects.

319

Actions You Can Take

- Choose not to smoke in your home or car and don't allow others to do so.

- Choose not to smoke in the presence of people with asthma.

- Choose not to smoke in the presence of children, who are particularly susceptible to the harmful effects of secondhand smoke.

- Do not allow babysitters, caregivers, or others in your home to smoke in your house or near your children.

- Talk to your children's teachers and daycare providers about keeping the places your children spend time smoke-free.

Five Keys for Quitting Smoking

Studies have shown that these five steps will help you quit and quit for good. You have the best chances of quitting if you use them together:

- Get ready

- Get support

- Learn new skills and behaviors

- Get medication and use it correctly

- Be prepared for relapse or difficult situations

Get Ready

- Set a quit date.

- Change your environment:

  - Get rid of *all* cigarettes and ashtrays in your home, car, and place of work.

  - Don't let people smoke in your home.

- Review your past attempts to quit. Think about what worked and what did not.

- Once you quit, don't smoke—*not even a puff!*

Get Support and Encouragement

Studies have shown that you have a better chance of being successful if you have help. You can get support in many ways:

- Tell your family, friends, and co-workers that you are going to quit and want their support. Ask them not to smoke around you or leave cigarettes out where you can see them.

- Talk to your healthcare provider (e.g., doctor, dentist, nurse, pharmacist, psychologist, or smoking cessation coach or counselor).

- Get individual, group, or telephone counseling. Counseling doubles your chances of success.

- The more help you have, the better your chances are of quitting. Free programs are available at local hospitals and health centers. Call your local health department for information about programs in your area.

Learn New Skills and Behaviors

- Try to distract yourself from urges to smoke. Talk to someone, go for a walk, or get busy with a task.

- When you first try to quit, change your routine. Use a different route to work. Drink tea instead of coffee. Eat breakfast in a different place.

- Do something to reduce your stress. Take a hot bath, exercise, or read a book.

- Plan something enjoyable to do every day.

- Drink a lot of water and other fluids.

Get Medication and Use It Correctly

Medications can help you stop smoking and lessen the urge to smoke.

The U.S. Food and Drug Administration (FDA) has approved seven medications to help you quit smoking:

- Bupropion SR—Available by prescription.
- Nicotine gum—Available over the counter.
- Nicotine inhaler—Available by prescription.
- Nicotine nasal spray—Available by prescription.
- Nicotine patch—Available by prescription and over the counter.
- Nicotine lozenge—Available over the counter.
- Varenicline tartrate—Available by prescription.

Ask your healthcare provider for advice and carefully read the information on the package.

All of these medications will at least double your chances of quitting and quitting for good.

Nearly everyone who is trying to quit can benefit from using a medication. However, if you are pregnant or trying to become pregnant, nursing, younger than eighteen years of age, smoking fewer than ten cigarettes per day, or have a medical condition, talk to your doctor or other healthcare provider before taking medications.

Be Prepared for Relapse or Difficult Situations

Most relapses occur within the first three months after quitting. Don't be discouraged if you start smoking again. Remember, most people try several times before they finally quit. The following are some difficult situations you may encounter:

- **Alcohol:** Avoid drinking alcohol. Drinking lowers your chances of success.

- **Other smokers:** Being around smoking can make you want to smoke.

- **Weight gain:** Many smokers will gain some weight when they quit, usually less than ten pounds. Eat a healthy diet and stay active. Don't let weight gain distract you from your main goal—quitting smoking. Some quit-smoking medications may help delay weight gain.

- **Bad mood or depression:** There are a lot of ways to improve your mood other than smoking. Some smoking cessation medications also lessen depression.

If you are having problems with any of these situations, talk to your doctor or other healthcare provider.

Section 25.8

What You Need to Know about Air Filters

What Do I Need to Know about Air Filters?

When we think of air pollution, we usually associate it with outdoor air. But with the growing epidemic of asthma in the United States in the last twenty years, especially among infants and children who spend most of their time inside, much attention has been given to indoor air. In fact, in 1990 the United States Environmental Protection Agency (EPA) ranked indoor air pollution as "a high-priority public health risk."

The EPA recommends three strategies for reducing indoor air pollution:

- controlling sources of pollution,

- ventilating adequately, and

- cleaning indoor air.

Before you make any changes to your indoor home environment or purchase any air filtration products, make sure to speak with a doctor who knows your personal medical history and current condition.

Will Air Filters Really Help My Asthma or Allergies?

Although the EPA recommends air filtration, controlling the sources of allergy-causing pollution and ventilation are more important. Air filters are worth considering, but not as a solution to your asthma or allergy problems by themselves. In fact, research studies disagree on whether or not filters give much added relief in a clean and well-ventilated home.

While many allergens and irritants are suspended in household air, there are far more resting on surfaces like rugs, furniture, and countertops. Keeping these areas clean is an important step in controlling your allergy and asthma triggers. However, the most effective step is to eliminate the source of these allergens and irritants in the first place.

Can Air Filters Protect Me from Secondhand Smoke?

The only effective way to eliminate environmental tobacco smoke (ETS)—also called "secondhand" smoke—is to eliminate the source of smoke: get smokers in your family to quit smoking. Some air cleaners may help to reduce secondhand smoke to a limited degree, but no air filtration or air purification system can completely eliminate all the harmful constituents of secondhand smoke. The U.S. Surgeon General has determined secondhand smoke to cause heart disease, lung cancer, and respiratory illness. Also, a simple reduction of secondhand smoke does not protect against the disease and death caused by exposure to secondhand smoke.

Are There National Health Standards for Air Filter Performance?

No. The Food and Drug Administration (FDA) has asked groups of experts to recommend national standards, but no federal standards have yet been adopted. So far they have concluded there isn't enough research data on the relationship between air filtration and actual health improvement to recommend national standards.

When you shop for air filters, you will find several rating systems that compare filters. But these are not health-related rating systems. They are standards used by manufacturers or manufacturers' organizations, and provide little guidance for the health-conscious shopper.

How Can I Find a Quality Air Filter?

Although the FDA has no health-related standards, it does consider some portable air filtration systems to be Class II medical devices. In the United States, nothing can claim this status without FDA approval. To get approval, a manufacturer must show two things: (1) that the device is safe, usually indicated by the Underwriters Laboratory (UL) seal, and (2) that it has a medical benefit. Look for both the UL seal and a statement of the FDA's Class II approval. If no FDA statement is available with the device, check the FDA's medical device listing before buying and always ask your doctor for guidance.

What is "Ozone" vs. "Ozone Byproduct"?

Most air filters have a normal "ozone byproduct." In fact, many of products already in your home make an ozone byproduct – kitchen mixers, ceiling fans, hair dryers, computers, TVs, copiers, and more. An acceptable level for ozone byproduct for certain household devices has been set in the Code of Federal Regulations (CFR) at a maximum 50 parts per billion (ppb), or lower. (This standard for acceptable levels of ozone byproduct is found in section 21:801.415 of the Code of Federal Regulations [CFR] and Underwriters Laboratory [UL] standard 867.) This maximum has also been voluntarily adopted by most air filter manufacturers and makers of other household electronics.

However, machines called "ozone generators" directly produce ozone (O_3) molecules—not as a byproduct, but as a direct product—and blow it into the room to "clean" the air. Unfortunately these "ozone generator" machines can produce ozone up to ten times more than the acceptable standard shown above. Therefore, the Asthma and Allergy Foundation of America (AAFA) and other groups recommend that you do not use "ozone generator" machines in your home.

Are there Different Kinds of Air Filters?

Yes. Many homes have whole-house air filtration, but there are also several types of single-room air filters on the market. Here are five basis types of room air filters.

Mechanical filters (fan-driven HEPA filters, for example): These force air through a special mesh that traps particles including allergens like pollen, pet dander, and dust mites. They also capture irritant particles like tobacco smoke. The fans in these types of devices produce ozone byproduct and are usually within the acceptable level. Make sure to ask for proof from the manufacturer that their product is within the acceptable level of ozone byproduct.

Electronic filters (ion-type cleaners, for example): These use electrical charges to attract and deposit allergens and irritants. If the device contains collecting plates, the particles are captured within the system. The ion chargers in these types of filters produce ozone byproduct, more than fans in mechanical filters, but may still be within the acceptable level. Make sure to ask for proof from the manufacturer that their product is within the acceptable level of ozone byproduct.

Hybrid filters: These contain the elements of both mechanical and electronic filters.

Gas phase filters: These remove odors and nonparticulate pollution like cooking gas, gasses given off by paint or building materials, and perfume. They cannot remove allergenic particles.

Ozone generators (not recommended—these types of "filters" are not reliable since their ozone levels usually exceed acceptable levels): Although ozone technically clears the air of some particles, most groups do not recommend these. (Note: these are not ion-type filters; see "Electronic Filters" above.) These devices all exceed the acceptable level for ozone.

If you have concerns about any air filter you own or are planning to buy, remember to talk to your doctor first, to find out if air filtration—and what type—is best for you.

What is a "HEPA" Filter?

A "HEPA" filter is a kind of mechanical filter that means it's a "high-efficiency particulate air" filter. HEPA was invented during World War II to prevent the escape of radioactive particles from laboratories. To qualify as a true HEPA filter, it must be able to capture at least 99.97 percent of all particles 0.3 microns in diameter or larger that enter it.

What Else Should I Consider Before Buying an Air Filtration System?

If your home is heated or air-conditioned through ducts, it may be possible to build filters into your air handling system. This has the advantage of the great force with which air will pass through the filter. And it eliminates a space-consuming appliance and an additional sound in your home. On the other hand, the filters may be more expensive and more difficult to handle; and they may need to be changed more often. Consult your doctor and your heating service on this alternative to a portable system.

Questions to Ask Before Purchasing an Air Filter

- What substances will the cleaner remove from the air in my home? What substances will it not?
- What is the efficiency rating of the cleaner in relation to the "true HEPA" standard?
- Will the unit clean the air in a room the size of my bedroom?

- How easy/difficult is it to change the filter? (Ask for demonstration.) How often does it have to be changed? How much do filters cost? Are they readily available throughout the year?

- How much noise does the unit make? Is it quiet enough to run while I sleep? (Turn it on and try it, even though you will probably be in a noisy place.)

Chapter 26

Managing Outdoor Asthma Triggers

Section 26.1

What Are the Health Effects of Outdoor Air Pollution?

"Air Pollution Sources, Effects, and Control," a fact sheet from the California Environmental Protection Agency Air Resources Board (www.arb.ca.gov), 2009. Reprinted with permission.

Where does air pollution come from? How does it affect people and the environment? How can we control, or better yet, prevent it? The following text summarizes the sources, effects, and prevention and control methods for ten of the most important air pollutants.

Ozone (O3)

Sources: Formed when reactive organic gases (ROG) and nitrogen oxides (NOx) react in the presence of sunlight. ROG sources include any source that burns fuels (e.g., gasoline, natural gas, wood, oil), solvents, petroleum processing and storage, and pesticides.

Effects: Breathing difficulties, lung tissue damage, damage to rubber and some plastics.

Prevention and control: Reduce motor vehicle reactive organic gas (ROG) and nitrogen oxide emissions through emissions standards, reformulated fuels, inspections programs, and reduced vehicle use. Limit ROG emissions from commercial operations and consumer products. Limit ROG and nitrogen oxide emissions from industrial sources such as power plants and refineries. Conserve energy.

Respirable Particulate Matter (PM10)

Sources: Road dust, windblown dust (agriculture), and construction (fireplaces). Also formed from other pollutants (acid rain, NOx, sulfur oxides [SOx], organics). Incomplete combustion of any fuel.

Effects: Increased respiratory disease, lung damage, cancer, premature death, reduced visibility, surface soiling.

Prevention and control: Control dust sources, industrial particulate emissions, wood-burning stoves and fireplaces. Reduce secondary pollutants which react to form PM10. Conserve energy.

Fine Particulate Matter (PM2.5)

Sources: Fuel combustion in motor vehicles, equipment, and industrial sources; residential and agricultural burning. Also formed from reaction of other pollutants (acid rain, NOx, SOx, organics).

Effects: Increases respiratory disease, lung damage, cancer, premature death, reduced visibility, surface soiling.

Prevention and control: Reduce combustion emissions from motor vehicles, equipment, industries, and agriculture, and residential burning. Precursor controls, like those for ozone, reduce fine particle formation in the atmosphere.

Carbon Monoxide (CO)

Sources: Any source that burns fuel, such as automobiles, trucks, heavy construction equipment, farming equipment, and residential heating.

Effects: Chest pain in heart patients, headaches, reduced mental alertness.

Prevention and control: Control motor vehicle and industrial emissions. Use oxygenated gasoline during winter months. Conserve energy.

Nitrogen Dioxide (NO2)

Sources: See carbon monoxide.

Effects: Lung irritation and damage. Reacts in the atmosphere to form ozone and acid rain.

Prevention and control: Control motor vehicle and industrial combustion emissions. Conserve energy.

Lead

Sources: Metal smelters, resource recovery, leaded gasoline, deterioration of lead paint.

Effects: Learning disabilities, brain and kidney damage.

Prevention and control: Control metal smelters, no lead in gasoline. Replace leaded paint with nonlead substitutes.

Sulfur Dioxide (SO2)

Sources: Coal- or oil-burning power plants and industries, refineries, diesel engines.

Effects: Increases lung disease and breathing problems for asthmatics. Reacts in the atmosphere to form acid rain.

Prevention and control: Reduce the use of high-sulfur fuels (e.g., use low-sulfur reformulated diesel or natural gas). Conserve energy.

Visibility-Reducing Particles

Sources: See PM2.5.

Effects: Reduces visibility (e.g., obscures mountains and other scenery), reduces airport safety, lowers real estate value, discourages tourism.

Prevention and control: See PM2.5.

Sulfates

Sources: Produced by the reaction in the air of SO2 (see SO2 sources), a component of acid rain.

Effects: Breathing difficulties, aggravates asthma, reduced visibility.

Prevention and control: See SO2.

Hydrogen Sulfide

Sources: Geothermal power plants, petroleum production and refining, sewer gas.

Effects: Nuisance odor (rotten egg smell), headache, and breathing difficulties (higher concentrations).

Prevention and control: Control emissions from geothermal power plants, petroleum production and refining, sewers, and sewage treatment plants.

Section 26.2

Dealing with Air Pollution

"Outdoor Air Pollution," U.S. Environmental Protection Agency,
October 5, 2010.

About Outdoor Air Pollution

Small particles and ozone come from things like exhaust from cars
and factories, smoke, and road dust. When inhaled, outdoor pollutants
can aggravate the lungs, and can lead to chest pain, coughing, shortness of breath, and throat irritation. Outdoor air pollution may also
worsen chronic respiratory diseases, such as asthma. On days when
ozone air pollution is highest, ozone has been associated with 10 to 20
percent of all respiratory hospital visits and admissions.

Watch for the Air Quality Index, or AQI, during your local weather
report. The AQI is a tool that offers you clear information every day on
whether air quality in your area could be a health risk. The AQI uses
colors to show how much pollution is in the air. Green and yellow mean
air pollution levels are low. Orange, red, or purple mean pollution is
at levels that may make asthma worse.

Actions You Can Take

State agencies will use television and radio to notify citizens of
ozone alerts. On days when your state or local air pollution control
agency calls an Ozone Action Day, people with asthma should limit
prolonged physical activity outdoors. Consider adjusting outdoor activities to early in the morning or later in the evening.

Also, on Ozone Action Days, you can do the following ten things to
help keep ozone formation to a minimum:

1. Instead of driving, share a ride, walk, or bike.

2. Take public transportation.

3. If you must drive, avoid excessive idling and jackrabbit starts.

4. Don't refuel your car or only do so after 7 p.m.

5.   Avoid using outboard motors, off-road vehicles, or other gasoline-powered recreational vehicles.

6.   Defer mowing your lawn until late evening or the next day. Also avoid using gasoline-powered garden equipment.

7.   Postpone chores that use oil-based paints, solvents, or varnishes that produce fumes.

8.   If you are barbecuing, use an electric starter instead of charcoal lighter fluid.

9.   Limit or postpone your household chores that will involve the use of consumer products.

10. Conserve energy in your home to reduce energy needs.

Section 26.3

Pollen and Asthma

What Is Pollen?

- Plants make tiny grains called pollen in order to reproduce.
- Pollen comes from trees, grasses, and weeds.
- These pollens are light and easily carried by the wind.
- Pollens are released at different times of the year:
  - **Trees:** April and May (spring)
  - **Grasses:** June and July
  - **Weeds:** August and September (fall)

- Pollen counts tend to be higher on warm, dry, windy days.
- Pollen counts tend to be higher in the morning.
- Pollen counts tend to be lower during cold, wet periods.

- You can find out pollen counts in your area on television or online.

Pollen Allergy

- Pollen is an outdoor allergen.

- An allergen is something you are allergic to.

- Pollen can trigger an allergic reaction or hay fever, causing sneezing; coughing; itchy eyes, nose, or throat; runny nose; and watery eyes.

- Ragweed pollen is a common asthma trigger.

- People with a pollen allergy may think that they have a spring or summer cold, but the symptoms last longer than two weeks.

- Symptoms that seem to occur at the same time each year may be caused by a pollen allergy. Talk to your doctor.

Avoidance Measures

- The more you avoid what you are allergic to, the fewer symptoms you will have.

- Keep home and car windows closed when pollen counts are high.

- Air conditioning may be helpful to keep pollen from coming indoors.

- Stay indoors in the morning when pollen levels are higher.

- If working outdoors, wearing a face mask to filter out pollen may be helpful.

- Avoid cutting the grass or doing yard work if it causes symptoms.

- Do not dry clothes outdoors. Pollen can stick to clothes.

Treating a Pollen Allergy

- Nasal symptoms can often be controlled with antihistamines and nasal steroid spray.

- If you have asthma, more controller medicine may be needed when the pollen count is high.

- Sometimes allergy shots are used for people with seasonal allergies to grass, tree, or weed pollen.

- Speak to your doctor to learn more about a pollen allergy.

Section 26.4

Avoidance Strategies for Common Pollens

"Pollen," National Institute of Environmental Health Sciences,
National Institutes of Health, June 9, 2010.

Ragweed Pollen

Ragweed and other weeds such as curly dock, lambs quarters, pig-weed, plantain, sheep sorrel, and sagebrush are some of the most prolific producers of pollen allergens.

Although the ragweed pollen season runs from August to November, ragweed pollen levels usually peak in mid-September in many areas in the country.

In addition, pollen counts are highest between 5 a.m. and 10 a.m. and on dry, hot, and windy days.

Preventive Strategies

- Avoid the outdoors between 5 a.m. and 10 a.m. Save outside activities for late afternoon or after a heavy rain, when pollen levels are lower.

- Keep windows in your home and car closed to lower exposure to pollen. To keep cool, use air conditioners and avoid using window and attic fans.

- Be aware that pollen can also be transported indoors on people and pets.

- Dry your clothes in an automatic dryer rather than hanging them outside. Otherwise pollen can collect on clothing and be carried indoors.

Grass Pollen

As with tree pollen, grass pollen is regional as well as seasonal. In addition, grass pollen levels can be affected by temperature, time of day, and rain.

Of the 1,200 species of grass that grow in North America, only a small percentage of these cause allergies. The most common grasses that can cause allergies are as follows:

- Bermuda grass

- Johnson grass

- Kentucky bluegrass

- Orchard grass

- Sweet vernal grass

- Timothy grass

Preventive Strategies

Specifically, do the following:

- If you have a grass lawn, have someone else do the mowing. If you must mow the lawn yourself, wear a mask.

- Keep grass cut short.

- Choose ground covers that don't produce much pollen, such as Irish moss, bunch, and dichondra.

In general, do the following:

- Avoid the outdoors between 5 a.m. and10 a.m. Save outside activities for late afternoon or after a heavy rain, when pollen levels are lower.

- Keep windows in your home and car closed to lower exposure to pollen. To keep cool, use air conditioners and avoid using window and attic fans.

- Be aware that pollen can also be transported indoors on people and pets.

- Dry your clothes in an automatic dryer rather than hanging them outside. Otherwise pollen can collect on clothing and be carried indoors.

Tree Pollen

Trees are the earliest pollen producers, releasing their pollen as early as January in the southern states and as late as May or June in the northern states.

Trees can aggravate your allergy whether or not they are on your property, since trees release large amounts of pollen that can be distributed miles away from the original source.

Of the fifty thousand different kinds of trees, less than one hundred have been shown to cause allergies. Most allergies are specific to one type of tree such as the following:

- Catalpa
- Hickory
- Pecan
- Walnut
- Elm
- Olive
- Sycamore

They may also be specific to the male cultivar of certain trees. The female of these species are totally pollen-free:

- Ash
- Cottonwood
- Maple (red)
- Phoenix palm
- Willow
- Box elder
- Date palm
- Maple (silver)
- Poplar

Some people, though, do show cross-reactivity among trees in the alder, beech, birch, and oak family, and the juniper and cedar family.

Preventive Strategies

- If you buy trees for your yard, look for species that do not aggravate allergies such as crape myrtle, dogwood, fig, fir, palm, pear, plum, redbud, and redwood trees or the female cultivars of ash, box elder, cottonwood, maple, palm, poplar, or willow trees.

- Avoid the outdoors between 5 a.m. and 10 a.m. Save outside activities for late afternoon or after a heavy rain, when pollen levels are lower.

- Keep windows in your home and car closed to lower exposure to pollen. To keep cool, use air conditioners and avoid using window and attic fans.

- Be aware that pollen can also be transported indoors on people and pets.

- Dry your clothes in an automatic dryer rather than hanging them outside. Otherwise pollen can collect on clothing and be carried indoors.

Section 26.5

Cold Air and Asthma Management

Cold air entering the lungs can cause airway constriction and is therefore a common trigger for asthmatics. The effects of cold air can be anticipated and prevented by some pre-planning. To help manage asthma in cold weather, consider these following tips:

- Keep your asthma well controlled at all times and carry your prescribed reliever medication with you.

- If cold air is a trigger for you, take your reliever medication ten to fifteen minutes before exposure to cold air.

- Check weather conditions before going out and dress for the weather conditions by covering up. Wear gloves, a scarf, and a hat.

- Breathe in through your nose. Your nose is designed to warm and humidify air.

- A scarf that covers both your nose and mouth will help keep the air you breathe warm and moist.

- Avoid outdoor exercise in extremely cold weather.

- Talk to your doctor about your asthma control.

Chapter 27

Managing Other Types of Asthma Triggers

Section 27.1

Food

Food allergies are more common among people with asthma and may contribute to asthma attacks, according to one of the most comprehensive surveys of food allergies ever undertaken. National Jewish Health Associate Professor of Pediatrics Andrew H. Liu and his colleagues also report in the November 2010 *Journal of Allergy and Clinical Immunology* that food allergies are more prevalent among children, males, and non-Hispanic blacks.

"Our study suggests that food allergies may be an important factor, and even an under-recognized trigger for severe asthma exacerbations," said Dr. Liu. "People with a food allergy and asthma should closely monitor both conditions and be aware that they might be related."

The researchers, funded by the National Institute of Environmental Health Sciences (NIEHS), analyzed data from 8,203 people, aged one to greater than sixty, who completed the National Health and Nutrition Examination Survey in 2005–2006, and had their blood tested for antibodies to four specific foods: peanuts, milk, eggs, and shrimp.

"This study is very comprehensive in its scope," said Darryl Zeldin, M.D., acting clinical director at the NIEHS and senior author on the paper. "It is the first study to use specific blood serum levels and look at food allergies across the whole life spectrum, from young children aged one to five, to adults sixty and older."

Depending on the immunoglobulin E (IgE) antibody levels found in participants' blood, they were categorized as sensitized to one or more of the foods or not sensitized. The sensitized participants were subdivided into those with an unlikely (10–20 percent), possible (50 percent), and likely (greater than 95 percent) chance of having food allergies.

Likely food allergies were twice as common among participants who had ever received an asthma diagnosis as among those with no asthma diagnosis.

The odds of having food allergies grew with increasing severity of asthma. Those who currently have asthma were 3.8 times as likely to have food allergies as those who had previously been diagnosed with the disease but no longer had it. Those who had visited an emergency department for asthma in the past year were almost 7 times as likely to have food allergies as those who had ever been diagnosed with asthma but not visited an emergency department. Overall, 15.8 percent of participants who had visited the emergency department for asthma had IgE levels indicating possible or likely food allergies.

Researchers could not determine if food allergies actually cause asthma attacks or if asthma and food allergies are both manifestations of a severe allergic profile. They speculated that food-allergic reactions might be triggered in some people with asthma only when combined with strenuous exercise.

Overall, the researchers estimate that 2.5 percent or 7.5 million Americans have food allergies. This estimate is lower than some estimates, but in line with many others. This study's analysis of actual IgE antibody levels to foods in a large nationally representative sample lent authority to the results. However, since the tests measure potential allergies to only four of the most commonly allergenic foods, the results may slightly underestimate overall prevalence of food allergies, wrote the authors.

Children ages one to nineteen were twice as likely to have food allergies as the general population. Non-Hispanic blacks were three times as likely to have food allergies, and males were twice as likely to have food allergies. Black male children were 4.4 times as likely to have food allergies.

Peanut allergy was the most common food allergy, affecting 1.3 percent of the surveyed population. Contrary to milk and egg allergies, which peaked in children under five, peanut allergies were highest among children ages six to nineteen (2.7 percent).

Section 27.2

Medications and Sulfites

"Some Medications and Food Additives Make Asthma Worse,"
Firestone Institute for Respiratory Health (www.firh.ca), © 2010.
Reprinted with permission.

Nonsteroidal Anti-Inflammatory Medications and Aspirin

Some people with asthma should not use acetylsalicylic acid (ASA) such as aspirin and Entrophen or products that contain ASA for fever, colds, or pain control.

There are many medications and products that can cause asthma attacks in people who react to aspirin. Some examples are Advil, Indocid, and Toradol.

If you need to take medication for fever, cold, or pain, talk to your doctor, asthma educator, or pharmacist for advice. Most people can take acetaminophen products such as Tylenol and Tempra without any reaction.

Beta-Blocker Medication

Beta-blocker medication makes asthma worse and should not be used by people with asthma. In pill form, this medication is used to treat high blood pressure, some heart problems, and migraine headaches. This medication is also used in eye drop form to treat glaucoma.

All forms of beta-blocker medication are dangerous for people with asthma and must not be used.

Sulfite Medication

Sulfites are sometimes added to foods such as wine, restaurant salads, dried fruits and vegetables, and many prepared foods and drinks. When you read a label, they are listed as sulfite metabisulfite or bisulfite. These can cause sudden worsening of asthma. Asthma symptoms often start within a few minutes or up to an hour after eating or drinking something with sulfites. You may also feel flushed or feel your neck is blocked. If you get any of these feelings, talk to your doctor and avoid the foods and drinks you think caused the problem.

Monosodium Glutamate or MSG Additive

Some people with asthma cannot eat monosodium glutamate, as it makes their symptoms worse. This is used in some Asian, Chinese, and Oriental restaurants. It is also in the product called Accent.

If you react to monosodium glutamate, you can have symptoms right away or many hours after. You may also have a headache or stomach upset.

Read the labels on all canned and preserved food to avoid problems. It can be listed as monosodium glutamate, glutamine, or glutamate.

Contact the doctor or healthcare provider who treats your asthma if you react to any of the above substances.

Section 27.3

Stress

It wasn't that long ago that asthma was considered a disease of the mind, a psychosomatic illness referred to in medical texts as asthma nervosa. In effect, the "blame" for having asthma was placed on the asthma sufferer: if only you were psychologically more well balanced, your breathing would be fine! And so too, according to some medical practitioners of the time, would your ulcers, your back pain, your headaches, and your colitis.

Modern science has made huge strides in understanding the biologic mechanisms of asthma, and more and more evidence indicates that the problem is in your breathing tubes, not in your head. We understand asthma to be a condition of the bronchial tubes, sensitized by an allergic type of inflammation, vulnerable to narrowing when stimulated by allergens, irritants, infections, or other triggers that provoke more swelling of the walls of the tubes and tightening of the muscles that surround the tubes.

Exploring the Mind-Body Connection

Still, the mind-body connection is strong, and as a person with asthma you may identify stress as one of those triggers that can make your asthma worse. Your breathing was fine until... (fill in the blank)... you had a fight with your boyfriend, your boss criticized you for something that could not be avoided, the bills piled up beyond your ability to pay them, or your day in divorce court loomed. Many people have had the experience that strong negative feelings such as fear, anger, deep sadness, or anxiety provoke their asthma symptoms of shortness of breath and tightness in the chest.

How might stress make your asthma worse? One might dismiss stress as mimicking asthma symptoms. Even those who don't have asthma can feel breathless and tight in the chest when heavily stressed, like that moment in childhood when you were asked to perform before a large audience for the first time! Or stress may compound the sensations of asthma: if you are wheezing and short of breath, stress will undoubtedly make you feel worse, whereas security and support will likely make your symptoms less intense. However, other explanations are possible: while sudden or brief stress may release in your body hormones that generally help your breathing (like cortisol and adrenaline), chronic stress may have negative effects on the healthy balance of these hormones. Our reaction to stress may also impact on our immune system and the nerve pathways through the body. And then there are the indirect ways in which stress can lead to worsened asthma control. For instance, it can make you more likely to smoke cigarettes, to overeat, to miss your doctor's appointments, or find the energy to take good care of your health in general.

Physical Violence as a Potent Form of Stress

Recently, researchers in Boston and elsewhere have wondered whether stress might contribute to the disproportionate burden of asthma severity found among the urban poor. Living in poverty imposes huge stresses on a daily basis, but one example seems to stand out from the rest: the stress of experiencing or witnessing physical violence. The frequency with which violence intrudes into the lives of children in our inner cities is shocking: in a study conducted at Boston Medical Center, 10 percent of children witnessed a knifing or shooting before six years of age; 18 percent witnessed shoving, kicking, or punching, and 47 percent heard gunshots. Exposure to the extreme stressor of physical violence may somehow—by mechanisms not well understood—contribute to difficult-to-control asthma, just like exposure to dust, animal danders, and cigarette smoke. Some have described this pervasive stress of family and community violence as a "social pollutant" that enters the body through the mind rather than the airways.

Psychological stress is here to stay. But it may be that stress reduction is an important part of asthma therapy, at least for some people. Young children in particular deserve the chance to live a childhood where stress is minimized, particularly the extreme and psychologically lingering form of stress that is physical violence and abuse.

Section 27.4

Weather

"Can the Weather Affect My Asthma?" June 2007, reprinted with permission from www.kidshealth.org. Copyright © 2007 The Nemours Foundation. This information was provided by KidsHealth, one of the largest resources online for medically reviewed health information written for parents, kids, and teens. For more articles like this one, visit www.KidsHealth.org, or www.TeensHealth.org.

There's a connection between asthma and weather. Some people find their asthma gets worse at certain times of the year. For others, a storm or sudden weather change may cause a flare-up.

Cold, dry air can be an asthma trigger, especially for people who do winter sports and who have asthma symptoms when they exercise. Hot, humid air can also trigger asthma symptoms. In some areas, heat and sunlight combine with pollution to make ozone (say: oh-zone), which is also an asthma trigger.

Wet weather and dry, windy weather can both be problems, too. And many people with asthma have symptoms during thunderstorms.

Your doctor can help you figure out if weather is causing some of your asthma symptoms. He or she can put this information into your asthma action plan. Once you know what your weather or seasonal triggers are, you can take steps to avoid them. You can:

- watch the forecast for pollen and mold counts as well as weather that might affect your asthma (an adult can help you do this);

- stay indoors on days when your triggers are strongest;

- wear a scarf over your mouth and nose outside during very cold weather;

- keep your windows closed at night (if it's hot, use air conditioning, which cleans, cools, and dries the air);

- stay indoors early in the morning (before 10 a.m.) when pollen levels in the air are at their highest;

- stay away from freshly cut grass and leaf piles;

- Keep your rescue medication with you all the time—whether the weather bothers you or not!

Chapter 28

Dealing with Co-Existing Respiratory Conditions

Chapter Contents

Section 28.1

Chronic Obstructive Pulmonary Disease (COPD)

"COPD and Asthma" and "Treatment of COPD and Asthma,"
© 2009 National Lung Health Education Program (www.nlhep.org).
Reprinted with permission.

COPD and Asthma

What Is COPD?

What does the term COPD mean? It stands for Chronic obstructive pulmonary disease and refers to a problem with breathing air out from your lungs. If you have difficulty breathing "used" air out of your lungs, not enough space is left for oxygen-rich air to enter your lungs.

Until recently, most people who had COPD were grouped together and considered to have one disease. We now know that several different diseases cause this difficulty in releasing air from the lungs. Asthmatic bronchitis, chronic bronchitis, and emphysema are three of the major diseases that are grouped together as COPD.

Asthmatic and Chronic Bronchitis

Both asthmatic and chronic bronchitis occur when the large airways or bronchi are inflamed and swollen. Imagine what happens to your skin when you've gotten an insect bite and it becomes swollen, red, and painful. This same idea can be applied to the swelling that occurs with bronchitis. The lining of the air tubes becomes swollen and produces large amounts of mucus. Because mucus clogs the airways, it complicates the problem, much like pus infects and irritates a wound and delays healing.

The muscles that surround the airways may tighten when they should not, causing bronchospasm. These narrowed airways prevent all the "used" air from leaving the lungs. Bronchospasm, inflammation, and swelling all make the space inside the airways smaller. This reduces the amount of air that can flow in and out of the lungs.

The first symptom of chronic bronchitis is a persistent cough that brings up mucus. This is often followed by wheezing, shortness of breath, and frequent chest infections. The symptoms of bronchitis can usually be relieved or improved with treatment.

Emphysema

Emphysema develops when many of the small air sacs or alveoli in the lungs are destroyed. This reduces their elasticity and decreases their ability to pass oxygen into the blood and remove carbon dioxide from the blood.

Shortness of breath is the major symptom of emphysema. At first, this difficulty in breathing may occur only with heavy exercise. Later it happens with light exercise and, still later, even when walking or engaging in other everyday activities. Many people who have emphysema also have chronic bronchitis. The mucus produced by these inflamed airways makes breathing even more difficult.

In most cases, a person's lungs can take a lot of abuse. It may be twenty or more years before someone who has emphysema notices a change in his or her health. However, when emphysema is diagnosed early, more can be done to treat it. By stopping smoking and using appropriate treatments or medication, persons with emphysema can generally lead a comfortable life.

What Causes COPD?

Asthmatic bronchitis, chronic bronchitis, and emphysema develop as a result of one or more of these factors:

- cigarette smoking,

- family susceptibility, or

- inhaling large amounts of dust at work or at home.

Conditions that can make these diseases worse are frequent colds or infections in the nose, sinuses, throat, or chest.

It is also known that emphysema can be hereditary. In some families this might be due to a lack of normal lung "defenses" that fight damage within the lung. It may also be because certain habits are passed along to other family members. For example, if parents smoke, there is a good chance that their children will smoke. Since smoking is the main cause of COPD, persons with family members who smoke are at greater risk of getting these diseases.

Treatment of COPD and Asthma

What can you do if you have chronic obstructive pulmonary disease (COPD)?

Certainly you should change any behavior that can make it worse. The single most important thing you can do for yourself is to stop smoking. In fact, if you don't stop smoking, none of your other efforts will be as effective as they could be, and your COPD will get worse.

As a COPD patient:

- You need clean air. Therefore, you should also avoid being around smokers and fume-laden air. During fog or smog, try to stay indoors with windows closed. If possible, use fumeless appliances for heating.

- Polluted air also can irritate your lungs. Try not to go out when the air quality is rated poor. But if you cannot avoid excessive air pollution, protect your mouth and nose with a mask.

- You should see your doctor on a regular basis—especially if you have a chest cold or any time you cough up mucus.

- It is also important to guard against catching the flu by getting an influenza vaccine each fall, well before winter starts. A pneumonia vaccine should also be given to anyone over age sixty, and all persons with COPD.

There are many different types of treatments that can help you cope with COPD and live your life to the fullest. Keep reading to find out more about COPD treatment—but remember that your doctor is the best person to direct your care and should be the one to select the treatment that will be most helpful to you.

Clearing Your Lungs

Coughing has an important "cleaning action" and is something you should practice every day—especially in the morning, when mucus may have settled in your lungs as you slept. You must learn to cough in such a way that you can clear your lungs of mucus with two or three coughs. Your doctor or the respiratory therapist will teach you the way that is best for your particular problem.

As an aid to this cleaning, your doctor may recommend breathing moist or humid air, and drinking plenty of fluids every day. Doing this may help thin out the mucus so that you can cough it up more easily.

Your doctor may also recommend that you use inhaled bronchodilating drugs or anti-inflammatory drugs to open your airways and help increase the normal flow of mucus out of your lungs (keep reading to find out more about these drugs).

Breathing Techniques

Learning to breathe properly is another very important lesson for people with COPD. If you have COPD, you usually work very hard to breathe. However, because you are not breathing properly, your hard work does not make you feel better and you become tired easily.

There are several things you can do to improve your breathing:

- Relax. Being tense makes it harder to breathe.

- Breathe out through pursed lips, like when whistling. This slows down your breathing and makes each breath do more good for you.

- Lean forward while exercising. This also helps control shortness of breath.

- "Belly breathing" may also help shortness of breath. This is done by allowing your belly to stick out while breathing in and then pulling your belly in while breathing out. Remember to purse your lips when breathing out!

Physical Activity

Often people make the mistake of believing that if they try to avoid becoming short of breath, they will protect their lungs and heart. *This is not true!* Remaining physically active will improve your breathing ability and help you feel better and enjoy life more.

You can exercise even if you have COPD. As we all know, muscles will become weak if we don't use them. This is true for the muscles of your chest, which are important in breathing, as well. Strengthening these muscles will help decrease shortness of breath.

Don't let COPD change your normal attitudes about exercise. You should walk every day, trying to do a little more than you did the day before. Start by walking in your house, then try walking out of doors (but not when there is poor air quality)—walking longer distances each time.

Your doctor will help you find the exercises that are best for you. Ask if there is a local pulmonary rehabilitation program, where you can learn more about your COPD and get advice and support to learn the best ways to exercise and control your COPD symptoms.

Oxygen

Supplemental oxygen is a very helpful treatment that enables many patients with severe COPD to lead a more normal and productive life.

Your doctor may order an oxygen test (by taking blood from an artery or by using an oximeter)—and if your oxygen level is low, the doctor will prescribe it for you. Portable devices will allow you to carry oxygen with you, or your doctor might tell you to use oxygen only at night during sleep when your oxygen level may drop because of shallow breathing. Liquid portable oxygen now comes in a very light device, making it the most practical ambulatory system. Your doctor will order the proper oxygen system, which can benefit you the most. The device supplier (often called a durable medical equipment company, or DME) must follow your doctor's prescription exactly as it is written. The DME will also instruct you in how to use your oxygen equipment safely. A respiratory therapist may also be called in to help you learn more about using supplemental oxygen. Follow the directions you are given carefully, as you would for any medication that is prescribed, and be sure to ask questions if you do not fully understand how to use your equipment!

Medications

Many different medications are used as treatment for COPD. Your doctor will decide which medicine is best for you based on your medical history, breathing tests, and other laboratory tests.

To help you breathe easier, your doctor may give you bronchodilator drugs. Bronchodilators relax the muscles that surround the breathing tubes and widen them, letting air travel in and out more easily.

Your doctor may also prescribe drugs to liquefy the mucus in your lungs or drugs called corticosteroids, which reduce the swelling in your breathing tubes. If you have an infection in your lungs, your doctor may prescribe antibiotics. Remember that it is never good to take an antibiotic as a protection against future infections—but when prescribed, take *all* of the medication exactly as directed by the doctor. If you have any questions about your medications and how they work, ask the doctor or your pharmacist!

Lung medications are available in many forms. In addition to pills or syrups that you swallow, your doctor may prescribe medication to be delivered through a metered-dose inhaler (MDI) or a dry powder inhaler (DPI), both of which deliver the medication in a "puff" that you breathe in. Liquid medications are delivered using a nebulizer, which turns the liquid into a mist that you breathe in. Directions for measuring your liquid medication and for using the cup and tubing that attach to the nebulizer should be given to you in written form (with pictures) by a respiratory therapist and/or the company that provides the nebulizer.

Metered-Dose Inhalers (MDIs) and Dry Powder Inhalers (DPIs)

Most of these devices which deliver medication to your lungs as a spray, mist, or fine powder require a prescription from your doctor. One MDI medication that can be bought without a prescription is called Primatene MistTM. Its main ingredient is adrenaline, a short-acting drug which may be dangerous for persons with heart disease. It is not appropriate for the treatment of COPD.

In order to get the maximum benefit from any medication, it is important to take it properly. This is especially true for medications that are inhaled.

Here are some good tips for using your MDI correctly:

- Remove the cap from the mouthpiece and shake the MDI well.

- Exhale slowly though pursed lips.

- Hold the inhaler upright and place it in front of your mouth. Keep your mouth slightly open. Breathe in deeply (and at the same time) press the inhaler between your thumb and forefinger. This forces the medication from the inhaler in a "puff" that you then inhale into your lungs.

- Remove the inhaler from your mouth, holding your breath for a few seconds. Then exhale slowly through pursed lips.

Most inhaler instructions ask you to take two puffs. You need to wait about two minutes before taking the second puff, using the same technique as described above.

A device called a spacer or holding chamber should always be used with your MDI inhaler. This device, which attaches to the mouthpiece of your MDI, catches the mist as it leaves the MDI, allowing you to get more medication without having to worry about coordination of your breathing when the "puff" comes out of the MDI.

Taking medication using a dry powder inhaler (DPI) is very differ-ent from using a metered dose inhaler MDI) Here are some do's and don'ts for using a DPI:

- _Do_ hold the device level when using it so that the powder does not fall out.

- *Do* store it in a cool, dry place so that the powder stays dry and does not cake up.

- *Don't* open the medication packet until you are ready to use it.

- *Don't* shake it before using!

- *Don't* breathe into your DPI, as that will blow the medication away or make it cake up.

- *Don't* use a spacer with your DPI.

Regardless of the type of medication your are taking, follow your doctor's directions carefully. Reread these instructions or the medication package insert often to make sure you are taking your medication the right way. Do not exceed the dose prescribed by your doctor. If you continue to have difficulty breathing, contact your doctor immediately.

Nebulizer Treatment

This type of treatment, which must also be prescribed by your doctor, delivers a mist of medication to your lungs by blowing air into the medication (liquid) in a cup attached to a small piece of tubing. When taking this treatment, here are some points to remember:

- Be sure you know the amount of medication and solution to use as well as the length and timing of your treatment. Follow your doctor's or respiratory therapist's instructions carefully about when each treatment should be scheduled and the length of time that it should be done.

- Relax and sit in a comfortable chair in an upright position.

- Make sure the tubing is not bent or dented, and that the liquid cup is level with your mouth.

- Put the mouthpiece in front of your teeth and keep your mouth slightly open.

- Take a deep, slow breath, activating the air control (if your machine has one). Your machine may make a mist constantly. Whichever type of machine you have, relax and take in slow deep breaths to allow the mist to fill your lungs. Hold your breath for about two seconds before exhaling. Remember to exhale slowly and completely each time.

If your mouth becomes dry during your treatment, don't be afraid to stop and drink some water. Also—and this is very important—if you bring up mucus during the treatment, turn your machine off and stop and cough it up. These treatments are helpful in eliminating mucus.

If you experience any discomfort after treatment, notify your doctor.

New Developments

Progress is continually being made in the treatment of COPD.

Beta agonists and anticholinergics are both bronchodilator medications. Many come in pill, liquid (for the nebulizer), or as MDIs or DPIs. Because these medications work in the lungs in different ways, they are often prescribed for use at the same time. Many are now available mixed together in the same MDI or DPI—meaning that you only need to use one device to get both medications if they are prescribed that way by your doctor.

A new treatment that may be effective in a rare hereditary form of emphysema is being tested on volunteers. A replacement for the inherited deficiency of alpha antitrypsin is commercially available. Although it restores a protective material in the lungs, its effectiveness in preventing the progress of emphysema remains to be proven.

Surgical approaches to improving dyspnea by removing areas of major lung damage from emphysema are called lung volume reduction surgery, (LVRS).

In selected patients, this operation can improve shortness of breath and quality of life. The mechanisms behind this improvement are complex. They include a restoration of the curvature of the diaphragm through a reduction in overinflation of diseased parts of the lung. These regions of excessive destruction are often in the upper parts of the lung, (apices). These areas contribute little to lung function, but they take up a lot of space for expansion of the rest of the lung, which is relatively normal. Extensive evaluations must be done through scans and tests of heart function to determine where the damaged parts of the lungs are and if you are a good candidate for this surgery.

Based on the results of a research study funded by Medicare, there is some reimbursement for this surgery. The study contrasted the results from surgery following a period of pulmonary rehabilitation compared to pulmonary rehabilitation alone. The study, called the National Emphysema Therapy Trial, (NETT), showed that only a small number of people with COPD will benefit from this surgery, while most will benefit from a full program of pulmonary rehabilitation (PR). Ask your doctor if there is a PR program in your area.

Section 28.2

Influenza

"Flu and People with Asthma," Centers for Disease
Control and Prevention, February 9, 2011.

What Is Asthma?

Asthma is a lung disease that is caused by chronic inflammation of the airways. It is one of the most common long-term diseases of children, but adults can have asthma, too. Asthma attacks occur when the lung airways become swollen and tighten due to airway inflammation. Asthma attacks can be caused by "triggers" such as airway infections, allergy particles, chemical irritants, and air pollution. During an attack, people with asthma experience symptoms such as wheezing, breathlessness, chest tightness, and nighttime or early morning coughing. Often, asthma attacks can be prevented by limiting one's exposure to triggers and by properly using asthma medications.

People with Asthma Are at Increased Risk of Severe Disease and Complications from Flu

Though people with asthma are not more likely to get the flu, influenza (flu) can be more serious for people with asthma, even if their asthma is mild or their symptoms are well controlled by medication. This is because people with asthma have swollen and sensitive airways, and influenza can cause further inflammation of the airways and lungs. Influenza infection in the lungs can trigger asthma attacks and a worsening of asthma symptoms. It can also lead to pneumonia and other acute respiratory diseases. In fact, adults and children with asthma are more likely to develop pneumonia after getting sick with the flu than people who do not have asthma. Asthma is the most common medical condition among adults and kids hospitalized with the flu.

If You Have Asthma, You Need to Take Steps to Fight the Flu

Everyone with asthma who is six months and older should get a flu vaccine to protect against getting the flu:

- Vaccination is the first and most important step in protecting against influenza. Even if you don't have a regular doctor or nurse, you can get a flu vaccine.

- Flu vaccines are offered in many locations including doctors' offices, clinics, health departments, pharmacies, college health centers, and increasingly by a number of employers and public schools.

- People with asthma should get flu vaccine made with inactivated (killed) flu virus. That kind of flu vaccine (commonly called a "flu shot") is given with a needle, usually in the arm. Persons with asthma should not use the nasal spray FluMist vaccine.

- Children, adults over sixty-five years of age, and people who have asthma should also get the pneumococcal vaccine to protect against pneumonia.

- Pneumococcal infections are a serious complication of influenza infections and can cause death. Pneumococcal vaccine may be given at the same time as influenza vaccine.

Take everyday preventive actions to stop the spread of flu:

- Cover your nose and mouth with a tissue when coughing or sneezing and throw the tissue away. If you do not have a tissue, cough or sneeze into your elbow or shoulder, not your bare hands.

- Wash your hands often with soap and water, especially after coughing or sneezing.

- Avoid touching your eyes, nose, or mouth (germs are spread that way)

- Stay home when you are sick, except to get medical care.

Follow an updated, written asthma action plan developed with your doctor:

- Follow this plan for daily treatment to control asthma long-term and to handle worsening asthma, or attacks.

- If your child has asthma, make sure that his or her updated, written asthma action plan is on file at school or at the daycare center. Be sure that the plan and medication(s) are easy to get to when needed.

- If you do get sick with flu symptoms, call your doctor and take flu antiviral drugs if your doctor recommends them.

- Treatment should begin as soon as possible because antiviral drug treatment works best when started early (within forty-eight hours after symptoms start).

- Antiviral drugs can make your flu illness milder and make you feel better faster. They may also prevent serious health problems that can result from flu illness.

- Oseltamivir (Tamiflu) is an antiviral drug that can be used to treat flu. To get Oseltamivir (Tamiflu), a doctor needs to write a prescription. This medicine fights against the flu by keeping flu viruses from making more viruses in your body.

- People with asthma should not use zanamivir (Relenza), a different antiviral drug, because there is a risk it may cause wheezing in people that already have asthma or other lung problems.

Section 28.3

Rhinitis

Excerpted from "Allergic Rhinitis and Your Asthma: What You Should Know," © 2006 National Asthma Council Australia. All rights reserved. Reprinted with permission. To view the complete text of this document, and additional information, visit http://www.nationalasthma.org.au. Reviewed by David A. Cooke, M.D., FACP, August 2011.

Allergic Rhinitis Facts

- Allergic rhinitis is becoming more common.

- It is most common among young to middle-age adults.

- Most people with asthma (up to 80 percent) have allergic rhinitis.

Rhinitis: A condition in which the lining of the nose, back of the mouth, and throat is inflamed. It becomes abnormally sensitive and can be irritated by cold air, fumes, strong odors, spicy foods, or tobacco smoke. A person with rhinitis may experience itching or soreness, and may have a blocked or runny nose.

Allergic rhinitis: Rhinitis that is caused by allergy. This means that the person's immune system reacts to specific substances (allergens) that do not bother most people. The most common allergens to cause allergic rhinitis when breathed into the nose are from house dust mites, pets, pollen, and molds.

How Allergic Rhinitis Can Affect Your Asthma

It is important to know if you or your child has allergic rhinitis, because allergic rhinitis can make asthma harder to control. Effective treatment for allergic rhinitis can reduce the chance of severe asthma attacks, and make the lungs work better. Allergic rhinitis can also cause problems with sleep and concentration at work or school.

Runny nose, blocked nose, and sneezing are caused by inflammation (swelling and irritation) of the lining of the nose and throat. The most effective treatments are corticosteroid nasal sprays: medications sprayed into the nose to prevent inflammation. The medications in these sprays are similar to inhaled preventers for asthma. People who have both asthma and allergic rhinitis should use both a preventer nasal spray and a preventer asthma puffer regularly.

People with asthma may not recognize that they also have allergic rhinitis, because the symptoms can be mistaken for asthma. International guidelines for doctors recommend that people with asthma should be checked for allergic rhinitis.

What Are the Symptoms of Allergic Rhinitis?

The most obvious and easily recognized type of allergic rhinitis is "hay fever." Hay fever causes itchy, runny nose and eyes during times of the year when people come into contact with pollens or other airborne allergens. But not everyone with allergic rhinitis has these symptoms. Symptoms of allergic rhinitis can be any combination of itching (in the nose, back of throat, and eyes), sneezing, runny nose or eyes, and a blocked nose. Allergic rhinitis can occur all year round when the allergen is dust mite or pet allergens.

Allergic rhinitis can cause any of these symptoms:

- Frequent sore throats

- Hoarse voice

- A frequently blocked nose with no other symptoms

- A frequent throat-clearing cough, especially in children

- Breathing through the mouth, especially in children

361

- Snoring

- A feeling of pressure over the sinuses (on the front of the face and head)

- Frequent unexplained headaches

- Frequent middle ear infections, especially in children

- Coughing, especially in children when they lie down at night

- Bad breath

- Loss of sense of smell

- Disturbed or unsatisfying sleep, with daytime tiredness and poor concentration

- Frequent unexplained respiratory symptoms in a person whose asthma is stable and well controlled with appropriate treatment.

What Causes Allergic Rhinitis?

The most common allergens for people with allergic rhinitis are pollens, house dust mites, pets, molds, and cockroaches.

Seasonal allergic rhinitis (hay fever) is usually triggered by wind-borne pollen from grasses, weeds, or trees. Symptoms are most common in spring and summer, but can occur at different times depending on the region and rainfall. In tropical regions, pollens can be in the air all year round. The amount of pollen in the air is highest:

- in the morning;

- outside;

- on windy days;

- after thunderstorms.

Allergic rhinitis that persists throughout the year (perennial allergic rhinitis) is typically caused by allergy to house dust mites, pets, or molds. Most people with allergic rhinitis are allergic to more than one substance (typically pollen and house dust mites), so many will have symptoms all year or for weeks to months at a time.

Food allergies do not cause allergic rhinitis. When the nose becomes runny or blocked as a reaction to food (e.g. spicy foods, wine), this is not due to allergy but may indicate irritation or a chemical intolerance. Rhinitis in response to fumes (e.g., fragrances and paints) is not an allergic reaction, though it may respond to the treatments for allergic rhinitis.

How Do Doctors Diagnose Allergic Rhinitis?

Doctors assess whether a person is likely to have allergic rhinitis by considering symptoms, finding out about the person's environment, doing a physical examination, checking asthma control, and investigating allergies. Usually, the doctor will check for rhinitis, then investigate whether this is caused by allergies. Most cases of rhinitis are due to allergy.

Your doctor may ask you about:

- when your symptoms started and whether they have become better or worse over time;

- whether you normally have symptoms at particular times of the year;

- anything that seems to trigger the symptoms or relieve them;

- allergic conditions (including asthma due to allergies, skin allergies) and whether family members have allergies;

- any medications you have tried (e.g. over-the-counter nasal sprays or tablets);

- your home environment, type of work, and leisure activities.

Your doctor may also:

- measure how well your lungs are working using a spirometer, or arrange for you to have this test. If you normally test your own lungs using a peak flow meter at home each day, bring your results.

- offer allergy tests—either skin-prick tests or blood tests, or arrange for you to have these tests done by a specialist.

- suggest that you try using a nasal spray for a few weeks.

- refer you to an allergy specialist or an ear, nose, and throat surgeon.

Allergy Tests

Skin prick testing and blood tests (radioallergosorbent test [RAST]) are often done to confirm which triggers will set off your rhinitis. The results of allergy tests provide useful information when analyzed together with information about your symptoms and other medical history.

Other methods that claim to test for allergies (e.g., cytotoxic food testing, kinesiology, Vega testing, pulse testing, reflexology, and hair analysis) are not useful tests and should not be used.

Avoid Things That Make Your Allergic Rhinitis Worse

People with allergic rhinitis should not smoke and should avoid other people's cigarette smoke. Smoking makes asthma and rhinitis worse, and can prevent medications from working properly. Campfires and wood smoke may worsen allergic rhinitis and asthma.

Often the same allergens will trigger both allergic rhinitis and asthma, so it is useful to identify triggers and avoid them if possible. Avoiding common allergens like pollens and house dust mites can be difficult and expensive.

What Is the Best Treatment for Allergic Rhinitis?

Corticosteroid (Anti-Inflammatory) Nasal Sprays

Most people with allergic rhinitis will benefit from using nasal sprays containing medications that reduce inflammation in the lining of the nose (corticosteroids). These medications are available over the counter and on prescription. Your doctor can advise which is best for you.

For best results, these medications are taken regularly and long term, just like preventers for asthma. Corticosteroid nasal sprays for allergic rhinitis have a good safety record, including in children and people of all ages with asthma.

It can take up to two weeks to experience the full effect of treatment, so your doctor or pharmacist may suggest that you also use another medication for a short time to relieve your symptoms immediately.

For people who experience allergic rhinitis symptoms only part of the year, and can predict when symptoms will occur, it is sometimes possible to take a corticosteroid nasal spray for six weeks or more, then stop.

Other Medications

- Antihistamine tablets (available over the counter) are effective against itching and sneezing. They can be used alone (for people who only need intermittent relief) or in combination with other medications including nasal sprays. Newer antihistamines are less sedating. Your doctor or pharmacist may advise you to take antihistamines before going anywhere that usually triggers your allergy symptoms.

- Antihistamine nasal sprays (available over the counter) can provide quick relief of itching and sneezing. They can be used as well as a corticosteroid nasal spray.

- Decongestant nasal sprays and tablets are used to unblock the nose. These should never be taken for more than a few days at a time.

- Saline irrigations: Your doctor may recommend that you use a salt water (saline) solution daily to help clear your nose and soothe the lining of the nose. Various types are available from pharmacies.

Other medications may be prescribed by your doctor or suggested by your pharmacist.

Before taking any medication for allergic rhinitis, you should tell your doctor or pharmacist if:

- you have any other medical conditions or are pregnant;

- you are taking other medications (including over-the-counter, complementary medicines, or food supplements);

- you have been experiencing nose bleeds.

I'm Pregnant—Can I Take Allergic Rhinitis Medications?

If you have troublesome symptoms of allergic rhinitis, or if effective medication for your allergic rhinitis helps control your asthma symptoms, your doctor might recommend that you take medication while you are pregnant.

Some corticosteroid nasal sprays have a good safety rating for pregnancy. There is also good evidence for the safety of these medications from very large numbers of pregnant women who have taken these same medications in an inhaled form (puffer) for asthma.

If you discover that you are pregnant while using medications for allergic rhinitis, tell your doctor. Most allergic rhinitis medications have no particular safety concerns for pregnant or lactating women, so the risk of harm to the fetus is very low. While medications are generally avoided in pregnancy, particularly during the first trimester, some allergic rhinitis medications have been taken by pregnant women with no evidence of harm.

How Is Allergic Rhinitis Treated in Children?

Treatments for allergic rhinitis in children are generally similar to those used in adults:

- Corticosteroid nasal sprays are appropriate in children who need long-term treatment, and some can be used in children as young as three years.

- Newer, less sedating oral antihistamines are effective for children whose symptoms are only mild or only need intermittent treatment. Some can be taken by children as young as twelve months. The older, more sedating antihistamines should be avoided.

What Is Immunotherapy (Desensitizing Therapy)?

Specific allergen immunotherapy (desensitization) is an effective treatment for allergic rhinitis in some people and can achieve lasting relief from symptoms. Over time, it reduces the immune system's tendency to overreact to an allergen.

Immunotherapy may be considered if your allergic rhinitis is mainly due to one allergen that you cannot avoid. To find out if this treatment option might work for you, you need to be referred to a specialist allergist.

Oral and injectable forms of immunotherapy are available. Injectable immunotherapy, which is by far the more common form, involves weekly to monthly injections over two to three years. Side effects can occur, including serious allergic reactions. It is not safe for people with severe or poorly controlled asthma. Oral immunotherapy involves daily treatment at home, and is expensive.

Follow-Up

After you have begun taking medication for allergic rhinitis, whether over-the-counter or prescribed by a doctor, tell your doctor so that your allergic rhinitis can be checked whenever you have an asthma check-up. You may need to visit a specialist or doctor with expertise in allergy if:

- your symptoms are severe or not responding to treatment;

- you think you may have to change jobs or move to improve your allergic rhinitis;

- the diagnosis is not certain.

Section 28.4

Sinusitis

Sinusitis is an inflammation or infection of one or more of the sinuses that drain into the nose. The lining of the nose and sinuses produce a protective layer of mucus to trap bacteria and inhaled particles. Tiny hairs called "cilia" project from the nasal and sinus lining and clear mucus from the sinuses.

Sinusitis often occurs when the lining of the nose and sinuses becomes inflamed and swollen, thereby blocking one or more openings that allow the sinuses to drain. Additionally, the cilia are unable to clear mucus from the sinuses. When the mucus cannot drain properly, it builds up in the sinus, allowing bacteria to multiply and cause an infection.

People with allergies are more likely to have problems with sinusitis because of the swelling and inflammation that can block the nose and sinuses. Viruses, such as colds or flu, and enlarged adenoids or polyps may also cause a blockage that prevents adequate sinus drainage. This increases the chance for sinusitis.

Sinusitis and Asthma

Chronic sinusitis may complicate asthma because of the chronic inflammation that can affect the entire airway including the nose and the lungs. An asthmatic with sinusitis may show peak flows that drop into the yellow zone. You may not have an acute asthma episode, but if you have a case of sinusitis, you may be more susceptible to exercise and irritant triggers. A sinus infection is often at the root of recurrent asthma attacks; preventing and controlling sinus disease is a key to managing asthma.

Do I Have a Sinus Infection?

Allergies are the most common cause of recurrent or chronic sinusitis and it might be difficult sometimes to differentiate between the two. Some of the chronic symptoms include:

- nasal congestion;
- several days of green or yellow nasal discharge;
- post-nasal drip;
- persistent cough, especially in the early morning or at night;
- bad breath;
- recurrent sinus headaches;
- dark circles or swelling under the eyes;
- sinus pressure;
- toothaches or facial pain;
- frequent asthma episodes.

If sinusitis is suspected, it is important that the ears, nose, and lungs are examined. Some people may have chronic sinusitis lasting for several months or more, with recurrent flare-ups. Your doctor may suggest a computed tomography (CT) scan to view the sinuses more effectively. The doctor may perform a rhinoscopy, where a small, flexible tube with fiber optics is placed inside the nose to view the sinuses, throat, and vocal cords.

Treatment

If the diagnosis of chronic sinusitis has been made, antibiotics are usually ordered for at least three weeks. A follow-up CT scan may be necessary to make sure the infection has completely cleared. Many allergy and sinus specialists will not order the first CT scan until at least a three- to four-week course of antibiotics has been tried. Decongestants, saline irrigations, and corticosteroid nasal sprays also may be used. For people with allergies, it is important to keep the allergies well controlled with avoidance measures, medication, and allergy injections for desensitization if necessary. Also, be sure that you keep asthma controlled by using the medications outlined by your asthma care plan.

Chapter 29

Dealing with Other Co-Existing Conditions

Chapter Contents

Section 29.1

Anaphylaxis

What Is Anaphylaxis?

- Anaphylaxis is a severe allergic reaction.
- Different parts of the body can be affected all at once.
- Anaphylaxis is most often caused by foods, medicines, or insect stings. It can be caused by other things, such as latex or exercise.
- This type of reaction usually occurs within a few minutes after contact.
- Anaphylaxis almost always occurs within an hour after contact, but can happen up to a few hours later.
- Antihistamine medicines will not prevent or stop anaphylaxis.
- Anaphylaxis is a medical emergency. Death can occur.

Asthma and Anaphylaxis

- Anaphylactic reactions can be worse if you also have asthma, especially if asthma is not well controlled.
- Trouble breathing can occur with both asthma and anaphylaxis. It usually comes on more quickly with anaphylaxis.
- Adrenalin (epinephrine) is needed to treat anaphylaxis.
- Asthma inhalers will not work for anaphylaxis.
- Some allergies, such as dog, can trigger asthma, but are unlikely to cause anaphylaxis.

Signs of Anaphylaxis

- Severe hives or itching that happen over minutes and affect most of the body

- Sudden swelling of the lips, tongue, throat, or face
- Drooling or trouble swallowing
- Sudden breathing problems such as cough, wheeze, or feeling short of breath
- Severe repeated vomiting
- Dizziness or fainting

Managing Anaphylaxis

- See an allergy doctor to confirm allergies.
- Learn how to avoid the things you are allergic to. Make sure to avoid them.
- Always carry your epinephrine auto-injector (EpiPen or Twinject). It can save your life.
- Check your auto-injector's expiry date. Replace it when it is expired. Review when and how to use it regularly.
- Use your auto-injector at the earliest sign of anaphylaxis. Do not wait for breathing problems.
- If in doubt, use the EpiPen or Twinject!
- As soon as it is used, call 911 or have someone take you to the nearest emergency department.
- Make sure that family, friends, and other caregivers know about your allergy and anaphylaxis plan.
- Make sure they know how to use the auto-injector.
- Wear a MedicAlert bracelet if you are at risk for anaphylaxis.

Section 29.2

Eczema

"Asthma and Eczema," © 2010 Children's Asthma Education Centre
(www.asthma-education.com). Reprinted with permission.

What Is Eczema?

- Eczema is a chronic disease which causes the skin to become red, swollen, and very itchy.

- Atopic (allergic) dermatitis (eczema) is the most common form of eczema.

- Eczema affects about 10 percent of children.

- In young children, eczema usually appears on the face, chest, back, and the outside of the arms and legs.

- In older children, eczema often appears on the hands, neck, ankles, behind the knees, and on the inside of the elbows.

- Eczema usually starts before age two. Often, eczema gets better by age five.

- Children have a 40 percent chance of outgrowing eczema by the time they become adults.

- You cannot catch eczema from someone else.

- Eczema can run in families. If one parent has eczema or another allergic disease (asthma, hay fever, or food allergy), the child has a greater chance of having eczema and other allergic diseases. The chances are even greater if both parents have eczema or allergies.

- Certain things can trigger eczema to get worse.

What Triggers Eczema?

Triggers are different from one child to the next but scratching is the most common problem.

Things that may make eczema worse are:

- dry skin;
- viral infections;
- irritants such as soaps, fabric softeners;
- some fabrics, such as wool or synthetic fabrics;
- stress;
- heat or sweating;
- dust or mold.

Scratching eczema will make it worse. Dry, itchy skin will cause the child to scratch and worsen eczema. Certain times of year, for example winter, may be worse.

Some allergies such as food, pets, or dust mites can worsen eczema. An allergist can help identify possible allergic triggers.

Skin infections can make eczema worse. Antibiotics are used to treat the skin infection.

Treatment and Control of Eczema

Learn what things trigger your child's eczema and avoid them. Dry skin makes eczema worse. To help keep skin moist:

- Use moisturizers every day.
- Give short baths in lukewarm water every day.
- Use as little soap as possible or mild unscented soaps when needed.
- Gently pat the skin.
- Use an unscented moisturizer immediately after a bath (and several times a day if needed).
- Medicated creams are sometimes needed. Follow your doctor's instructions on how to apply them.
- Keep your child's fingernails short.

Dress your child in cotton clothing. Wash the clothes in mild unscented detergent and double rinse with clean water. Do not use fabric softeners in the dryer.

Keep your home cool.

Asthma and Eczema

- Childhood eczema is associated with other allergic diseases such as hay fever, food allergies, and asthma.

- Eczema may be the first sign of allergies in a child. Half of children with asthma also have eczema.

- Eczema does not cause asthma or other allergic diseases.

- Speak to your doctor if your child shows possible signs of asthma.

Common Signs of Asthma in Children

- Frequent colds that last longer than seven to ten days

- Coughing, often at night, early in the morning, or with exercise

- Wheezing

- Chest tightness or difficulty breathing

Section 29.3

Gastroesophageal Reflux Disease

A nagging question for patients with poorly controlled asthma and for their doctors is the following: might acid reflux be playing a role in making the asthma difficult to control, and might treatment of acid reflux help to control asthma? New information from a well-done experiment is available to help answer this question.

Nearly everyone has experienced an episode of reflux at least once. We are speaking of the regurgitation of stomach contents—stomach "juices"—from the stomach back up the esophagus (swallowing tube) into the chest. Reflux is typically experienced as a burning sensation behind the breastbone, or the regurgitated liquid may suddenly appear in the back of the throat, bringing with it a bitter or sour taste or the taste of recently eaten food.

A muscle that rings the esophagus at its end where it meets the stomach is meant to tighten, preventing food, stomach acid, and digestive juices from returning back "the wrong way" out of the stomach. However, in some people this muscle sphincter is unusually lax and allows frequent return of stomach contents into the esophagus, particularly when one lies down and gravity no longer helps to keep material in the stomach. Stomach acid that is repeatedly splashed onto the lining of the esophagus can cause serious problems and is considered a disease: gastroesophageal reflux disease, or GERD. People with GERD may experience severe chest pain and think that they are having a heart attack. Or they may have a vague sense of tightness in their chest, feeling unable to get a full, satisfying breath, not too dissimilar to an asthma attack. It is even possible to have stomach acid reflux all the way up the esophagus to one's throat, where small amounts can be unknowingly breathed onto the bronchial tubes. You can imagine that aspiration of even tiny amounts of stomach acid onto the breathing tubes will be bad for asthma!

Silent Reflux

To make matters more complex, it is possible to have acid reflux and not know it. It is said that as many as half the people with reflux may have no symptoms at all, so-called silent reflux. If one measures for the regurgitation of stomach acid into the esophagus (using an instrument called a pH probe to record the acidity or pH of the liquid in the esophagus), one finds abnormally frequent reflux of stomach acid occurring in people without any symptoms. How often does this happen in people with asthma? It depends who is doing the testing and in which patients, but anywhere from one-third to two-thirds of asthmatic patients tested had abnormal acid reflux.

It is clear that asthma and acid reflux are both common and interrelated. It is possible for severe and symptomatic GERD to cause asthma to worsen, as well as to cause chest symptoms that feel like one's asthma is acting up. And poorly controlled asthma, along with some of the medicines used to treat it, can cause more frequent reflux. But what is the role of "silent" or minimally symptomatic reflux in causing asthma to worsen? If your asthma is not well controlled despite appropriate treatment, should you be worried that acid reflux is playing a role, even in the absence of symptoms of heartburn?

That specific question was addressed in a research study recently published in the *New England Journal of Medicine*. Doctors investigated the role of silent or minimally symptomatic reflux in approximately four hundred persons whose asthma remained poorly controlled despite taking their controller medication (an inhaled steroid) every day. All of the subjects in the study were tested for acid reflux; and half were given an intensive treatment to neutralize stomach acid (esomeprazole or Nexium taken twice daily), whereas the other half received an identical-looking placebo tablet to be taken twice daily. The outcome: 40 percent of the subjects had asymptomatic acid reflux, but treatment with a powerful therapy to treat their "silent reflux" had no impact on their asthma. Their asthma was not better controlled if they took esomeprazole rather than placebo. They did not feel better, they did not have better lung function (peak flow tests), and they did not experience fewer flare-ups of their asthma.

So, now we know. If you have asthma and troublesome symptoms of GERD, it is worthwhile treating the acid reflux. You will feel better, protect your esophagus from harmful effects of stomach acid, and perhaps help to get your asthma under control. But if you have asthma and are not troubled by symptoms of acid reflux, then it is not worthwhile taking treatments for acid reflux on the possibility that silent reflux is making your asthma worse. Asymptomatic reflux is not the cause of poorly controlled asthma; it is necessary to look elsewhere.

Section 29.4

Obesity

Is it my weight or is it my asthma that is causing my symptoms?

Research into the link between increasing levels of obesity and asthma still hasn't come up with a definite answer. There is a recognized association between increasing body mass index (BMI) and increased levels of diagnosed or reported asthma in both children and adults, and it's possible that there are other factors, e.g., genetic or environmental that may lead to both conditions. We do know that being obese makes asthma a lot more of a problem.

People who are obese are more likely to have asthma, to have more severe asthma, and to need more medication to control it.

Obesity can lead to people being breathless and wheezy without having asthma, so it's important that you get a proper diagnosis from your doctor. Once you have that, and the right medications, you should be able to increase your activity levels without getting too breathless, and start living an active life.

Why does obesity make asthma worse?

Having a larger amount of fat on the body means there's more pushing onto and into the chest, so there's less room for the lungs to move. This causes the muscles around the airways to contract more, causing more asthma symptoms.

Airways in obese people with asthma are more likely to stay closed in normal breathing, so there's less oxygen exchange able to happen.

Obesity causes general inflammation in the body, which makes asthma symptoms worse.

People who are obese are more likely to have problems with reflux and obstructive sleep apnea (where you stop breathing while asleep), both of which can make asthma worse.

There has been some suggestion in research studies that people who are obese might have less response to some asthma medications. The reason for this is not clear, and more research is needed to clarify this.

Will losing weight really help my asthma?

Losing weight can have a big impact on your asthma; it can improve your symptoms and reduce your need for medication. In fact if you are overweight or obese, losing weight might have a greater impact on your asthma control than increasing medication. If you have asthma and are overweight or obese you should discuss weight control and healthy lifestyle with your doctor as part of your asthma management.

Remember: it is important that you don't change your medication without speaking with your doctor first.

Having a healthy lifestyle with regular activity and a balanced diet is important for everyone.

Section 29.5

Depression

Research has shown that there is a link between depression and asthma. In fact, having severe asthma more than doubles the risk of developing depression. Around one in five women and one in eight men will experience depression in their life, and these numbers are even higher in people with asthma. As with other chronic illnesses, research shows that having severe asthma more than doubles the risk of developing depression.

What is depression?

Depression is a serious health condition, not just a low mood. People with depression can have trouble doing normal activities, and it can have serious effects on mental and physical health.

How can depression and asthma affect each other?

Having both depression and asthma worsens health more than either condition alone.

Having depression makes it less likely that people will be treated for asthma effectively. This may be because of poor memory and problem-solving skills with a shortened attention, making it harder to recognize the need to get medical help.

People with depression have trouble concentrating or staying motivated. This may make them less likely to get help with their asthma, keep appointments, and take medication.

Having uncontrolled asthma can make it harder to join in with fun activities such as playing sports or other recreational activities. This can make people with depression further isolated and low in motivation.

Stress can be a trigger for both asthma and depression.

How do I know if I'm depressed?

There are different checklists on the internet you can check to get a better idea if you or someone you know may have symptoms of depression. Depression is more than just stress and needs proper diagnosis by a health professional. You should talk to your doctor to learn more and get correct treatment.

What can I do?

Both depression and asthma can be treated, but first need to be recognized and diagnosed by a health professional. There are a number of treatments for depression, both therapy and medication-based. It is important to have a treatment plan that monitors both the symptoms of depression and asthma in order to find the treatment that works best for you. Some things you can do yourself include:

- Learn relaxation techniques.
- Get your asthma well controlled so you can take part in activities without being limited by your symptoms.
- Learn as much as you can about both conditions.
- Get help and support from family and friends.
- Visit a doctor regularly to review both your asthma and your depression.

Chapter 30

Lifestyle Modification for Asthma Control

Chapter Contents

Section 30.1

Exercise and Asthma

"Asthma and Exercise," © 2010 Children's Asthma Education Centre (www.asthma-education.com). Reprinted with permission.

Exercise Facts

- Exercise makes your heart and lungs stronger.
- Exercise increases muscle strength.
- Exercise improves posture and makes you more flexible.
- Exercise improves self-esteem, confidence, and gives you energy.
- Feeling short of breath may be normal when you exercise. But when you stop exercising, the shortness of breath should go away.

Asthma Facts

- Asthma is a chronic disease of the airways in the lungs.
- Children with asthma can lead healthy, active lives.
- Asthma can be different for each person.
- Asthma cannot be cured, but it can be controlled.

Asthma and Exercise

- Regular exercise is important for everyone, especially if you have asthma.
- People with asthma should be able to do any exercise or play any sport.
- More than one in ten Olympic athletes have asthma.
- Exercise may trigger asthma symptoms during or five to ten minutes after you start exercising.
- Well-controlled asthma should not limit exercise.

- If asthma stops you from being active, your asthma is out of control. See your doctor.

- The only exercise people with asthma should not do is scuba dive.

Asthma Symptoms during Exercise

- Don't start exercising if you are having asthma symptoms.

- Asthma symptoms may include cough, wheeze, shortness of breath, or a tight feeling in the chest.

- You may have other symptoms such as tiring easily or not being able to keep up with your friends.

- Prolonged exercise (e.g., running, soccer, hockey) is more likely to cause symptoms than short bursts of exercise such as volleyball or tennis.

- Exercising in a warm, humid setting (e.g., swimming) may be less likely to cause symptoms.

- If you have asthma, exercise can cause symptoms, but exercise does not cause asthma.

Prevent symptoms by:

- Keeping your asthma under control.

- Starting to exercise slowly. Work up to a more demanding exercise.

- Always warming up before exercising and cooling down after.

- Using your reliever medicine ten to fifteen minutes before exercise.

- Breathing through your nose, if possible, instead of your mouth when you exercise.

- Avoiding exercising outside when air pollution is bad or pollen counts are high. Exercise indoors instead.

- Covering your mouth and nose with a scarf or neck warmer when exercising outside in cold air.

Section 30.2

Nutrition and Asthma

The best diet for asthma is one that follows the dietary guidelines for general good health. Some people may need to avoid some foods if they get asthma symptoms after eating them.

Foods That Are Good for Asthma

Although no food will cure asthma, reports from around the world show that people who eat plenty of fresh fruits and vegetables, lean meat, and fish have healthier lungs.

Body Weight and Asthma

If you are overweight or obese, losing weight can reduce symptoms of asthma.

Food Allergy and Asthma

People who have both food allergy and asthma are at greater risk of having a fatal reaction and must eliminate the food completely. An accredited practicing dietitian can provide expert advice on how to avoid and replace the food with suitable alternatives.

Food Chemicals and Asthma

Foods are made of many different chemicals. Some chemicals are natural and some are added to foods. A few food chemicals can cause symptoms of asthma. Fortunately, only a small number of people with asthma have symptoms after eating these food chemicals. If food chemicals are suspected of causing symptoms, an accredited practicing dietitian can assist in identifying the food chemicals responsible and provide the advice and support needed to maintain a healthy diet.

Dairy Products and Asthma—A Common Myth

You may have been told that dairy products "make mucus" and that they are not good for asthma. This is false for most people with asthma and dairy products are well tolerated by the majority of people with asthma.

If you suspect that food is causing symptoms of asthma, first consult your doctor. An accredited practicing dietitian can assist in the investigation of adverse food reactions and provide expert advice on how to best meet nutritional needs.

Chapter 31

Traveling with Asthma

Chapter Contents

Section 31.1

Tips for Traveling with Asthma

The fun of traveling is being in a completely different place. But if you have asthma, a new environment can seem less fun because there's always the worry that something unexpected may cause an asthma flare-up. But you can take steps to help avoid problems while you're away from home—so you can concentrate on the fun.

Before You Go

Before you leave, make sure your asthma is well controlled. If it has been flaring up, check with your doctor before you head off on your trip. He or she may need to adjust your medicine or ask you to come in for a visit.

When packing, remember all medicine you're taking for your asthma, including rescue and controller medicines. Keep your medications in your carry-on bags so they're always with you. It's also a good idea to pack a little extra medication, so you don't run out while you're on the road.

If you'll be leaving the country, it can help to have a letter from your doctor that describes your asthma and your medicines. This can help you with airport security or customs. You also might want to know the generic names of your medicines. These are the chemical names of the medicine, not the brand name the drug company has given it. If you need to get a refill in another country, the medication might have a different brand name. You can get the generic names from your doctor's office or pharmacist.

Other things to pack include your peak flow meter (if you use one), a copy of your asthma action plan, your health insurance card, and your doctor's phone number.

Windows Up or Down?

Trains, buses, and even your family car might have dust mites and mold trapped in the upholstery or the ventilation system. You can't do much about a bus or train (except make sure you've taken your controller medication and have your rescue medication handy).

But if you're traveling by car, ask the driver to run the air conditioner or heater with the windows open for at least ten minutes. If pollen or air pollution trigger your asthma and counts are high during your trip, travel with the windows closed and the air conditioner on.

Finding the Friendly Skies

Although smoking on airplanes used to be common, it is now banned on all commercial flights of U.S. airlines. It is also banned on foreign airline flights into and out of the United States.

But smoking is still permitted by law on charter flights. If you find yourself on a charter flight, ask about their smoking policy and ask to be seated in the nonsmoking section.

The air on planes is also very dry, and this can trigger an asthma flare-up. Make sure you have your rescue medications handy and try to drink a lot of water.

Home Away From Home

If you're staying in a hotel, you may find that something in the room triggers your asthma. Requesting a sunny, dry room away from the hotel's pool might help. If animal allergens trigger your asthma, ask for a room that has never had pets in it. And you should always stay in a nonsmoking room. If it's possible, bringing your own blanket and pillow can help prevent a flare-up.

If you're staying with family or friends, tell them in advance about your triggers. They won't be able to clear away all dust mites or mold, but they can dust and vacuum carefully, especially in the room you'll sleep in. You also can ask them to avoid using scented candles, potpourri, or aerosol products, if those bother you.

Just like at home, you'll want to avoid tobacco smoke. Ask anyone who smokes to step outside, especially if you're sharing a room. Wood fires in the fireplace or woodstove also could be a problem for you.

Traveling on Your Own

If possible, carry a copy of your asthma action plan so people who are traveling with you (or the people you're staying with) can help if you have any breathing trouble. If you don't have a copy of your plan, let these people know which medicines you take, what the dosages are, and the number where your parents and your doctor can be reached, in case of an emergency.

Without your parents along, you will have more responsibility for your asthma. Keep your triggers in mind and take steps to avoid them. If pollen bothers you, find out what the readings are on a day when you'll be going for a hike or taking part in other outdoor activities. If air pollution bothers you, make sure you keep that in mind when you're visiting a smoggy city. Cities like Los Angeles make information on air pollution levels available through their weather services.

If you're planning to take part in any new activities while you're away, talk to your doctor about them before you leave. And whatever you do, make sure your rescue medication is nearby in case you need it.

Of course, you'll want to forget about your asthma and have fun while you're away. And the best way to do this is by planning ahead and having your medication with you—so you don't have to worry if you do have a flare-up. If you ignore your asthma completely by not taking precautions, there's a chance you could end up in the emergency department. And that's no way to spend a vacation.

Section 31.2

Asthma Travel Checklist

Create an asthma travel pack to ensure you have all of the medicines and instructions you need in one, easily accessible place. When creating your asthma travel pack consider including:

- copies of your asthma action plan;

- an extra written prescription in case medication is lost or destroyed;

- insurance card and healthcare provider contact information;

- both quick-relief and controller medications (make sure there is enough to get you through your stay, and extra in case you get held over unexpectedly);

- a spacer/chamber;

- a peak flow meter.

Chapter 32

Asthma and the Law: The Americans with Disabilities Act

Americans with Disabilities Act: How It Affects You

Has your child been rejected by a preschool or excluded from a field trip because a teacher was afraid to use his or her EpiPen? Does a moldy carpet at work or school make you sick? Does stale smoke in offices, hotel rooms, or conference centers make it hard for you to take part in routine business activities?

The Americans with Disabilities Act (ADA) is a civil rights law that gives you the right to ask for changes where policies, practices, or conditions exclude or disadvantage you. As of January 26, 1992, public entities and public accommodations must ensure that individuals with disabilities have full access to and equal enjoyment of all facilities, programs, goods, and services.

The ADA borrows from Section 504 of the Rehabilitation Act of 1973. Section 504 prohibits discrimination on the basis of disability in employment and education in agencies, programs, and services that receive federal money. The ADA extends many of the rights and duties of Section 504 to public accommodations such as restaurants, hotels, theaters, stores, doctors' offices, museums, private schools, and child care programs. They must be readily accessible to and usable by individuals with disabilities. No one can be excluded or denied services just because he or she is disabled or based on ignorance, attitudes, or stereotypes.

"Americans with Disabilities Act," reprinted with permission from the Asthma and Allergy Foundation of America, www.aafa.org, © 2005. All rights reserved. Reviewed by David A. Cooke, M.D., FACP, May 2011.

Does the ADA Apply to People with Asthma and Allergies?

Yes. In both the ADA and Section 504, a person with a disability is described as someone who has a physical or mental impairment that substantially limits one or more major life activities, or is regarded as having such impairments. Breathing, eating, working, and going to school are "major life activities." Asthma and allergies are still considered disabilities under the ADA, even if symptoms are controlled by medication.

The ADA can help people with asthma and allergies obtain safer, healthier environments where they work, shop, eat, and go to school. The ADA also affects employment policies. For example, a private preschool cannot refuse to enroll children because giving medication to or adapting snacks for students with allergies requires special staff training or because insurance rates might go up. A firm cannot refuse to hire an otherwise qualified person solely because of the potential time or insurance needs of a family member.

In public schools where policies and practices do not comply with Section 504, the ADA should stimulate significant changes. In contrast, the ADA will cause few changes in schools where students have reliable access to medication, options for physical education, and classrooms that are free of allergens and irritants.

How Will the ADA Work?

In most cases, employees and employers, consumers and businesses, and administrators and students will work together to improve conditions and remove barriers to promote equal access and full inclusion.

Marie Trottier, Harvard University's administrator of disability services, explains that her role includes educating nonallergic managers, colleagues, and coworkers about the needs of people with environmental sensitivities. She also trains staff in education and employment policies, benefits, and procedures.

"Changes depend as much on interpersonal consideration as they do on legal rights," she says. "It shouldn't be uncommon for people with asthma and allergies to get the same respect for their needs as people with more visible disabilities."

When Ms. Trottier arranges for accommodations in offices, classrooms, and student housing, she considers the nature of the disability and the specifics of each situation. She might install an air conditioner or arrange for an office with a window that opens. She has relocated a microwave oven and reorganized office spaces to help people with allergies avoid cooking odors.

Employees might need prior notice of renovation or lawn care projects so they can modify their schedules to avoid the irritants and allergens.

Professors may ask students not to wear scented products to class. Students affected by dust, paper fibers, or ink can have someone borrow library materials for them or they can use an online computer system. Ms. Trottier says that "all of these options for students and employees require time and energy, flexibility and creativity, more so than money." A sign in her office underscores her point, "Attitudes are the real disabilities."

Making the ADA Work for You

If you or your child would like consideration due to asthma or allergies, speak with a school administrator, manager, employer, human specialist, or disabilities service coordinator. He or she should know the procedure for collecting necessary information and planning appropriate changes, aids, or services. You can call on a variety of sources for advice and creative practical ideas.

Under Section 504, public schools and programs cannot avoid their responsibility by claiming to have limited funds or resources. Nor can they impose a "disparate impact" on people with disabilities. The ADA requires public accommodations to make changes, except in cases where an "undue burden" would result.

The law does not define "undue burden." It depends on the organization's size and the real costs of the changes. The business or program must show that it properly assessed the individual's needs and tried to find the necessary changes.

Don't be Afraid to Speak Up

The ADA prohibits retaliation, harassment, or coercion against individuals who exercise their rights or assist others in doing so. If you feel you have been treated unfairly, you may file a complaint with the U.S. Attorney General, who refers complaints to the appropriate agency. The attorney general can bring lawsuits to seek money damages and civil penalties in cases of general public importance, or where there is a "pattern or practice" of discrimination.

Individuals can also file a private suit to get a court order requiring a business or program to make necessary changes and to pay attorney's fees. Other remedies may include reinstatement in your job and back pay.

The ADA Is Evolving

Court decisions and rulings will slowly define how the ADA will affect us. The real momentum for change will come as we work creatively together to promote the inclusive attitudes and environments that fulfill the promise of the ADA for ourselves and our children.

Part Five

Pediatric Asthma

Chapter 33

Basic Facts about Asthma in Children

Asthma is a chronic inflammation of the airways with reversible episodes of obstruction, caused by an increased reaction of the airways to various stimuli. Asthma breathing problems usually happen in "episodes" or attacks but the inflammation underlying asthma is continuous.

Asthma is one of the most common chronic disorders in childhood, currently affecting an estimated 7.1 million children under eighteen years; of which 4.1 million suffered from an asthma attack or episode in 2009.[1]

An asthma episode is a series of events that results in narrowed airways. These include: swelling of the lining, tightening of the muscle, and increased secretion of mucus in the airway. The narrowed airway is responsible for the difficulty in breathing with the familiar "wheeze."

Asthma is characterized by excessive sensitivity of the lungs to various stimuli. Triggers range from viral infections to allergies, to irritating gases and particles in the air. Each child reacts differently to the factors that may trigger asthma, including:

- respiratory infections, colds;

- allergic reactions to allergens such as pollen, mold, animal dander;

- feathers, dust, food, and cockroaches;

- exposure to cold air or sudden temperature change;

- cigarette smoke;

- excitement/stress;

- exercise.

Secondhand smoke can cause serious harm to children. An estimated four hundred thousand to one million asthmatic children have their condition worsened by exposure to secondhand smoke.[2]

Asthma can be a life-threatening disease if not properly managed. In 2006, 3,613 deaths were attributed to asthma. However, deaths due to asthma are rare among children. The number of deaths increases with age. In 2006, 131 children under fifteen died from asthma compared to 653 adults over eighty-five.[3]

Asthma is the third leading cause of hospitalization among children under the age of fifteen. Approximately 32.7 percent of all asthma hospital discharges in 2006 were in those under fifteen, however only 20.1 percent of the U.S. population was less than fifteen years old.[4]

In 2005, there were approximately 679,000 emergency room visits were due to asthma in those under fifteen.[5]

Current asthma prevalence in children under eighteen ranges from 5.2 percent in South Dakota and Idaho to 14.4 percent in Delaware.[6]

Since 1999, mortality and hospitalizations due to asthma have decreased and asthma prevalence has stabilized, possibly indicating a better level of disease management.

Asthma medications help reduce underlying inflammation in the airways and relieve or prevent airway narrowing. Control of inflammation should lead to reduction in airway sensitivity and help prevent airway obstruction.

Two classes of medications have been used to treat asthma—anti-inflammatory agents and bronchodilators. Anti-inflammatory drugs interrupt the development of bronchial inflammation and have a preventive action. They may also modify or terminate ongoing inflammatory reactions in the airways. These agents include inhaled corticosteroids, cromolyn sodium, and other anti-inflammatory compounds. A new class of anti-inflammatory medications known as leukotriene modifiers, which work in a different way by blocking the activity of chemicals called leukotrienes that are involved in airway inflammation, have recently come on the market.

Bronchodilators act principally to dilate the airways by relaxing bronchial smooth muscle. They include beta-adrenergic agonists, methylxanthines, and anticholinergics.

The annual direct healthcare cost of asthma is approximately $15.6 billion; indirect costs (e.g., lost productivity) add another $5.1 billion, for a total of $20.7 billion. Prescription drugs represented the largest single direct cost, at $5.9 billion.[7]

Asthma is one of the leading causes of school absenteeism;[8] in 2008, asthma accounted for an estimated 14.4 million lost school days in children with an asthma attack in the previous year.[9]

Notes

1. Centers for Disease Control and Prevention: National Center for Health Statistics, National Health Interview Survey Raw Data, 2009. Analysis by the American Lung Association Research and Program Services Division using SPSS and SUDAAN software.

2. California Environmental Protection Agency: Respiratory Health Effect of Passive Smoking, June 2005.

3. Centers for Disease Control and Prevention. National Center for Health Statistics. Final Vital Statistics Report. Deaths: Final Data for 2006. April 17, 2009. Vol 57 No 14.

4. Centers for Disease Control and Prevention: National Center for Health Statistics, National Hospital Discharge Survey, 2006. Unpublished data provided upon special request to the NCHS.

5. Centers for Disease Control and Prevention: National Center for Health Statistics, National Hospital Ambulatory Medical Care Survey, 2005. Unpublished data provided upon special request to the NCHS.

6. Centers for Disease Control and Prevention: National Center for Health Statistics, National Survey of Children's Health through State and Local Area Integrated Telephone Survey, 2007. Analysis by the American Lung Association Research and Program Services Division using SPSS and SUDAAN software.

7. National Heart, Lung and Blood Institute Chartbook, U.S. Department of Health and Human Services, National Institute of Health, 2009.

8. Centers for Disease Control and Prevention. National Center for Chronic Disease Prevention and Health Promotion.

Healthy Youth! Health Topics: Asthma. August 14, 2009. Accessed on February 9, 2010.

9. Centers for Disease Control and Prevention: National Center for Health Statistics, National Health Interview Survey Raw Data, 2008. Analysis by the American Lung Association Research and Program Services Division using SPSS and SUDAAN software.

Chapter 34

Asthma and Babies

In babies, it is often difficult to distinguish asthma from other more common airway conditions that cause cough and wheeze; however, most other airway conditions are less likely than asthma to persist.

What Is Asthma?

Asthma is a condition in which the airways are over-reactive, resulting in them narrowing and restricting airflow. This narrowing comes about because:

- the smooth muscle in the airway walls tightens (contracts);

- the cells lining the airways become inflamed and swollen; and

- extra mucus builds up in the airways.

In adults, asthma usually causes breathlessness, a feeling of chest tightness, wheeze, and coughing. In a severe asthma attack breathing can be very difficult.

In babies younger than twelve months, the airways are already small so it doesn't take much inflammation or contraction to cause symptoms. A recurring wheeze can be the first indication that a baby might have asthma. However, the presence of a cough alone does not tend to indicate asthma, as only very rarely is coughing the only symptom of asthma.

What's Causing My Baby's Coughing and Wheezing?

It is not always easy for doctors to tell whether a baby has asthma or another condition causing similar symptoms, especially before twelve months of age. There are many other causes of wheezing in babies apart from asthma that must be considered.

Bronchiolitis is a common condition of babies under six months old. Most cases occur between late autumn and early spring. Caused by a virus, bronchiolitis starts like a cold, then the baby often wheezes, coughs, and breathes quickly. There may also be a fever. Bronchiolitis generally lasts about ten days; the cough, however, may last for weeks. In some infants, especially young babies, bronchiolitis can be severe, occasionally requiring hospitalization.

Other conditions apart from asthma and bronchiolitis that can cause cough and/or wheeze in babies under twelve months are:

- respiratory viruses; and

- croup, an infection mainly affecting the larynx (voice box) and trachea (windpipe), causing the baby to have a harsh, barking cough.

And, less commonly:

- cystic fibrosis;

- lung development problems, including those due to a premature birth;

- milk aspiration (milk flowing into the airways instead of the stomach during feeding);

- a foreign body in the airways; and

- heart problems.

Most babies who have recurrent wheezing grow out of it by early childhood, and do not end up with asthma. Several things may suggest to your doctor that asthma is likely:

- several respiratory symptoms; for example, cough, shortness of breath, and wheeze;

- frequent wheezing;

- severe wheezing spells, especially after six months of age;

- close relatives having a history of asthma, eczema, or urticaria;

- premature birth;

- being exposed to cigarette smoke either before or after birth; and

- improvement when given an inhaled asthma medicine.

However, a definite diagnosis of asthma may not be possible until your child is old enough for lung function tests—usually seven years old or older.

Can I Stop My Baby Getting Asthma?

Asthma seems to be a product of the complex interplay between a baby's genes and a baby's environment, both before and after birth, especially in the first year of life.

The most important thing you can do to help prevent asthma is not smoke while pregnant or after your baby is born. Tell your partner, other family members, and friends not to smoke inside the house or anywhere near the baby.

In terms of other measures that are sometimes suggested to reduce the risk of a child developing asthma, the National Asthma Council gives the following advice:

- Breastfeeding should be encouraged, as it has many benefits for your baby. Breastfeeding may reduce the risk of asthma in early childhood, but as yet there is no evidence that breastfeeding protects against asthma for longer than this.

- If you are not breastfeeding, hydrolyzed milk formulas seem to be associated with a slightly lower risk of childhood asthma than other formulas, including those made from soy.

- Giving your baby omega 3 fatty acid supplements does not appear to reduce the risk of childhood asthma or wheeze.

- Taking probiotics during late pregnancy and while breastfeeding (or giving probiotics to formula-fed babies) does not seem to prevent asthma.

- Avoiding potential allergens in the diet (e.g. eggs, milk, nuts, and shellfish) while pregnant or breastfeeding, or omitting these foods from an older baby's diet, does not appear to prevent asthma. (However, the National Health and Medical Research Council [NHMRC] recommends that whole cow's milk is introduced only from about twelve months of age.)

405

- Avoiding house dust mites does not seem to prevent asthma in young children.

- At present, it is not clear whether having a pet in the house protects against asthma or increases the risk of asthma in children.

It is recommended that you do not go on a restriction diet during pregnancy or when breastfeeding—unless you need to do so for a definite food allergy that you have had diagnosed—as this appears to have no influence over your baby developing asthma, and it may lead to you eating a diet that is poor for both you and your developing baby. Always check with your doctor or dietitian before making changes to your diet during pregnancy or breastfeeding or to your baby's diet.

Treating Asthma in Babies

If your baby needs asthma medicine, your doctor will explain how to give this to the baby. A reliever medicine with or without a preventer medicine may be prescribed; both are likely to be inhaled (breathed in) rather than swallowed.

For babies and very young children, the inhaler is attached to a small spacer chamber, which is attached to a face mask. The inhaler is pressed by the parent or doctor to dispense the medicine into the holding chamber, and the baby's own breathing then draws in the medicine from the spacer via the face mask.

Alternatively, a nebulizer may be used with a face mask. A nebulizer is a device that makes a liquid medicine into a fine vapor, ready for inhalation.

If your baby has been treated with asthma medicine and gets better on this treatment your doctor may wish you to continue with this approach. You will need to have your baby checked regularly by the doctor as changes in treatment are likely as your baby grows.

If your baby continues to cough or wheeze despite a trial of asthma medicine, this may mean that your baby needs to be reassessed as another condition may be causing their symptoms.

If your baby has been diagnosed with asthma, your doctor will teach you how to know when your baby's asthma is getting worse, and will give you an asthma action plan that tells you which medicine to give if this happens, and when to contact your doctor or a hospital.

The asthma action plan is an important part of keeping your baby's asthma well controlled. It is also important to make sure your baby has regular check-ups and is given any prescribed medicine regularly.

Chapter 35

Benefits of Breastfeeding in Preventing Childhood Asthma: A Controversial Issue

Chapter Contents

Section 35.1

Study Shows Link Between Breastfeeding and Lower Incidence of Asthma in Children

A Sunderland academic has discovered a link between breastfeeding and a lower incidence in asthma in young children.

Dr. Mohammad Shamssain and his research team recently completed a two-phase study into the prevalence and severity of asthma in children in the North-East. Their research focused specifically on the positive benefits of breastfeeding in the prevention of asthma, and also the effect of obesity on the prevalence of asthma among young children.

Dr. Shamssain and his team analyzed seven thousand schoolchildren in the region aged six to fifteen years.

The team discovered that children who had been breastfed for six months or more had a significantly reduced risk of asthma—particularly among young boys.

Dr. Shamssain says: "Breastfed children showed lower prevalence rates of asthma, rhinitis, and eczema, and the effect of breastfeeding was more evident in boys than girls. Asthma and wheeze were resolved significantly earlier in breastfed children than those who were not breastfed."

The University of Sunderland team discovered that breastfeeding lowers the incidence of allergic disorders, and that children breastfed from four to nine months had a significantly lower risk of asthma. Those breastfed up to seven to nine months had lower instances of persistence wheezing and coughing.

Dr. Shamssain says: "Breastfeeding is a cost-effective approach to a significant prevention of allergic disease in children. Our research demonstrates that exclusive breastfeeding prevents the development of allergic diseases in children."

In the second part of the study Dr. Shamssain's team discovered that both boys and girls in the highest body mass index (BMI) percentile, and therefore classified as obese, have higher prevalence rates of asthma and respiratory symptoms (wheeze, cough, breathlessness, and exercise-induced wheezing) than non-obese children.

Dr. Shamssain says: "The association between overweight and exercise-induced wheezing is stronger in boys than girls. In boys, the risk of being overweight is associated with exercise-induced wheezing, lifetime asthma, and current wheeze. In girls, the risk of being overweight is mainly associated with exercise-induced wheezing."

"These results demonstrate that obesity is a definite risk factor in asthma among young children, and there are gender differences regarding the respiratory risk of obesity."

Dr. Shamssain presented his findings at the European Respiratory Society in Berlin in October 2008.

Section 35.2

Study Reports Breastfeeding Does Not Protect Against Asthma

"Breastfeeding Does Not Protect Against Asthma, Allergies,"
September 12, 2007. © McGill University (www.mcgill.ca).
Reprinted with permission.

Breastfeeding does not protect children against developing asthma or allergies, says a new study led by McGill University's Dr. Michael Kramer and funded by the Canadian Institutes of Health Research (CIHR). The findings were pre-published online September 11, 2007, by the *British Medical Journal*.

Dr. Kramer—James McGill Professor of Pediatrics, Epidemiology and Biostatistics at McGill University and Scientific Director of CIHR's Institute of Human Development, Child and Youth Health—and his colleagues followed 13,889 children who had been selected at birth from thirty-one Belarussian maternity hospitals in the randomized Promotion of the Breastfeeding Intervention Trial (PROBIT). The follow-up took place from December 2002 to April 2005, when the children were 6.5 years old.

In the survey, a control group of maternity hospitals and affiliated polyclinics was randomized to continue their traditional practices, while those in the experimental group were trained to teach better breastfeeding techniques and to encourage mothers to breastfeed as long and as exclusively as possible. At the end of the trial, the researchers concluded that breastfeeding does not provide any protection against asthma or allergies. "We found, not only was there no protective effect," said Dr. Kramer, "but the results even suggested an increased risk of positive allergic skin tests."

PROBIT was led by Dr. Kramer in collaboration with Drs. Robert Platt and Bruce Mazer of McGill and colleagues from the Belarussian Maternal and Child Health Research Institute. The study was conducted in Belarussian maternity hospitals because the former Soviet republic had not yet adopted many of the so-called "baby-friendly" innovations now common in most western countries. "At the time we began this trial in the mid-1990s, the former Soviet countries still had very rigid rules, like the maternity services offered here thirty years ago," explained Kramer. "In a western country, we just wouldn't have been able to make a large difference between the control and the experimental groups."

"Belarus, like most former Soviet and other Eastern European countries, has much lower rates of allergy and asthma than places like Canada, and there's considerable debate as to why that is." explained Dr. Kramer. "However, our results are similar to those found in nonrandomized cohort studies in New Zealand, where allergy and asthma are even more common than they are in Canada. This suggests that there is nothing unusual about the setting that would explain our results."

Dr. Kramer remained positive about the benefits of breastfeeding. "In the first phase of our project, we observed reductions in gastrointestinal infections and atopic eczema for the first year of life. I urge mothers to continue to breastfeed."

Chapter 36

Diagnosing Asthma in Children

Chapter Contents

Section 36.1

Special Issues in Diagnosing Asthma in Children

Excerpted from "How Is Asthma Diagnosed?" National Heart Lung and Blood Institute, National Institutes of Health, February 2011.

Most children who have asthma develop their first symptoms before five years of age. However, asthma in young children (aged zero to five years) can be hard to diagnose.

Sometimes it's hard to tell whether a child has asthma or another childhood condition. This is because the symptoms of asthma also occur with other conditions.

Also, many young children who wheeze when they get colds or respiratory infections don't go on to have asthma after they're six years old.

A child may wheeze because he or she has small airways that become even narrower during colds or respiratory infections. The airways grow as the child grows older, so wheezing no longer occurs when the child gets colds.

A young child who has frequent wheezing with colds or respiratory infections is more likely to have asthma if:

- one or both parents have asthma;
- the child has signs of allergies, including the allergic skin condition eczema;
- the child has allergic reactions to pollens or other airborne allergens;
- the child wheezes even when he or she doesn't have a cold or other infection.

The most certain way to diagnose asthma is with a lung function test, a medical history, and a physical exam. However, it's hard to do lung function tests in children younger than five years. Thus, doctors must rely on children's medical histories, signs and symptoms, and physical exams to make a diagnosis.

Doctors also may use a four- to six-week trial of asthma medicines to see how well a child responds.

Section 36.2

Lung Function Testing in Children

Lung (or pulmonary) function tests are performed for a variety of reasons in children. They may help with making the diagnosis and determining the severity of respiratory disease, and also help with monitoring response to treatment.

What Types of Tests Are Available?

The more commonly used tests in older children include spirometry and peak flow measurement. Other tests, which are available at respiratory departments in teaching hospitals, include exercise testing and measurement of lung volumes.

There are also some more specialized tests that have mainly been used in research but are now beginning to be used in clinical practice.

Spirometry

Spirometry is a test of lung function that measures the amount of air breathed in and out. Children older than seven years are usually able to perform spirometry. They may be tested with a spirometer in their doctor's surgery or local laboratory.

Spirometry gives a measure of the maximum amount of air a person can breathe out (after taking in a deep breath) and how much they can breathe out in one second.

Spirometry is commonly used in older children to help make a diagnosis of asthma, to determine how severe asthma is, and monitor the success of treatment. It is also part of the routine management of people with respiratory diseases that get worse with time (such as cystic fibrosis) or progressive neuromuscular conditions (such as Duchenne muscular dystrophy).

Peak Flow Measurement

Peak flow meters measure the greatest speed reached when a person breathes out through the meter as hard and fast as possible (having taken a deep breath in first). Peak flow measurement is not the recommended test for diagnosing asthma.

A peak flow meter is a small portable device that can generally be used by children older than seven years. Your doctor may suggest using a peak flow meter at home as part of monitoring the status of your child's asthma and the success of their treatment, but spirometry is the best test to determine the severity of asthma at any given point in time.

Other Tests

Lung volume measurements are used for distinguishing between people with obstructive airways disease and air trapping (such as may occur in cystic fibrosis) and people with restrictive lung disease (such as in some neuromuscular diseases).

Exercise testing may be used to assess older children (older than eight years) who complain of shortness of breath, often associated with exercise. It can help to determine whether the diagnosis may be asthma, restrictive lung disease, anxiety, or lack of fitness.

Section 36.3

Pediatric Allergy Testing

"Allergy Testing in the Pediatric Specialty Clinic," © 2005 the
University of Iowa (www.uihealthcare.com). Reprinted with permission.
Reviewed by David A. Cooke, M.D., FACP, August 2011.

Allergy testing may be done during your child's clinic visit.

We believe it is important to know what your child may be experiencing in order that you and your child are better able to prepare for the visit. As a parent you are best able to choose the most appropriate way to inform your child. In general, most children can be told one to two days before the visit. If your child is an anxious child or a very young child, you may want to wait until the day of or until shortly before the start of the procedure.

Be honest about the day's destination and purpose, and assure your child that you will be with him or her throughout the testing.

Why perform allergy testing?

An allergy test helps to identify things in your environment that may be causing your child's symptoms and enable the doctors to decide what type of medications, if any, may be needed to treat your child's condition. By identifying these things, changes can be made in your living space to potentially improve your child's health. For instance, if the test identifies your child is allergic to feathers; feather pillows could be replaced with a different type of pillow.

What happens during allergy testing?

The most common types of allergy tests used are the puncture and intradermal allergy tests. Your child's physician will decide which type of testing will be used. In many cases, both types are combined to provide the most useful information.

Puncture allergy testing: A child having this test will be asked to remove his or her shirt and lie on his or her stomach while the test is applied on the back. A nurse will write letters on the child's back with an ink pen to label the areas where the test will be applied. The area is then cleaned. Drops of an allergen solution are placed on the spokes of a plastic test applicator. An allergen is a thing in your child's environment that may cause an allergic reaction. The applicator is then pressed on the child's back. Patients have described this sensation as feeling "like a hair brush being pressed on their back." Once the test is placed, each test location will have a drop of wet liquid. The patient will then be asked to lie very still for approximately fifteen minutes to keep the drops of liquid from running together. This is important to keep the drops of different allergens from running together. Children may be tested for as many as thirty environmental allergens during this test. (The number could be higher if the child is being screened for food allergies in addition to the environmental allergens if food allergy testing is necessary. Individual cases vary at the discretion of the physician).

Intradermal allergy testing: A child having this test will be asked to remove his or her shirt, and sit upright as the test is applied to the upper arms. (If you are comfortable doing so, the child may sit on a parent's lap during the test application).

A nurse will write letters on the child's arms with an ink pen to label the areas where the test will be applied. The area is then cleaned. Small amounts of allergen are injected with a small needle syringe just below the surface of the skin. A child having this test can be tested for up to fourteen allergens, each requiring individual injections.

A small reaction (similar to a mosquito bite) will appear within approximately fifteen minutes if the test is positive. To be sure the test is effective, a control solution (histamine) will be applied. A positive reaction at this test site indicates the test is accurate.

A nurse will measure areas of reaction with a small ruler after test time has elapsed. Your child may experience some mild discomfort with "itching" from the testing. Applying a cool wet cloth following the reading of the test often relieves this discomfort.

What do I say if my child wants to know if allergy testing will hurt?

Each child is different in his or her ability to tolerate pain or discomfort. It is important to let your child know that they will probably experience some discomfort-especially during the intradermal testing. It is very important to be honest in answering their questions. Be honest about medical events at all costs. A child who has been deceived may lose trust with the medical team, and with you as a parent. Trust is a very difficult thing to rebuild. Finding out that testing is necessary may lead to some tears at the time of the discussion, but in the long run is healthier for your child's ability to cope.

Chapter 37

Issues in Treating Asthma in Children

Chapter Contents

Section 37.1

What to Ask Your Doctor about Your Child's Asthma Care

Asthma is a problem with the airways that bring oxygen to your lungs. A person with asthma may not feel symptoms all the time. But when an asthma attack happens, it becomes hard for air to pass through your airways. The symptoms are coughing, wheezing, chest tightness, or shortness of breath.

Below are some questions you may want to ask your doctor or nurse to help you take care of your child's asthma.

- Is my child taking asthma medicines the right way?

  - What drugs should my child take every day (called controller drugs)? What should I do if my child misses a day?

  - Which drugs should my child take when he or she is short of breath (called rescue drugs)? Is it okay to use these rescue drugs every day?

  - What are the side effects of these medicines? For what side effects should I call the doctor?

  - How will I know when the inhalers are getting empty? Is my child using the inhaler the right way? Should my child be using a spacer?

- What are some signs that a child's asthma is getting worse and that I need to call the doctor? What should I do when my child feels short of breath?

- What shots or vaccinations does my child need?

- How do I find out when smog or pollution is worse?

- What sort of changes should I make around the home?

  - Can we have a pet? In the house or outside? How about in the bedroom?

- Is it okay for anyone to smoke in the house? How about if my child is not in the house when someone is smoking?

- Is it okay for me to clean and vacuum when my child is in the house?

- Is it okay to have carpets in the house?

- What type of furniture is best to have?

- How do I get rid of dust and mold in the house? Do I need to cover my child's bed or pillows?

- Can my child have stuffed animals?

- How do I know if I have cockroaches in my home? How do I get rid of them?

- Can I have a fire in my fireplace or wood-burning stove?

- What does my child's school or daycare need to know about my child's asthma?

  - Do I need to have an asthma plan for the school?

  - How can I make sure my child can use the medicines at school?

  - Can my child participate fully in gym class at school?

- What types of exercises or activities are better for a child with asthma to do?

  - Are there times when my child should avoid being outside?

  - Are there things that I can do before my child starts exercising?

- Does my child need tests or treatments for allergies? What should I do when I know my child will be around something that triggers their asthma?

- What type of arrangements do I need to make when we are planning to travel?

  - What drugs should I bring? How do we get refills?

  - Who should I call if my child's asthma gets worse?

Section 37.2

Inhaler or Nebulizer: Which One Should My Child Use?

November 2009, reprinted with permission from www.kidshealth.org. Copyright © 2009 The Nemours Foundation. This information was provided by KidsHealth, one of the largest resources online for medically reviewed health information written for parents, kids, and teens. For more articles like this one, visit www.KidsHealth.org, or www.TeensHealth .org.

Some kids who need asthma medicine start out using a nebulizer. Others are given an inhaler with a spacer and face mask. Some older kids use only an inhaler, with no spacer attached. So which is the best way to deliver asthma medicine to the lungs?

Studies show that the device used really doesn't matter, as long as it's used properly. All methods work just as well when the correct technique is used.

Of course, there are pros and cons to each type of device. Inhalers are smaller and require no power source. And because they deliver the medicine much more quickly than a nebulizer, they may be preferred by some parents.

The age of the child also makes a difference in how an inhaler is used. Metered dose inhalers (MDI) are the most widely used, but they require coordination. The child must be able to activate the device and breathe in at the same time. This can be a bit tough and can generally only be mastered by older kids. That's why many doctors recommend attaching the metered dose inhaler to a spacer.

Almost anyone (from infants to the elderly) can use a metered dose inhaler when it's attached to a spacer. Some experts say that everyone with asthma, even adults, would benefit by using a spacer with their metered dose inhaler.

Dry powder inhalers (DPI) are easier to use than metered dose inhalers because they don't require coordination. The force of the child's inhaled breath delivers the aerosolized powder into the lungs. Most kids over five or six years old are able to use a dry powder inhaler, although they must be able to inhale quickly and strongly.

However, some people may feel like they get a better treatment from a nebulizer because they can see and feel the mist coming from the machine.

Your doctor will work with you and your child to decide which device is most appropriate. Besides your child's age and abilities, the decision also will be based on what type of medication is needed. Your child may try several different types of devices before you find the right one.

Used properly, though, any device will be effective. Talk with your doctor if you have any questions, especially if you're concerned that your child isn't getting the proper dose of medicine.

Section 37.3

Helping Your Child Cooperate While Using a Nebulizer

"How Can I Help My Child Cooperate While Using the Nebulizer?" October 2010, reprinted with permission from www.kidshealth.org. Copyright © 2010 The Nemours Foundation. This information was provided by KidsHealth, one of the largest resources online for medically reviewed health information written for parents, kids, and teens. For more articles like this one, visit www.KidsHealth.org, or www.TeensHealth.org.

A nebulizer is an electric- or battery-powered machine that turns liquid asthma medicine into a fine mist that's inhaled into the lungs. Nebulizers are often used with young kids because they require little effort on the child's part. But the child does need to stay in one place and cooperate. And if you have a young child, you know how challenging that can be.

Most nebulizers come equipped with a face mask (they're also available with a mouthpiece). A child wears the mask and breathes normally for five to ten minutes until the medicine is gone. A child who doesn't stay still and cooperate may not get a proper dose of the medicine. For instance, if the mask is held a half inch (1.27 centimeters) away from the face, half of the medicine won't reach the lungs. Increase that distance to an inch (2.54 centimeters) and 80 percent of the medicine is lost.

It might seem as though a crying child takes deeper breaths, which can lead a parent to think that the child will inhale the medication more deeply when crying. In fact, the opposite is true. Crying is a long exhalation followed by a very rapid inhalation to catch one's breath. Almost none of the medication will make it to the lungs if given while the child is crying.

For an infant, you may be able to use the nebulizer while your child is sleeping or your child might be cooperative while being held. But what about older babies and toddlers? They might be frightened by the face mask and are sure to resist sitting still.

Here are some suggestions for making nebulizer use easier and more enjoyable:

- Make it part of your daily routine. Use the nebulizer at the same time (or times) each day, so your child knows what to expect.

- If your child is afraid of the mask, you can talk about how it's a "pilot mask" or a "space mask." You might even buy a video about pilots or astronauts and use some of the lingo like "start your engines" before you turn the nebulizer on. You also can buy masks shaped like dragons and other animals.

- Allow your child to decorate the nebulizer machine with stickers.

- Try having your child sit in a highchair. If that doesn't work, your little one might prefer sitting in your lap.

- Make the time your child has to sit still as fun as possible. Read stories, sing songs, or pull out some special toys only available during nebulizer time.

- Watch a short DVD or video together.

- If your child is old enough, encourage him or her to help you put the mask on, hold the tubing, and turn the machine on.

- Praise your child for a job well done!

Section 37.4

What to Do When Your Child Doesn't Take His or Her Asthma Medication

"What If My Child Doesn't Take His or Her Asthma Medication?" November 2009, reprinted with permission from www.kidshealth.org. Copyright © 2009 The Nemours Foundation. This information was provided by KidsHealth, one of the largest resources online for medically reviewed health information written for parents, kids, and teens. For more articles like this one, visit www.KidsHealth.org, or www.TeensHealth.org.

One of the best ways to help kids manage asthma, besides avoiding triggers, is to make sure they take their medicine as prescribed. The effect of skipping medication will vary depending on what kind it is.

What Controller Medications Do

Also called preventive or maintenance medications, controller medicines work over time to reduce airway inflammation and help prevent asthma symptoms from occurring. Kids need to take these medicines regularly, even when feeling fine.

If One or More Doses Is Skipped

Although skipping a dose appears to have no immediate effect, it allows the lungs to slowly get more irritated, putting a child at increased risk of an asthma flare-up.

When taking controller medicine as directed, kids may be better able to tolerate triggers, such as a cold or tobacco smoke, without getting a flare-up. But if they're not taking the controller medicine correctly, the lungs won't be functioning as well and these irritants can cause an asthma flare-up.

What Rescue Medications Do

Also called quick-relief or fast-acting medications, rescue medicines work immediately to handle asthma symptoms when they occur. These types of medicines are often inhaled directly into the lungs, where they open up the airways and relieve symptoms such as wheezing, coughing, and shortness of breath, often within minutes.

If One or More Doses Is Skipped

If a child doesn't use his or her rescue medications during an asthma flare-up, the airways can continue to tighten until the child ends up in the emergency department. So it's important for kids to always have rescue medication available and to take it as directed by the doctor.

Involving kids in their asthma treatment can help ensure that they take the asthma medications appropriately. Explain how the medicines work and how much your child needs to take. Having an asthma action plan can help both of you learn what you need to know.

It's also important to stress these two key concepts to kids:

- They should take their controller medication as directed, even when feeling well.

- Rescue medication should be kept on hand, no matter where the child is.

You can help by prompting your child to take controller medications and reminding him or her to take rescue medication along when leaving the house. Also make sure that your child doesn't run out of medicine.

Resist the temptation to adjust medication dosages above or below the prescribed amounts. If you're noticing that your child seems to be doing better or worse, talk with the doctor about whether changes are needed. Also be sure to talk with the doctor if side effects are a concern. He or she may be able to adjust the dosage or prescribe a different medication.

Section 37.5

Safety of Inhaled Steroids for Children with Asthma

"Inhaled Steroids Safe and Effective for Children with Asthma,
NHLBI Study Shows," National Institutes of Health, October 11, 2000.
Editor's note added by David A. Cooke, MD, FACP, May 2011.

Inhaled corticosteroids are safe and effective for the long-term treatment of children with mild to moderate asthma, according to the "Childhood Asthma Management Program (CAMP)," a five-year, eight-center study funded by the National Heart, Lung, and Blood Institute (NHLBI) of the National Institutes of Health. The study appeared in the October 12, 2000, *New England Journal of Medicine (NEJM)*.

CAMP is the longest and largest controlled study of treatments for childhood asthma to date. It showed that inhaled corticosteroids provide superior asthma control. Their only side effect was a temporary one—a small reduction in the children's rate of growth observed just in the first year of treatment. The inhaled corticosteroids significantly reduced airway hyper-responsiveness, the heightened sensitivity in the airways that leads to asthma symptoms following exposure to certain irritants and allergens. However, their use did not result in the anticipated improvements in measures of lung function.

"Although asthma experts around the world have recognized the effectiveness of inhaled corticosteroids in treating asthma, their long-term effects in children were not clear, and questions have been raised about their possible effects on growth," said NHLBI Director Dr. Claude Lenfant. "CAMP confirms their effectiveness while providing reassuring evidence about their safety."

"We hope these results will convince more physicians, and parents as well, that treating children with mild to moderate asthma with inhaled corticosteroids will result in better asthma control and improved quality of life, " he added.

Asthma is the most common chronic respiratory disease of childhood throughout the world, and its prevalence has been increasing in epidemic proportions worldwide. In the United States, asthma affects close to five million children, approximately 30 to 40 percent of whom are estimated to have mild to moderate asthma (symptoms more than twice a week). Childhood asthma is a leading cause of school absences—resulting in more than eleven million lost schooldays a year. It is currently estimated to cost the U.S. economy nearly $2 billion each year.

CAMP involved more than one thousand children ages five to twelve with mild to moderate asthma. The children were randomly assigned to receive either budesonide, an inhaled corticosteroid; nedocromil, a nonsteroidal anti-inflammatory medication; or a placebo. All children were also provided with a beta-agonist for use, as needed, to relieve symptoms.

CAMP showed that the inhaled corticosteroid provided superior asthma control. Compared to children on placebo, children treated with the steroid had 45 percent fewer urgent care visits; 43 percent fewer hospitalizations; 45 percent less use of oral steroids, which are used to treat severe exacerbations; 30 percent fewer days in which additional asthma medication was needed; and 22 percent more episode-free days. The nedocromil group had 27 percent fewer urgent care visits and 16 percent less use of oral steroids, compared to the group on placebo, but there was no difference between the nedocromil and placebo groups in hospitalizations, use of additional medications, or episode-free days.

The only side effect from the inhaled corticosteroids was a slight, but temporary, reduction in growth rate. In the first year of the study, the average increase in height in the children treated with budesonide was about three-eighths of an inch less than that of the other children. However, after the first year and throughout the remaining four years of the study, the children on budesonide grew at an identical rate to the other children. Wrist x-rays taken at the end of the study suggest that the adult height of these children will be the same as that of the children taking nedocromil or placebo. (A second study in the October 12, 2000, *NEJM*, which followed children with asthma into adulthood, found that the children with asthma who received long-term treatment with budesonide attained normal adult height.)

Said Lenfant, "We recognize that even a slight slowing of growth may be a concern for parents. But this effect was short term and temporary—after the first year, the growth rates were the same in all groups. And there are substantial long-term benefits of enabling a child with asthma to be active at play and school, to sleep through the night, and to stay away from the emergency department and hospital."

"We will continue to observe CAMP participants for another four years, by which time most of them will have reached puberty. This will give us a complete picture of the effects of inhaled corticoster-oids on both final adult height and maximum adult lung function," he added.

Several recent smaller studies have suggested that childhood asthma may be associated with impairments in lung growth and a steady decline in lung function. The CAMP investigators hypothesized that treating children with asthma with anti-inflammatory medication might improve lung growth and reduce lung function decline. However, at the end of the study, there were no differences in lung function in any of the groups, when measured after administration of a bronchodi-lator to relax the airways. It is possible that the children had already experienced an irreversible decline in lung function by the time they enrolled in CAMP, and treatment was not started early enough to ef-fect change. Future NHLBI studies will examine asthma treatments in younger children.

The NHLBI's 1991 "Guidelines for the Diagnosis and Management of Asthma," with their emphasis on inflammation, rather than bron-chospasm, as the underlying cause of asthma, marked the beginning of a new approach to treating asthma. The Guidelines recommended anti-inflammatory medications for long-term asthma control in people with frequent asthma symptoms, although data on their long-term effects in children were limited. Since the CAMP study started, new asthma medication have become available, including long-acting beta agonists and leukotriene modifiers, but data on their long-term effects in children are not yet available.

Said Lenfant, "CAMP provides scientific evidence regarding the long-term effectiveness and safety of inhaled corticosteroids for chil-dren. Physicians, other healthcare professionals, and parents should feel comfortable using them to help children with mild to moderate asthma participate fully in childhood activities."

[Editor's Note: Several additional trials have produced results simi-lar to the CAMP trial, supporting the safety of inhaled corticosteroid use in children.]

Section 37.6

Corticosteroids and Chickenpox

Most people think of chickenpox as a common harmless childhood disease. However, children with chickenpox usually have a high fever, feel ill for several days, and develop a rash. The rash includes tiny, clear blisters that start on the chest, back, or belly. Normally, these blisters form scabs and begin to heal in three to four days. In rare cases, chickenpox may result in serious complications, even death.

Are Asthmatic Children Treated with an Oral Steroid at Extra Risk?

Some asthmatic children are treated for months or years with an oral steroid. Other asthmatic children may never receive oral steroid treatment, while others may be treated with a short "burst" of an oral steroid for five to seven days. A burst is prescribed in an emergency situation when asthma is suddenly worse. Children receiving oral steroid treatment rarely have complications from chickenpox.

Are Asthmatic Children Treated with an Inhaled Steroid at Extra Risk?

No. There is no evidence that an inhaled steroid poses an increased risk for asthmatic children exposed to chickenpox. Inhaled steroids reduce asthma symptoms and the need for extra medicine such as oral steroids.

May I Stop My Child's Steroid Therapy to Prevent the Risk of Side Effects from Chickenpox?

No. Stopping prescribed asthma treatment is much more dangerous to the child than the potential risk from chickenpox.

How Do I Prevent My Child from Getting Chickenpox?

Current medical guidelines recommend that almost all children should receive the vaccine. Vaccination helps prevent most cases of chickenpox. Even if a vaccinated child develops chickenpox, the disease should be milder and less likely to have severe complications.

How Do I Know If My Child Has Been Exposed to Chickenpox?

When cases of chickenpox are reported at school, find out if the infected children are in your child's class. If so, your child has been exposed to chickenpox. If your child's playmate becomes infected with chickenpox, your child has been exposed.

What Should I Do After My Child Has Been Exposed?

Check every day for fever and for the tiny chickenpox blisters. Incubation for chickenpox is two to three weeks. Check your child every day for three weeks.

If your child is treated with an oral or injected steroid, call your doctor immediately. Tell the doctor that your child has been exposed to chickenpox. If exposure occurred within the last two days, the doctor may prescribe a shot called Varicella Immune Globulin (VZIG). If your child is being treated with an inhaled steroid but not with an oral steroid, VZIG is not necessary. A special antibiotic, acyclovir, also is available for treatment of asthmatic children with chickenpox.

What Do I Do If My Child Is Receiving or Has Recently Received Oral or Injected Steroids and Becomes Infected with Chickenpox?

Inform your physician *immediately*. Do not wait for a problem to develop.

Remember

Steroid use in asthmatic children under a doctor's care is safe and effective. Complications due to chickenpox exposure are rare. The key to preventing chickenpox complications for children is to vaccinate them with the chickenpox vaccine before they become infected.

Section 37.7

Do Inhaled Steroids Stunt Your Growth?

"Do Inhaled Steroids Stunt Your Growth?" by David A. Cooke, M.D.
© 2004 Omnigraphics, Inc. Updated November 2011.

Teens may worry whether medication used to treat their asthma
will make them shorter as adults. A great deal of research has been
performed on this subject; this section will look at the basis of these
concerns, and describe what the evidence tells us.

What Are Corticosteroids and Why Are They Used?

Corticosteroids are a group of hormones that have widespread effects in the human body. Cortisol is produced in the adrenal glands.
Among many other functions, it influences immune function, metabolism, blood pressure, and bone growth. A number of synthetic hormones
with effects similar to cortisol have been developed to treat a variety of
disease conditions. Commonly used corticosteroids include prednisone,
prednisolone, triamcinolone, beclomethasone, budesonide, mometasone,
ciclesonide, flunisolide, and fluticasone.

Asthma is a disease where chronic airway inflammation is present
throughout the lungs. This inflammation leads to airway narrowing
through muscle spasm, swelling, and excess mucus production. Reducing the inflammation is essential to treating asthma.

Corticosteroids have potent anti-inflammatory effects. In asthma,
they are used to reduce airway swelling and spasm and stop excess
mucus production. This results in less wheezing, less shortness of
breath, and increased ability to participate in everyday activities.

Because the inflammation in asthma is mainly confined to the lungs,
corticosteroids are most often given as an inhaled mist or powder. This
delivers the medication directly to where it is needed.

Important Terms

- **Adrenal Glands:** A pair of yellow, triangle-shaped glands; one
  sits on top of each kidney. They produce many different important hormones.

- **Adult Height:** How tall you are when you stop growing. Most teens stop growing between age fifteen and nineteen; a few may stop sooner or grow longer.

- **Bronchodilators:** Medications that open airways and relieve shortness of breath. Albuterol is one commonly used bronchodilator medication. Most give quick relief, but they don't treat the inflammation that causes asthma.

- **Corticosteroids:** Hormones made in the human body that reduce inflammation. Many are used as medications.

- **Growth Velocity:** How quickly a person is growing. For example, growing one inch taller per year.

- **Inflammation:** Irritated and swollen tissue, packed with angry white blood cells.

- **Leukotriene Modifiers:** Medications which reduce inflammation in a different way than corticosteroids or mast cell stabilizers. Montelukast, zafirlukast, and zileuton are the most commonly used forms. They are also less powerful than corticosteroids, but may be helpful when corticosteroids alone don't stop asthma symptoms.

- **Mast Cell Stabilizers:** Medications to prevent certain cells from releasing hormones that cause more inflammation. Cromolyn and nedocromil are the most commonly used mast cell stabilizers. They have anti-inflammatory effects, but are weaker medications than corticosteroids.

- **Methylxanthines:** An older type of asthma medication that helps open airways. Theophylline is an example. They do not treat inflammation. They are not used often today because of side effects and tricky dosing.

Why Are There Concerns about Corticosteroid Use in Children and Teens?

While corticosteroids reduce inflammation, they have many other effects. When given in high doses, corticosteroids reduce bone growth. In growing children and teens, this might lead to slowed growth and shorter heights as adults.

There is little question that these negative effects of corticosteroids are seen when they are given in high doses for months or years by oral or intravenous routes. Inhaled corticosteroids are given in much lower

433

doses, and they are delivered mainly to the lungs. Some of the inhaled medication is absorbed into the bloodstream from the lungs, however, and could have effects elsewhere in the body.

It's a Fact

Taking your corticosteroid inhaler daily helps prevent:

- wheezing;
- shortness of breath;
- needing to use your "emergency" inhaler;
- emergency department visits;
- hospitalization;
- death.

If Corticosteroids Might Have These Risks Why Don't We Use Other Kinds of Medications?

A number of medications have been developed for treatment of asthma. These include bronchodilators (such as albuterol), mast cell stabilizers (such as cromolyn), leukotriene modifiers (such as montelukast), and methylxanthines (such as theophylline). Each of these medication types have their roles in asthma therapy, and are often used in addition to inhaled corticosteroids.

It has become very clear from clinical studies, however, that corticosteroids are the most effective medications for treating all but the mildest cases of asthma. Many comparative studies between corticosteroids and other medications have been performed. These studies consistently show that corticosteroids are superior to other medications. Corticosteroids improve airflow and ability to exercise, and reduce wheezing, shortness of breath, hospitalizations, and death more than any other medications tested to date.

Accordingly, corticosteroids have become the cornerstone of asthma therapy. There is universal agreement among experts and medical organizations that corticosteroids should be first-line treatment for asthma.

Do Corticosteroids Slow Growth?

A number of studies have looked at rates of growth in children and teens with asthma. Determining the effects of corticosteroids can be difficult for a number of reasons. Severe asthma itself can affect growth, although in general, asthmatic children do not end up shorter than those without asthma. Because corticosteroids are so important in controlling asthma, it is ethically and practically difficult to study severely asthmatic people who do not receive inhaled corticosteroids. Therefore, nearly all studies have been performed in people with mild to moderate asthma symptoms.

The majority of studies have shown a small but significant reduction in growth velocity among children receiving inhaled steroids for asthma. This seems to be greatest in the first one to two years of use, and decreases as time goes on. Some studies have suggested that this effect may be stronger with some drugs than others. However, most experts feel that all inhaled corticosteroids have the potential to slow growth.

So, Does This Mean Corticosteroids Will Make Me Shorter as an Adult?

Interestingly, the answer appears to be no. Although the rate of growth may be somewhat slower with inhaled corticosteroids, multiple studies have concluded that there are little or no effects on final adult height.

Many studies have reported no difference in final height between asthmatic children who received inhaled corticosteroids and those who did not. Among those that did find a difference, the difference was very small: about one centimeter (less than half an inch).

It's a Fact

Inhaled corticosteroids change your adult height by less than a half-inch.

If Corticosteroids Slow Growth Velocity, Why Doesn't This Mean Shorter Adult Height?

This does seem like a contradiction. The studies don't tell us why treated children don't end up shorter, but there are some theories.

While children or teens initially grow more slowly on inhaled corticosteroids, it may be that they later "make up" for the lost growth near the start of treatment. It is also possible that teens on inhaled corticosteroids stop growing at a later age, so that slower growth is balanced by more time for growth.

What's the Bottom Line? Will Inhaled Steroids Stunt My Growth?

The evidence strongly indicates that inhaled corticosteroid use has little, if any, effects on their height as adults. Inhaled corticosteroid use will not stunt your growth.

Each person is different, and your treatment will need to be tailored to your individual needs. If your asthma requires high doses of inhaled corticosteroids, talk to your doctor about making regular growth measurements. Still, for the vast majority of asthmatics, the health benefits of inhaled corticosteroids far outweigh any known or theoretical risks.

Remember

- If you get short of breath more than twice a week, you probably need an inhaled corticosteroid.

- In people with asthma, the benefits of inhaled corticosteroids almost always outweigh their risks.

Chapter 38

Dealing with Asthma Flare-Ups in Children

Chapter Contents

Section 38.1

Handling an Asthma Flare-Up

Flare-ups can be dangerous, so if your child is having them often and using rescue medication more than a couple of times a week, talk to your doctor. It's possible that your child's asthma action plan needs to be adjusted.

Predicting Flare-Ups

The severity and duration of asthma flare-ups vary from person to person and even from attack to attack. They might happen without warning, with sudden coughing, shortness of breath, and wheezing. But because people with asthma have inflamed airways that worsen with gradual exposure to triggers, flare-ups can also build up over time, especially in those whose asthma isn't well controlled.

Flare-ups can and should be treated at their earliest stages, so it's important to recognize early warning signs. These clues are unique to each child and might be the same or different with each asthma flare-up. Early warning signs include:

- coughing, even if your child has no cold;
- throat clearing;
- rapid or irregular breathing;
- unusual fatigue;
- trouble sitting or standing still;
- restless sleep.

A peak flow meter can help predict when a flare-up may be on its way.

Preventing Flare-Ups

Managing your child's asthma includes doing all you can to avoid flare-ups. That means working with your child to:

- take all medication as the doctor prescribed;
- keep rescue medicine on hand at all times;
- take peak flow meter readings as recommended by the doctor;
- avoid triggers, such as allergens.

If Your Child Has a Flare-Up

Not all flare-ups can be prevented, and because they can be life threatening, they demand immediate attention. Your child might need to take rescue medication, visit the doctor, or even go to the hospital. For that reason, you should have an asthma action plan.

Work with the doctor to write this plan, which provides instructions on how to handle changes in your child's breathing. This will help you know exactly what to do, even in an emergency.

Section 38.2

When to Go to the Emergency Room If Your Child Has Asthma

One of the main goals of parents whose kids have asthma is avoiding trips to the emergency room (ER) for breathing problems. But it's also important to know when going to the ER is the right choice.

You'll be better prepared to make that decision if you discuss it with your child's doctor before your child has a severe flare-up. The doctor's instructions should be included in your child's asthma action plan, which also will list peak flow meter readings or specific symptoms that are your cue to go to the ER. If old enough, your child also should know what these signs are.

When to Seek Help

Some general signs that indicate you should seek help very quickly by getting to the doctor (or if the doctor isn't available, going to the ER or calling an ambulance) include:

- if there are changes in your child's color, like bluish or gray lips and fingernails;
- if your child is having trouble talking;
- if the areas below the ribs, between the ribs, and in the neck visibly pull in during inhalation (called retractions);
- if your child uses rescue medications repeatedly for severe flare-up symptoms that don't go away after five or ten minutes or return again quickly;
- if your child's peak flow reading falls below 50 percent and doesn't improve with medication.

Making ER Trips Less Stressful

Advance planning can make trips to the ER less stressful for you and your child. Here are some ways to make it a little easier:

- Know the location of your closest emergency room. If there's a children's hospital ER nearby, go there and have the address and phone number readily accessible (it can be written on your child's action plan).

- If you have other kids, try to make arrangements with a relative or other caregiver who can take them in an emergency situation. But don't let the lack of a babysitter delay your trip to the ER. Someone can always come to the hospital later to pick up your other children.

- Take a copy of your child's asthma action plan or a note with the names and dosages of any medications your child takes to share with the medical staff at the ER.

Following Your Child's Asthma Action Plan

Well-managed asthma is rarely life threatening. People who have died from asthma usually haven't taken their medications as prescribed and have a history of repeated severe asthma flare-ups and emergency care. If you and your child take asthma seriously and work to manage it, you can reduce the chances that your child will need to go to the emergency room.

It's important to monitor your child's asthma using the written asthma action plan your doctor helps you create. This plan will outline your child's day-to-day treatment, list symptoms to watch for, and give detailed, step-by-step instructions to follow when your child has a flare-up.

Some key points of a plan are:

- **Avoiding triggers:** The doctor should be able to help you identify the triggers that can cause asthma flare-ups. These may include animals, dust mites, mold, tobacco smoke, cold air, exercise, and infections.

- **Taking the controller medications:** Your child should take his or her controller medications as prescribed by the doctor, even when feeling fine. Skipping doses can cause the lungs to become more inflamed, which can lead to a decrease in lung function. (This can happen without your child even experiencing any symptoms.) It also puts your child at risk for more frequent and severe flare-ups.

- **Keeping rescue medications on hand:** Many kids go to the ER simply because they didn't have their rescue medications handy. Your child should have rescue medication accessible at all times.

Make Your Child a Partner in Asthma Management

As soon as your child is old enough, make sure he or she understands the asthma action plan and the importance of following it. Some kids with asthma, especially teens, resist taking controller medications and rely instead on their rescue medications to help them on an as-needed basis. This is never a good idea and will increase your child's chances of needing emergency care.

Know the Early Signs of a Flare-Up

Everyone's asthma is different. Some kids cough only at night, while others have flare-ups whenever they get a cold or exercise outside. As you manage your child's asthma, pay attention to what happens before a flare-up so that you know the early warning signs. These signs might not definitively mean that a flare-up will happen, but they can help you to plan ahead.

A peak flow meter is an essential tool in helping to predict a flare-up. Your doctor will give you specific number ranges to watch for.

Other early warning signs of a flare-up can include:

- coughing, even if your child doesn't have a cold;
- tightness in the chest;
- throat clearing;
- rapid or irregular breathing;
- inability to stand or sit still;
- unusual fatigue;
- restless sleep.

Communicating with the Doctor

Be sure to call your doctor at the earliest sign of a flare-up or if you have any other concerns. Being prepared means you might prevent your child's symptoms from worsening and thus can make a trip to the doctor's office instead of to the emergency room.

Section 38.3

Helping Children Cope with Hospitalization

Excerpted from "When a Child Is Hospitalized: Tips and Resources for Parents," © 2011 Vanderbilt Kennedy Center (http://kc.vanderbilt.edu). Reprinted with permission. To view the complete text of this document, including a list of Vanderbilt and other resources, along with recommendations for additional reading, visit http://kc.vanderbilt.edu/site/services/disabilityservices/tipsheets.aspx.

Talking about Going to the Hospital

Whether for a check-up with a pediatrician or an overnight surgery stay, going to the hospital can be a frightening and confusing experience for children of all ages. A difficult thing for many children to understand is why something has to hurt or make them feel badly in order to make them feel better. Not talking with the child at all about going, or telling them too much can make the situation more difficult.

Child Life Specialists

At the hospital, you may encounter a child life specialist, who is an expert in child development. Their job is to help your child cope with hospitalization in the best way possible, through play, preparation, education, and expressive activities like arts and crafts. They are there to provide informational and emotional support for your child and your family, making sure to aid your child's development along the way. In other words, they help your child maintain the best outlook possible on medical experiences—an outlook that they can carry with them for medical experiences in the future.

Although a child life specialist will be available to you once your child enters the hospital, there are several things you can do to help your child cope with the situation at home. Here are some tips organized by age group.

0–3 Years

- If possible, plan doctor's visits or procedures around your child's normal routine.

443

- Bring your child's pacifier, bottle, teddy bear, blanket, or other comforting objects from home.

- Ask friends and family members for their support. Try to be sure that you or one of them is with your child at all times—this can be especially helpful when you need a short break.

- Reassure your child that you will be with them as much as possible.

- Spend time reading to your child about going to the doctor or visiting the hospital.

3–6 Years

- Start preparing your child one or two days in advance.

- Allow them to pack their own overnight bag, choosing which pajamas to bring and other items to include. When packing, have the child include some familiar objects from home, such as favorite toys, blankets, dolls, or stuffed animals.

- If the child will be hospitalized for an extended length of time, it might be helpful to bring a new toy, just to give them something fresh and engaging to lift their spirits along the way.

- Read books about hospitalization or doctor's visits with your child.

- It can be fun and beneficial to play doctor or nurse with your child beforehand, using pretend medical equipment.

6–12 Years

- Start preparing your child four or five days before the appointment if possible.

- Bring favorite toys or games.

- Be honest and up front about the hospital visit.

- Respect your child's questions and concerns and encourage them to express to you what they are thinking or questioning.

- This age group is growing interested in privacy, so you will want to emphasize that their privacy will be respected while in the hospital. As a parent, you also should be ready to advocate for your child's privacy to medical staff.

12–18 Years

- Teenagers understand more information about their hospitalization, but that doesn't mean they understand everything. Encourage them to ask questions—if not to you, then to a doctor or nurse.

- Be sure they are included in decisions that need to be made regarding treatment or the hospital stay.

- They may be worried about their privacy, especially when they may be facing surgery. Ensure them that their privacy will be respected.

- Familiar objects such as their iPod, favorite DVDs, or journals can be helpful.

- Encourage visits or communication from friends and peers, whether via phone, email, or in person.

Chapter 39

Helping Your Child Get a Good Night's Sleep with Asthma and Allergies

Nocturnal asthma. Many parents know all too well the coughing, choking, wheezing, and congestion that can keep their children—and the rest of the family—awake at night.

"When my three-year-old's asthma acts up, it definitely disrupts his sleep and mine," says Allergy and Asthma Network Mothers of Asthmatics (AANMA) member Rachel Gerke. "I know it is bothering him when he is really restless at night, crying or moaning and hitting the sides of the bed when rolling. And when I go in to listen to him he is either breathing faster, usually from his belly, his chest not rising, or I hear a whistle at the end of his breaths."

Rachel's family is not alone. More than twenty million Americans are affected by nocturnal asthma—also called nighttime or sleep-related asthma. The condition has been reported in medical literature for centuries.

AANMA consulted sleep experts—including parents!—for advice to help you and your family get a good night's sleep.

Why We're Losing Sleep

When you breathe in, the lungs transport oxygen into the bloodstream, where it's carried to the rest of the body. When you breathe out, they transport the waste product—carbon dioxide—out of the bloodstream. How well this process works varies throughout the day as part of the body's natural circadian rhythm—an internal clock that regulates body mechanics over a twenty-four-hour period. Lungs work best during the day, with peak lung function at about 4 p.m. Several studies show that twelve hours later—around 4 a.m.—lung function is at its lowest. The fluctuation is usually less than 10 percent. However, people with asthma can have up to a 50 percent difference between daytime and nighttime lung function.

In addition to rhythmic fluctuations, other factors contribute to worsening asthma symptoms during sleep. According to Eli Meltzer, M.D., of the Allergy and Asthma Medical Group and Research Center in San Diego, California, "these factors include changes in the degree of inflammation, the amount of allergen exposure, and the responsiveness patients have to their medications. Not only do short-acting bronchodilators wear off while patients are asleep, their effect over the four to six hours of their activity is less at night than in the day. These conditions result in patients waking up short of breath because they need to take another dose."

Gastroesophageal reflux (often called acid reflux or reflux), a backwash of stomach acid into the esophagus, is also a contributing factor to sleep disturbance. AANMA member Carol O'Leary found reflux to be the cause of her son's sleep problems. "After two and a half years of sleepless nights, my son's acid reflux was finally diagnosed and treated. An effective treatment plan helped our whole family start sleeping better."

Researchers aren't sure exactly how reflux and asthma interact, but they do see a connection—adult studies suggest as many as 75 percent of adults with asthma also have reflux. Reflux can set off asthma symptoms. Because reflux is more common when a person is lying down, people with asthma may have more difficulty during sleep.

Another sleep-related condition that can worsen nighttime asthma is sleep apnea. This sleep disorder causes repeated pauses in breathing throughout the night—a serious problem in itself, but also one that can set off or worsen asthma symptoms. A recent study by the Cincinnati Children's Hospital Medical Center showed that women with asthma are twice as likely to have symptoms of sleep apnea as women without asthma.

"Please don't rule out sleep apnea as a cause of poor sleep—even in children!" says AANMA member Laurie Soares. "My ten-year-old son has asthma and allergies. He snored, was a mouth breather at night, was tired a lot, and had poor height and weight growth. His father has sleep apnea, so with all those factors present we had my son's tonsils and adenoids removed. Since then, he sleeps quietly, is gaining weight, and reports that he now has dreams!"

Allergens—like pollen or mold that cause allergic reactions—can also play a role in sleep problems. Exposure to allergens during the day may set off a chain reaction in the immune system that produces symptoms hours later, as can allergens in the bedroom like dust mites or animal dander.

Studies show that postnasal drip and congestion from allergies can cause multiple nighttime "micro-arousals." These awakenings are so brief that the sleeper doesn't even remember them, but they affect alertness the following day.

The Next Day

The effects of nighttime asthma and allergy symptoms reach beyond the bedroom. Children with nighttime asthma miss more time from school—and their parents more time from work—than healthy children. School and work performance can suffer when the family can't sleep. Children whose rest is disturbed by asthma symptoms have a higher incidence of psychological problems and poor school performance. Studies show that these children score lower on memory and time-limited tests. The most obvious signs that asthma is disturbing someone's sleep are fatigue, irritability, and reduced alertness the following day. According to Dr. Meltzer, other signs to look for include morning headaches, depression, and impaired concentration.

Doctors use the term "allergic fatigue" to describe the tiredness and general lack of energy experienced by people with nasal allergies. This condition is often blamed on antihistamine medications, many of which cause sedation. But recent studies show that, in addition to other factors, poor sleep quality contributes to the exhaustion people with allergies may feel all day long.

Clean Sleep

Eliminating allergens and potential asthma triggers in the bedroom can make a big difference in your child's quality of sleep. Allergy testing, combined with your child's symptom history, will help your doctor determine which specific allergens are triggering your child's asthma or allergy symptoms. Then you can focus your efforts on eliminating exposure to those specific allergens.

AANMA member Rachel Clarke reports, "We were amazed at the huge difference in our children's quality of sleep once we removed our carpeting and installed wooden floors. It was expensive—but well worth it."

Jan Frey concurs. After finding out her son was allergic to dust mites and mold, she says, "We ripped out carpeting, removed drapes and stuffed animals, and got rid of the clutter that collects dust. We allergy-proofed not only his bed but also his brother's bed in the same room and our bed. We were amazed at the immediate improvement. His nightly wheezing and asthma flare-ups cleared and he now sleeps more deeply and soundly."

Christine Noriega took a multi-step approach to helping her son get a good night's sleep. "My son's eczema would flare up and keep him scratching all night and his asthma would get worse. First, we found out he had food allergies and eliminated those foods. This helped calm his eczema. We also found he was allergic to dust mites. We put dust mite covers on his mattress and pillows, wash his bedding frequently in *hot* water, and put a high-efficiency particulate air (HEPA) filter in his room. When he comes in after playing outdoors, we get him into the bath right away to get rid of the pollen and other allergens. Then we rub Vaseline all over his body and put on cotton pajamas. This helps his eczema. All of these steps are helping calm his asthma and he's finally getting a good night's sleep."

If cleaning up the bedroom isn't enough to curb allergy symptoms, work with an allergist on treatment options, including immunotherapy (allergy shots), oral and nasal antihistamines, and nasal corticosteroids. Children twelve and older can also be tested to see if they qualify for a medication that reduces the number of antibodies responsible for allergic reactions.

Ensuring Sleep

If you think your child is having trouble sleeping due to asthma or allergies, monitor his symptoms, encourage him to report any problems to you, and keep a sleep journal (this can be part of his daily symptom diary). Talk to your child's doctor about nighttime problems. "We need to control asthma both during the day and at night to maximize a patient's health-related quality of life," emphasizes Dr. Meltzer. If you notice excessive napping or drowsiness, school problems, hyperactivity, or distractibility, ask your doctor to assess your child's nighttime symptoms. Talk about your child's sleep schedule, sleep environment, sleep-related symptoms, and behavioral issues. You should also carefully monitor your child's use of medication: Is he taking all doses on time? Adept at using a metered-dose inhaler or nebulizer? Check his inhaler technique at the next medical appointment and talk to the doctor about other medical conditions—like reflux and sleep apnea—that could be contributing to sleep problems.

Rachel Gerke says, "It has taken us all three years of his life, but we've finally started to get my son's asthma symptoms under control." Rachel makes regular appointments for her son with his allergist and asthma program coordinator. "He's had fewer asthma symptoms now that we fine-tuned his medication plan, put wood flooring in his room, removed all stuffed animals, started washing his bedding frequently, and put dust mite–proof covers on his mattress and pillow cases. I also think that it made a difference to take the diaper wipes warmer out of his room—it gave off a scent from the wipes that I believe irritated his airways. It is all those little things that a lot of people don't think about doing in their sleeping environment that make a world of difference."

Asthma and allergies don't have to keep your family from getting the sleep you need. Work with your child's medical care team to determine what's causing sleep problems and how you can solve them.

Dealing with Dust Mites

Most children and even teenagers have well-loved stuffed animals that are full of dust mites. How do you get rid of those dust mites? You could turn the hot water heater up to 130° F on laundry day. Or you can make your child's stuffed animals "allergy friendly" by sticking them in the freezer overnight. This tip was first reported by AANMA president and founder Nancy Sander in "A Parent's Guide to Asthma" in 1989. After the deep freeze, wash and dry the stuffed animals to get rid of dust mite body parts and fecal pellets.

What's on Your Bed?

With all the mattress and pillow options available today, are some better than others for people with asthma and allergies? It depends on what's causing your sneezing and wheezing.

If you have dust mite allergy, the keys to a good night's sleep are using mattress and pillow encasements and monitoring humidity levels. Dust mites need two things to thrive: water (which they absorb from the air) and food (which they get from you in the form of dead skin cells). Keeping your bedroom's humidity below 50 percent will deprive dust mites of their water source, and a special cover over your mattress and pillow will deprive them of food. The mattress and pillow encasements will also protect you from allergens in mite body parts and poop.

A word about mattress and pillow encasements: Old-style pillow and mattress encasements were made of plastic; they didn't allow air to flow through, so you'd end up sweaty, and they made a lot of noise when you rolled over. New encasements are made of tightly woven fabric that's soft and silent. Small pores allow air to pass through but are too small for dust mites and allergens to get through. When shopping for encasements, look for bound seams and a pore size (the amount of space between fabric threads) of ten microns or less. Avoid coatings or lamination that can wear off in the wash.

New allergy-free and hypoallergenic pillows may not solve your slumber problems. According to the American Academy of Allergy, Asthma and Immunology, both synthetic pillows and feather pillows promote dust mite growth. And allergy to feathers is actually very rare. So select the pillow that's most comfortable for you and use a tightly woven pillow encasement.

Chapter 40

If Your Child Has Asthma, Can He or She Keep a Pet?

Austin loves watching TV with his dog, Max. They hang out on the sofa together for hours on rainy days. Sometimes, Austin lies with his head right on Max's soft furry belly. What a pillow!

But Austin just found out he's allergic to animal allergens. That means he's allergic to stuff animals produce. This stuff is found in:

- animal dander, or skin flakes (kind of like animal dandruff);

- animal saliva (spit);

- animal urine (pee).

Because he's allergic to this stuff, spending time with Max is probably making his asthma worse. Lots of kids with asthma are allergic to animals—and not just furry animals. Feathered animals, too, can cause allergic reactions.

Aside from carrying dander, saliva, or urine, animal fur or feathers also can collect:

- dust mites (tiny bugs);

- pollen (from plants);

"If I Have Asthma, Can I Keep My Pet?" October 2010, reprinted with permission from www.kidshealth.org. Copyright © 2010 The Nemours Foundation. This information was provided by KidsHealth, one of the largest resources online for medically reviewed health information written for parents, kids, and teens. For more articles like this one, visit www.KidsHealth.org, or www.TeensHealth.org.

- mold (like the stuff that makes your basement smell);

- other stuff that causes allergies.

And any animal that lives in a cage—from birds to gerbils—will have droppings that get mold and dust mites on them too.

Finding out that you're allergic to animals can be sad because, if your asthma is really bad, you may have to find a new home for your pet. Because that's such a tough thing to do, your doctor might suggest that you try allergy medicine or shots first. Those, in addition to your regular asthma medicines, can help control your asthma flare-ups.

You also can take these steps to keep your bedroom free of allergens and reduce the allergens in your home:

- Keep your pet out of your room. If possible, keep your pet outside.

- Even if it's a small pet, like a bird or gerbil, don't keep the animal in your room.

- For caged animals, have someone else clean the cage.

- If there's a pet in your classroom, let your teacher know about your allergies.

- Play with your pet, but try not to hug or kiss the animal.

- Wash your hands when you're done playing with your pet.

- Get rid of any rugs or wall-to-wall carpeting in your room.

- Clean your room so it's free of household dust.

- Have someone else wash and brush your pet every week (cats as well as dogs).

If you try all these things and are still having lots of asthma flare-ups, you may need to find another home for your pet. This might make you feel a lot of different feelings. At first, you may feel nothing at all. Or you may feel like crying. You may feel lonely or mad. All of these feelings are OK.

You might want to talk to your parents about how you're feeling. They might be feeling sad and missing your pet, too. Talking can help you start feeling better. You might decide to write a poem or make a scrapbook to remember your pet.

It takes months for all of the allergens to leave the house, so your allergies might not get better right away. Even if you don't have animals at home, you'll probably still come in contact with them from time to time.

When going over to a friend's house where there is a pet, be sure to take your allergy medicine before going over. Also, bring your asthma inhaler along, just in case.

If you're missing your pet, it may take a long time before you want a new one. But if you do, consider getting a few fish, which are less likely to cause allergies.

Chapter 41

Dealing with Asthma at School

Chapter Contents

Section 41.1

School and Asthma: The Basics

An estimated seven million U.S. kids under age eighteen have been
diagnosed with asthma and more than thirteen million days of school
are missed each year because of the condition, according to the American Academy of Allergy, Asthma, and Immunology.

But well-managed asthma is far less likely to result in a sick day.
When kids' asthma is under control, they have a minimum of flare-ups
and fewer problems between them.

Other benefits of proper asthma control include helping kids to:

- sleep well at night and focus at school during the day;

- spend time at school in the classroom, not the nurse's office;

- avoid anxiety or embarrassment about flare-ups and asthma
  symptoms;

- study, run, play sports, and fully participate in all school activities.

Creating an Asthma Action Plan

So how do you get your child's asthma under control? The first step
is to work with your doctor to create and implement a written asthma
action plan that may include a list of:

- the medications your child takes and their dosages;

- your child's asthma triggers;

- early symptoms of a flare-up;

- what to do if your child is having a flare-up, including when to
  seek emergency care.

The plan might also include instructions for peak flow monitoring and recommendations for dealing with exercise-induced asthma.

Communicating with Your Child's School

Once you and the doctor have completed the asthma action plan, make sure to give your child's school a copy. A meeting with your child's teacher and other school staff at the start of every school year can also be helpful for making sure that arrangements are in place.

You should talk about:

- the history of your child's asthma;

- how independently your child is able to manage the asthma;

- how to reach you and your child's doctor;

- plans for handling treatment during any off-site activities, such as field trips;

- what the school's rules are about medication for kids old enough to handle monitoring and treatment at school (can kids keep an inhaler on hand or do they have to go the health office to use it?);

- who handles asthma medications at the school if your child isn't old enough to take care of monitoring and treatment. Someone on the school's staff should know how to work the peak flow meter and how to administer medications if your child can't do it alone. Ideally, a health professional at the school will do this. If not, find out who will.

A supportive environment that helps kids assume responsibility for their own care is an important part of asthma management. Without it, kids might avoid taking their medications or using their peak flow meters. Encourage the school's staff to help your child settle into a routine that's efficient and low-key.

Handling Flare-Ups at School

Ideally, rescue medication should always be immediately available to kids. This means that for kids who aren't old enough to self-administer the medicine, the teacher will have it in the classroom or it will be readily available (not under lock and key) in the school nurse's office.

Once kids are old enough to recognize symptoms and know how and when to take their medication, they should carry it at all times, if the school permits. Your doctor can help you determine at what point your child can be responsible for the medication.

Talk to school administrators and find out what they're willing to allow. Stress the importance of immediate treatment during an asthma flare-up. Administrators may allow your child to self-medicate, but might ask you to sign an "asthma contract," indicating that you've given permission for this to happen and also listing which school personnel are permitted to give your child medication.

Kids who have exercise-induced asthma should have their rescue medication available before any strenuous play or exercise. So they might need permission to go to the nurse's office before recess or gym class, which may be embarrassing and cumbersome for older kids. Again, it might be better for these kids to carry the rescue medication with them.

Is your child responsible and organized enough to carry the inhaler at all times and to use it when necessary? If so, you can help by reminding your child to have it on hand. Keep track of how much medicine is left in the inhaler, and consider asking to keep extra rescue medication in the nurse's office, just in case.

Dealing with Triggers at School

Kids are likely to encounter these possible asthma triggers at school:

- mold;
- dust mites;
- cockroaches;
- chalk dust;
- perfumes;
- cleaning products or other chemicals;
- animal dander, saliva, or urine.

You should let the school's staff know if any of these will trigger your child's asthma. You might also want to make some suggestions, such as:

- Ask teachers to use "dustless" chalk or dry-erase boards.
- Ask the staff to avoid using perfumed cleaning products or soaps.

- Propose the use of air conditioners and dehumidifiers.

- Ask that any classroom where art supplies are used and locker rooms where mold can grow be well ventilated.

- Make sure that the school is vacuumed and dusted regularly, that it's routinely treated by a pest control company, and that it's completely smoke free.

Section 41.2

Using an Asthma Action Plan at School

"Asthma and School, " © 2011 A.D.A.M., Inc. Reprinted with permission.

Children with asthma need a lot of support at school. They may need help from school staff to keep their asthma under control and to be able to do school activities.

You should give the school staff an asthma action plan that tells staff how to take care of your child's asthma. Ask your child's doctor to write one.

The student and school staff should follow this asthma action plan. Your child should be able to take asthma medicines at school when needed.

School staff should know what things make your child's asthma worse. These are called "triggers." Your child should be able to go to another location to get away from asthma triggers, if needed.

What Should Be in Your Child's School Asthma Plan

Your child's school asthma plan should include:

- a brief history of your child's asthma;

- asthma symptoms to watch out for;

- phone numbers or e-mail addresses of your child's doctor, nurse, and parent or guardian;

- a list of triggers that make your child's asthma worse:

- Smells from chemicals and cleaners
- Grass and weeds
- Smoke
- Dust
- Cockroaches
- Rooms that are moldy or damp
- the student's personal best peak flow reading;
- a list of the student's asthma medicines and how to take them:
  - Medicines your child takes every day to control asthma
  - Quick-relief asthma medicines when your child has symptoms
- what to do to make sure your child can be as active as possible during recess and physical education class.

Your child's doctor and parent or guardian's signatures should be on this action plan.

Who Should Have a Copy of the Action Plan

The following people should have a copy of the plan:

- Your child's teacher
- The school nurse
- The school office
- Gym teachers and coaches

References

Bruzzese JM, Evans D, Kattan M. School-based asthma programs. *J Allergy Clin Immunol.* 2009 Aug;124(2):195–200. Epub 2009 Jul 16.

Guidelines for the Diagnosis and Management of Asthma. Rockville, MD. National Heart, Lung, and Blood Institute, US Dept of Health and Human Services; 2007. NIH publications 08-4051.

Section 41.3

Asthma in the Classroom: What Schools Can Do

Excerpted from "Managing Asthma in the School Environment,"
U.S. Environmental Protection Agency, August 2010.

Asthma in Schools

Each day, one in five Americans occupies a school building. The majority of these occupants are children. Environmental asthma triggers commonly found in school buildings include respiratory viruses; cockroaches and other pests; mold resulting from excess moisture in the building; dander from animals in the classroom; and dander brought in on clothing from animals at home. Secondhand smoke and dust mites are other known environmental asthma triggers found in schools. Children with asthma may be affected by other pollutants from sources found inside schools, such as unvented stoves or heaters and common products including chemicals, cleaning agents, perfumes, pesticides, and sprays. In addition, outdoor environmental asthma triggers, like ozone and particle pollution, or bus exhaust, can affect children with asthma while at school.

Students with uncontrolled asthma often miss more school and have poorer academic performance than healthy students. With the help of strong school asthma management programs, students with asthma can have equally good school attendance. When asthma is well controlled, students are ready to learn.

Effectively managing a child's asthma is best accomplished through a comprehensive plan that addresses both the medical management of the disease and the avoidance of environmental triggers. Because children spend most of their time in schools, day care facilities, or at home, it is important to reduce their exposure to environmental asthma triggers as much as possible in each of these environments. This section focuses on steps that schools can take to help children breathe easier.

Develop an Asthma Management Plan in Your School

The components described below form the foundation for an effective asthma management plan:

- Establish management and support systems for asthma-friendly schools.

- Provide appropriate school health and mental health services for students with asthma.

- Provide asthma education and awareness programs for students and school staff.

- Provide a safe and healthy school environment to reduce asthma triggers.

- Provide safe, enjoyable physical education and activity opportunities for students with asthma.

- Coordinate school, family, and community efforts to better manage asthma symptoms and reduce school absences among students with asthma.

It is important to identify all students with asthma through monitoring morbidity associated with asthma, for example, frequent episodes at school, health room visits, limited physical activity, needing to leave school early, or absenteeism. This can help to assess which programs or monitoring activities your school or district should implement. Focus resources on students whose asthma is not well controlled in order to promote improved school attendance and performance.

In order to identify what works and how you can improve the design and delivery of your school asthma management plan, it is essential to monitor program effectiveness.

Reduce Environmental Asthma Triggers

Help manage asthma in your school with the following tips for controlling environmental asthma triggers.

Control Animal Allergens

Classrooms often adopt animals as classroom pets or science projects. Any warm-blooded animals, including gerbils, birds, cats, dogs, mice, and rats, may trigger asthma. Proteins, which act as allergens in the dander, urine, or saliva of warm-blooded animals, can cause allergic reactions or trigger asthma episodes in people sensitive to animal allergens.

The most common sources of animal allergens in schools are in the air and on the clothing of staff and children who handle pets. If an animal is present in the school, there is a possibility of direct, daily exposure to the animal's dander and bodily fluids. It is important to realize that, even after extensive cleaning, pet allergens may stay in the indoor environment for several months after the animal is removed. In addition, animal allergens can readily migrate to other areas of the school environment through the air and on the clothing of staff and children who handle pets.

The most effective method to control exposure to animal allergens in schools is to keep your school free of warm-blooded animals.

Control Cockroach and Pest Allergens

Cockroaches and other pests, such as rats and mice, are often found in the school setting. Certain proteins that act as allergens in the waste products and saliva of pests can cause allergic reactions or trigger asthma symptoms in some individuals.

Pest problems in schools may be caused or worsened by a variety of conditions, such as plumbing leaks, moisture problems, and improper food handling and storage practices. To manage and avoid pest problems, it is important to control water and food sources. Integrated pest management—IPM—is composed of commonsense practices that should be used throughout the entire school.

There are four key IPM methods for reducing exposure to pests in the school setting:

- Look for signs of pests.

- Do not leave food, water, or garbage exposed.

- Remove pest pathways and shelters.

- Use pest control products such as poison baits, traps, and pesticide sprays, as needed and as allowed by state law. However, do not rely on widespread, indiscriminate use of pesticides to control pests.

- Track cockroach populations by using small sticky traps or monitoring traps that contain no pesticide.

- Rather than using bait, trap rats and mice.

- Use pesticide sprays in classrooms only as a last resort.

Clean Up Mold and Control Moisture

Molds can be found almost anywhere; they can grow on virtually any substance if moisture is present. Molds produce tiny reproductive

465

spores that travel through the indoor and outdoor air continually. When mold spores land on a damp spot indoors, they digest available material to survive and grow. When mold growth occurs in buildings, it may be followed by reports of health symptoms from some building occupants, particularly those with allergies or respiratory problems. Potential health effects and symptoms associated with mold exposures include allergic reactions, asthma exacerbations and other respiratory complaints.

If excessive moisture or water accumulates indoors, mold growth may occur, particularly if the moisture problem remains undiscovered or unaddressed. Moisture problems in school buildings can be caused by a variety of problems, including roof and plumbing leaks, condensation and excess humidity. Some moisture problems in schools have been linked to changes in building construction practices. For example, tightly sealed buildings may not allow moisture to escape as easily. Moisture problems in schools also are associated with delayed or insufficient maintenance, sometimes due to budget constraints. Temporary structures in schools, such as trailers and portable classrooms, have also frequently been associated with moisture and mold problems.

To prevent mold from being a problem in your school, take the following actions:

- Eliminate sources of moisture by reducing indoor humidity.

- Prevent moisture condensation through the proper use of insulation.

- Inspect the building for signs of mold, moisture, leaks or spills.

- Respond promptly when you see signs of moisture and/or mold or when leaks or spills occur.

Because moisture is the key to mold control, it is essential to clean up the mold and get rid of excess water or moisture. If the excess water or moisture problem is not fixed, mold will most likely grow again, even if the area was completely cleaned. Clean hard surfaces with water and detergent and dry quickly and completely. Absorbent materials such as ceiling tiles may have to be discarded.

Control Sources of Indoor Air Pollutants

Usually the most effective way to improve indoor air quality is to eliminate individual sources of pollution or to reduce their emissions.

Common sources of indoor pollution include secondhand smoke, school bus diesel exhaust coming into the school building, the off-gassing of furnishings and flooring, and chemicals from cleaning products. The following pollutant sources are especially important to control:

- **Secondhand smoke:** Secondhand smoke is an irritant that may trigger an asthma episode, and evidence suggests that secondhand smoke may cause asthma in children. The U.S. Environmental Protection Agency estimates that exposure to secondhand smoke exacerbates asthma symptoms in 200,000 to 1,000,000 children. It is imperative for school districts to develop and pass comprehensive tobacco-free school policies, and then enforce these policies at all times. In addition, it is recommended that schools educate staff, students, and the community on the effects of secondhand smoke and its relation to asthma.

- **School bus exhaust:** Passing no-idling policies near the school building can reduce the indoor air pollution from school bus exhaust.

- **Cleaning products:** Choosing the least toxic cleaning methods and selecting appropriate products are important components of pollutant control. Fumes from cleaning products can linger long after they have been applied, which can exacerbate asthma symptoms and expose students and staff to potentially harmful substances.

Reduce Exposure to Dust Mites

Dust mite allergens play a significant role in triggering asthma. They may cause an allergic reaction or trigger an asthma episode in sensitive individuals. In addition, there is evidence that dust mites cause new cases of asthma in susceptible children.

Dust mites are too small to be seen but are found in schools in carpeting, upholstered furniture, stuffed animals or toys, and pillows. Their food source is dead skin flakes and these tend to accumulate in porous fabric materials.

It is important to keep classrooms free of clutter, to dust regularly and to wash items frequently that attract dust. When using pillows, cover them with dust-proof, allergen impermeable, zipped covers. If stuffed toys are necessary, choose ones that can be washed in hot water. People with asthma or dust mite allergies should leave any area while it is being vacuumed. Vacuums with high-efficiency filters or central vacuums may be helpful.

Section 41.4

Can Your Child Carry an Inhaler at School?

When asthma is well managed, a child should not need to use "quick-relief" or "rescue" medicines often. But families and schools must always be prepared for an asthma emergency. Access to quick-relief inhalers at school is critical for children with asthma, as this medicine will immediately open the airways during an asthma attack and can be life-saving. The longer it takes to administer quick-relief medications, the worse the asthma attack may become.

Many localities now have laws or policies in place that allow students with asthma to carry and self-administer asthma quick-relief inhalers and other life-saving medicines. If self-carry/self-administration is not allowed in your school, find out why. Also, make sure the school has a plan that ensures immediate access to quick-relief medicine. For example, inhalers cannot be locked in the school nurse's office, with only a few staff members able to get at them. Such a situation could result in a lack of access to the medicine in an emergency.

You may wonder if your child is mature enough to carry and self-administer asthma inhalers at school. Even young children can be encouraged to learn to manage their own asthma, including avoiding their triggers, recognizing their signs and symptoms, and taking their medicine appropriately. Work with your child's healthcare provider and school to determine if this is the best option for your child.

Things to consider:

- Does your child want to be able to carry and self-administer asthma medications?

- Can your child identify warning signs and symptoms of asthma?

- Does your child understand which medicine to take when?

- Does your child use correct technique when using the inhaler?

- Is your child aware of medication side effects and what to report?

Is your child willing to comply with school's rules about use of medicine at school, which might include:

- keeping the asthma inhaler with him or her at all times;

- notifying a responsible adult (e.g., teacher, nurse, coach, playground assistant) during the day when a quick-relief inhaler is used;

- not sharing medication with other students or leaving the medicine unattended;

- not using a quick-relief asthma inhaler for any other use than what is intended.

Contact your school officials and ask about the self-carry/self-administration policy in your school district. Working with your child, his or her healthcare provider, and the school is the best way to keep your child healthy, in school, and ready to learn.

Section 41.5

When to Keep a Child with Asthma Home from School

Some days it can be hard to decide whether a child with asthma symptoms should go to school or not. Your goal is always zero missed school days due to asthma, but that can be difficult to achieve when your child's treatment plan is still in development, you're not sure what environmental factors are causing his asthma symptoms, or he's in a transition period.

Your can send your child to school with:

- a stuffy nose but no wheezing (listen to his chest);
- peak flow meter readings at or near his target number after medication;
- the ability to participate in expected daily school activities;
- no difficulty breathing.

Keep your child home with:

- evidence of infection, sore throat, or swollen, painful neck glands;
- a fever above 100° F; face hot and flushed;
- peak flow meter readings that are not near his target number after medication;
- wheezing that continues to be labored thirty minutes after medication;
- weakness or tiredness that makes it hard to take part in usual daily activities;
- difficulty breathing.

Good communication among teachers, parents, and students will enable a child to attend school on marginal days. Notify teachers that your child is in pre- or post-asthma flare stages but controlled with medications. If possible or if needed, go to the school to check on your child just before the next dose of medication is due.

When a Child Needs Help

The key to keeping kids in school is keeping them healthy. Children with high absentee rates need medical help. Children who can't participate in physical activities need medical help. Children who are frequently in crisis need medical help. These are signs that a child's asthma or allergy management plan is not working. Parents and teachers should take the time to identify why the child is missing school and unable to participate fully in school activities.

Parents should consider:

- Is the child under the care of an asthma or allergy specialist?

- Is the asthma or allergy management plan individualized and in writing?

- Are home and school environments free of allergens and irritants?

- Is the school environment a healthy place for the child to breathe?

If the answer to any of these questions is "no," your child may miss more school than necessary. If you answered "yes" to all of these questions and your child is still having problems at school with asthma or allergies, further investigation by your child's physician or perhaps a second medical opinion would be helpful.

Helping your child stay in school is an important part of helping him overcome, not just cope with, asthma and allergies.

471

Chapter 42

Exercise and Children with Asthma

Chapter Contents

Section 42.1

Physical Activity in Children with Asthma: Tips for Parents and Caregivers

Excerpted from "Physical Activity: What If My Child Has Asthma? Advice for Parents and Carers," © British Heart Foundation National Center for Physical Activity and Health, 2011. All rights reserved. Reprinted with permission. This text does not replace the advice that health professionals involved in the care of your child may give, as they know more about your child's condition. This text explains why it is good for your child to be physically active, provides information to help you make it easy and enjoyable for your child to be active safely, and aims to make sure your child is not put off being active. To view the complete text of this document, including resources for further information, visit www.bhfactive.org.uk.

Is It Safe for My Child to Do Physical Activity?

Yes. There are very few children and young people who will be advised not to do any physical activity. Many people wrongly think that physical activity is not safe for anyone with asthma because it can trigger their asthma symptoms.

For some children and young people, physical activity may be the only trigger of their asthma. This is known as "exercise-induced asthma." For others, physical activity may be one of several triggers. And for others, physical activity is not a trigger at all.

If physical activity is a trigger for your child, it is understandable that you may worry about them taking part in physical activity and getting out of breath. But as long as your child's asthma is under control, they can take part in any physical activity they enjoy.

Every child is different and most children and young people who have asthma will know their triggers and limitations. However, you might want to get advice about your child's condition before encouraging your child to become more active. Your child's healthcare professionals should be able to advise you if there are any particular activities that your child should avoid.

How Much Physical Activity Should My Child Do?

To improve health, experts recommend that all children and young people aged 5 to 17 years should do at least 60 minutes of moderate to vigorous-intensity physical activity every day. This applies to all children and young people, including those who have asthma.

Moderate-intensity activity is activity that may raise your child's pulse, and make them breathe slightly faster and feel a little warmer—for example, brisk walking, steady cycling, roller-skating, or active play.

Vigorous-intensity activity is activity that makes your child 'huff and puff' and makes them feel sweaty—for example, organised games such as football and basketball as well as activities such as running, fast cycling, swimming laps, and jumping and climbing over obstacles.

The 60 minutes of activity doesn't have to be done all at once. It can be spread across the whole day by doing several shorter amounts of activity—for example, two short bouts of 15 minutes of activity running around in the playground, combined with a longer bout of programmed activity such as physical education or supervised recreational activity.

If your child is currently inactive, they should gradually increase the amount of physical activity they do, and should aim to eventually achieve the 60 minutes a day target. If your child is currently not doing any physical activity, doing some activity—even if it's below the recommended level—will bring more benefits than doing no physical activity at all. Any physical activity is better than none, and generally the more the better.

What Are the Benefits of Regular Physical Activity for My Child?

There is lots of evidence that children and young people benefit from being physically active. This applies to all children and young people, including those with asthma.

Regular physical activity can:

- promote healthy growth and development
- help keep the heart and lungs healthy
- help develop strong muscles and bones
- improve balance and flexibility

- help achieve and maintain a healthy body weight
- make them feel good, improve their mood, and help them cope with the stresses of everyday life
- improve self-esteem and body image
- provide opportunities to make friends
- build confidence and help develop social skills.

In addition, regular physical activity has the following important benefits for children and young people with asthma.

- It can help improve lung function by strengthening the breathing muscles in the chest. This can have important long-term effects on breathing and asthma control.
- It can help your child to manage their asthma better during periods of physical activity, as they have increased lung capacity and better fitness.
- It can help your child to cope better with everyday activities, as they will have more stamina.
- It helps reduce any anxieties your child may have about their asthma, and give your child confidence to manage their condition.
- It can help your child reach or keep to a healthy weight. This is particularly important, as children and young people who are overweight often need to take more medicine to control their asthma, and their asthma is usually less well controlled.

What Can I Do to Help?

All children and young people should try to do regular physical activity. However, if your child's asthma is poorly controlled, they should see their doctor or asthma nurse before they start becoming more active.

We can all play a vital role in supporting and encouraging children and young people to be more active.

Be Positive about Your Child's Condition

- Don't let asthma be an obstacle to your child being active. Many Olympic athletes, professional soccer players, and other high-level sportspeople have asthma.

476

Make Sure Your Child Is Adequately Prepared for Physical Activity

- Make sure your child takes their asthma medicine correctly and regularly. Explain to them why this is important.

- Make sure your child has their reliever inhaler, and their spacer if they use one, close by them during physical activity.

- If your child's asthma is triggered by physical activity (exercise-induced asthma), make sure they take their reliever inhaler about 5 minutes before they begin the activity. The symptoms of exercise-induced asthma may start shortly after physical activity begins and usually get worse about 15 minutes after the physical activity has stopped. Taking their reliever inhaler before doing the activity can help prevent them getting these symptoms.

- Teach your child to stop being physically active as soon as they experience any symptoms of asthma, and to take their reliever inhaler. They can return to light activity once they feel fully recovered. They should wait at least 5 minutes. Sometimes high doses from the reliever can slightly increase the child's heartbeat or result in mild muscle shakes, but these effects are harmless and generally wear off after a short time.

Try a Range of Different Activities

There are lots of different ways to be active and most children and young people will be keen to try out new activities.

- Encourage your child to try a range of different physical activities to find out which ones they enjoy and which ones they can cope with better.

- Trying out different activities will help your child understand how their body responds to various types of physical activity. This is all part of them learning how to manage their asthma.

Try to Be More Active as a Family

Children and young people who have physically active parents are more likely to be active themselves.

- Be a good role model for your child. For example, simply walking more often can help your child see that you value physical activity.

477

- Make time to be active and have fun as a family. For example, go for a walk, play Frisbee, play in the garden or local park, or perhaps go swimming together. Providing opportunities for your child to be active with you may help build their confidence about being physically active with friends, and reassure them that it is safe for them to be active.

Teach Your Child to Warm Up and Cool Down

Your child should always warm up for at least 10 minutes before physical activity and cool down gradually afterwards.

- Warming up means beginning physical activity slowly and building up gradually. Cooling down means taking time to slow down and not stopping physical activity suddenly.

- An extended warm-up and gradual cool-down are important. They help slow the change of air temperature in the airways. This may help reduce the likelihood of your child developing asthma symptoms and will help keep their symptoms under control.

Try to Reduce Your Child's Exposure to Triggers

It can be difficult to identify exactly what triggers your child's asthma.

- If you're aware of any triggers to your child's asthma, teach your child how they can avoid these. For example, in cold weather, make sure your child covers their nose and mouth with a scarf. In summer, avoid outdoor activities when pollen levels are high or during grass cutting.

- Avoiding triggers applies not just to when your child is being active. It also includes things like avoiding pets if your child is allergic to them, and avoiding cigarette smoke.

Keep a Record of What Triggers Your Child's Asthma

It may be a good idea for your child to keep a diary of any symptoms (such as wheezing, coughing, tightness in the chest, or difficulty breathing) together with any potential triggers they have been exposed to (such as pollen, traffic fumes or pets, or if they have a cold or cough). If your child is too young to do this themselves, you could keep a diary for your child. You may find it helpful to bring this diary along to the regular asthma reviews your child has.

Arrange Regular Asthma Reviews with Your Child's Doctor or Asthma Nurse

- Arrange a regular asthma review with your child's doctor or asthma nurse. Your child should have a review at least once every six months, depending on their condition and how well their asthma is controlled.

- Make sure you have an asthma action plan for your child.

- You may find it useful to fill in the action plan with the help of your child's doctor or asthma nurse, and to give this to your child's daycare, school, or physical activity leaders.

Are Some Types of Physical Activity Better than Others for People with Asthma?

You may need to think about the **type** of physical activity that your child can do, especially if your child is very limited by their asthma symptoms. Certain types of physical activity may be better suited to your child than others. But as long as your child's asthma is under control, they can take part in any physical activity they enjoy.

Dynamic aerobic activities—such as walking, cycling, swimming, dancing, fitness classes, and adapted team games—are generally better for children and young people with asthma, as these can be done at low intensity and intermittently.

Also, children and young people with asthma tend to cope better with **'interval-type activities.'** That means activities that require bursts of activity interspersed with spells of activity at a slower pace—for example, relay races, tag, or chasing or jumping games. With this type of activity, the child or young person can rest in between bursts of activity. Interval-type activities can be used to slowly improve your child's stamina, without causing them discomfort. At first your child may need longer rest periods, but these can be made shorter as their stamina improves.

Activities with rest periods should still involve some movement, but at a slower pace. This is known as "active rest." Complete rest in between bursts of activity is not recommended.

Indoor Swimming

Recreational indoor swimming is an excellent activity for children and young people with asthma, as they can do it at their own pace. Also, the warm, humid air in the swimming pool is less likely to trigger

479

your child's asthma symptoms. However, your child should take care in heavily chlorinated or very cold pools, as these can be a trigger to asthma symptoms for some children and young people.

Team Games

Team games such as football, hockey, basketball, or volleyball are good activities for children and young people with asthma because they tend to involve brief bursts of playing at a higher intensity followed by active rest periods, so they are less likely to cause asthma symptoms. Some children and young people with asthma may struggle to complete a full game, but may be able to cope with an adapted game—for example, having more players on each team, or using a smaller play area.

Racquet and Net Games

Racquet and net games such as badminton or table tennis are ideal activities for children and young people with asthma, as they involve brief bursts of activity. Badminton is ideal, as the shuttlecock travels slowly and the court is quite small. Tennis and squash usually involve more constant activity and are faster paced. Your child may struggle to cope with a full game of tennis, but may find short tennis easier.

Striking and Fielding Games

Activities such as cricket, softball, and baseball may be ideal for children and young people with asthma. These games tend to include brief bursts of activity followed by short breaks. Also, the pace of the game can be adapted to suit different abilities.

Gymnastics and Dancing

Children and young people with asthma rarely experience any difficulties with gymnastics, aerobic dance, or dancing. These are ideal activities, as they lend themselves to brief bursts of activity. Your child can set their own pace and can include active rest periods. Complete rest in between bursts of activity is not advised, as this can trigger exercise-induced asthma.

Yoga, Pilates, and T'ai Chi

These are excellent activities for children and young people with asthma, as they relax the body and may help with breathing.

Cycling, Rollerblading, and Skateboarding

These activities can be great fun. They are perfect for children and young people with asthma, as they can control how fast or how slow they want to go!

Every child's and young person's condition is different. If you have any concerns or queries about your child being active, always ask your child's doctor or asthma nurse.

Are There Any Types of Physical Activity That My Child Should Avoid?

Some types of physical activity may present problems for some children and young people with asthma due to the environment in which they take place—for example, long-distance or cross-country running, adventure sports, or outdoor activities.

- Long-distance or cross-country running can be a strong asthma trigger because they are done outside, sometimes in cold air and without rest breaks. There is also less opportunity to see how the child or young person is coping with the activity.

- Some adventure sports or outdoor activities may bring on asthma symptoms. This is more likely to be related to emotional or environmental factors associated with the activity than the activity itself—for example, excitement, anxiety, stress, weather, high pollen count, and altitude.

It is recommended that you should contact your child's doctor and seek advice before your child takes part in any adventure sports.

What about taking part in physical education, sports, and physical activity at school?

Taking part in physical education (PE) and other physical activities at school is important for your child, both for their long-term health and well-being and to make sure they are fully involved in school life.

Here are some things you can do to help:

- Teach your child the importance of taking part in PE and physical activity at school and in after-school clubs. Encourage them to take part at their own pace and within their own limitations.

481

- Remind your child to take their medicines regularly, especially their preventer inhaler, and to keep their reliever inhaler and spacer with them at all times.

- Make sure that the school always has a spare reliever inhaler and spacer for your child. Check the expiration date on inhalers regularly and replace them when needed.

- Keep your child's teachers and physical activity leaders (for example, after-school club leaders or sports coaches) informed about your child's asthma, particularly about what triggers their asthma and how best to avoid those triggers. Make sure your child's daycare, school, or physical activity leader has written information about your child's triggers and symptoms, their inhaler, your emergency contact details, and how to recognise if your child is having an asthma attack and what to do about it.

- Let your child's teachers and physical activity leaders know about any recent asthma attacks your child has had, or changes in their condition or medicines. Make sure their asthma action plan is updated.

- It might help put your mind at rest if you discuss any concerns you have regarding your child's involvement in PE with your child's teacher or school nurse.

- Ask about the school's asthma policy (or their medical conditions policy). For example, you might want to ask about their policy on access and storage of pupils' inhalers; whether staff have had training in asthma awareness (knowing what to do if a child has an asthma attack, and how to avoid asthma triggers); or whether teachers will always let parents or caregivers know if a child has an asthma attack or has needed to use their reliever inhaler more often than usual during school time.

What are the symptoms to look out for when my child is active?

It's ok and "normal" for your child to feel warm, breathe harder, look 'flushed,' and feel his or her heart beat faster during physical activity.

Your child should stop doing the activity if he or she:

- starts coughing or wheezing

- starts to become short of breath

- feels tightness in the chest

- has difficulty speaking in short sentences

- is unusually quiet and quite still

- has tummy ache (sometimes in younger children)

- has cyanosis (a blue tinge to the skin or lips), which is a sign of a lack of oxygen in the blood, and indicates the need for urgent medical attention

Your child may not have all of these symptoms. Also, how severe the symptoms are and how long they last may vary greatly between separate asthma attacks.

If you notice any of the preceding signs or symptoms, you should:

- Get your child to stop and rest immediately.

- **Never** push your child to continue their activity. Asthma symptoms will often get worse once activity is stopped, so insisting that your child keeps going until they are forced to rest can be dangerous.

- Give your child one or two puffs of their reliever inhaler immediately, preferably through a spacer.

- Sit your child up and slightly forward. **Don't** lie them down or hug them.

- Encourage them to take slow, steady breaths.

- Loosen tight clothing.

- Stay with them and reassure them.

- If there is no immediate improvement, continue to make sure your child takes two puffs of their reliever inhaler every 2 minutes, taking up to 10 puffs.

- If your child's symptoms don't improve after 10 puffs, or if you are worried at any time, call 911 for an ambulance.

- If an ambulance does not arrive within 15 minutes and your child is not improving, give further doses of their reliever inhaler. Make sure your child takes two puffs of their reliever every two minutes, taking up to 10 puffs.

What else can I do to encourage my child to be active?

- Teach your child to slowly build up the amount of physical activity they do.

- Encourage your child to be physically active throughout the day, aiming for at least 60 minutes of physical activity every day.

- Choose physical activity carefully. Try to match activities to your child's likes, needs, and abilities, so they don't become disheartened over any difficulties and discomforts.

- Remember that your child doesn't have to be 'sporty' or join a team or a gym in order to take part in physical activity. Walking or dancing to their favorite music are excellent forms of physical activity and cost nothing.

- Find different ways of keeping your child active, and encourage them to take part in activities they enjoy.

- Encourage your child to try out new activities with their friends.

- Try to limit the amount of time that your child spends on sitting-down activities—such as watching TV or DVDs, or playing computer games—to no more than two hours a day.

- Set a good example and try to be more active as a family. Where possible, allow your child to walk or cycle to the shops and school.

- Praise and reward your child for being active. Be positive about their achievements, big or small, and reward them for persistence and taking part.

Remember: It's important to encourage your child to take part in physical activities that are appropriate for them. Activities should be enjoyable and offer variety. Some physical activity is better than nothing at all. Generally the more the better.

Section 42.2

Exercising and Asthma at School

Excerpted from "Asthma and Physical Activity in the School," National Heart, Lung, and Blood Institute, National Institutes of Health, NIH Publication No. 95-3651, September 1995. Reviewed by David A. Cooke, M.D., FACP, May 2011.

What Is Asthma?

Asthma is a chronic lung condition with ongoing airway inflammation that results in recurring acute episodes (attacks) of breathing problems such as coughing, wheezing, chest tightness, and shortness of breath. These symptoms occur because the inflammation makes the airways overreact to a variety of stimuli including physical activity, upper respiratory infections, allergens, and irritants. Exposure to these stimuli—often called triggers—creates more swelling and blocking of the airways. Asthma episodes can be mild, moderate, or even life threatening. Vigorous exercise will cause symptoms for most students with asthma if their asthma is not well controlled. Some students experience symptoms only when they exercise. However, today's treatments can successfully control asthma so that students can participate fully in physical activities most of the time.

Asthma varies from student to student and often from season to season. This is why physical education teachers and coaches need to understand what asthma is and what the individual needs of their students are. At times, programs for students with asthma may need temporary modification, such as varying the type, length, and/or frequency of activity. At all times, students with asthma should be included in activities as much as possible. Remaining behind in the gym or library or frequently sitting on the bench can set the stage for teasing, loss of self-esteem, unnecessary restriction of activity, and low levels of physical fitness.

Helping Students Control Their Asthma

Getting control of asthma means recognizing asthma triggers (the factors that make asthma worse or cause an asthma episode), avoiding or controlling these triggers, following an asthma management plan, and having convenient access to asthma medications. It also means modifying physical activities to match the students' current asthma status.

Asthma Triggers

- Exercise (running or playing hard), especially in cold weather

- Upper respiratory infections (colds or flu)

- Laughing or crying hard

- Allergens:

  - Pollens from trees, plants, and grasses, including freshly cut grass

  - Animal dander from pets with fur or feathers

  - Dust and dust mites in carpeting, pillows, and upholstery

  - Cockroach droppings

  - Molds

- Irritants:

  - Cold air

  - Strong smells and chemical sprays, including perfumes, paint, and cleaning solutions, chalk dust, lawn and turf treatments

  - Weather changes

  - Cigarette and other tobacco smoke

Each student with asthma has a list of triggers that can make his or her condition worse—that is, that increase airway inflammation and/or make the airways constrict, which makes breathing difficult.

Avoid or Control Asthma Triggers

Some asthma triggers—like pets with fur or feathers—can be avoided.

Others—like physical exercise—are important for good health and should be controlled rather than avoided.

Here are some actions to consider:

- Identify students' known asthma triggers and eliminate as many as possible. For example, keep animals with fur out of the classroom. Consult the students' asthma management plans for guidance (see the next section).

- Use wood, tile, or vinyl floor coverings instead of carpeting.

- Schedule maintenance or pest control that involves strong irritants and odors for times when students are not in the area and the area can be well ventilated.

- Adjust schedules for students whose asthma is worsened by pollen or cold air. A midday or indoor physical education class may allow more active participation.

- Help students follow their asthma management plans. These plans are designed to keep asthma under control.

Follow the Asthma Management Plan

A student's asthma management plan is developed by the student, parent/guardian, and healthcare provider. Depending on the student's needs, the plan may be a brief information card or a more extensive individualized health plan (IHP). Following is a list of what asthma plans typically contain. A copy of the plan should be on file in the school office or health services office, with additional copies for the student's teachers and coaches. The plan—as well as the student's asthma medications—should be easily available for all on- and off-site activities before, during, and after school.

An asthma management plan typically contains the following things:

- A brief history of the student's asthma

- A description of asthma symptoms

- Information on how to contact the student's healthcare provider and parent or guardian

- Physician and parent or guardian signatures

- A list of factors that make the student's asthma worse

- The student's personal best peak flow reading if the student uses peak flow monitoring

- A list of the student's asthma medications

- A description of the student's treatment plan, based on symptoms or peak flow readings, including recommended actions for school personnel to help handle asthma episodes

Winners with Exercise-Induced Asthma

Supporting and encouraging each student's efforts to follow his or her asthma management plan is essential for the student's active participation in physical activities. Students with asthma need understanding from both teachers and students in dealing with their asthma. If students with asthma are teased about their condition, they may be embarrassed, avoid using their medication, or cut class. If students with asthma are encouraged to "tough it out," they may risk health problems or just give up.

Here are some actions to consider:

- Get a copy of each student's asthma management plan. Review the plan to identify the role of the teacher and coach in the student's asthma management plan.

- Teach asthma awareness and peer sensitivity. As students learn more about asthma, they can more easily offer support instead of barriers to their classmates with asthma.

Ensure That Students with Asthma Have Convenient Access to Their Medications

Many students with asthma require two different medications: one for daily control and prevention, the other to treat and relieve symptoms. These medications are usually taken using a metered-dose inhaler. Preventive asthma medications are taken daily and usually can be scheduled for before and after school hours. However, some students may need to take preventive daily medication during school hours. All students with asthma need to have their medication that relieves symptoms available at school in case of unexpected exposure to asthma triggers, or an asthma episode. In addition, students with asthma often benefit from using their inhaled medication five to ten minutes before exercise. If accessing the medication is difficult, inconvenient, or embarrassing, the student may be discouraged and fail to use the inhaler as needed. The student's asthma may become unnecessarily worse and his or her activities needlessly limited.

Here are some actions to consider:

- Provide students with asthma convenient access to their medications for all on- and off-site activities before, during, and after school. These medications prevent as well as treat symptoms and enable the student to participate safely and vigorously in physical activities.

- Enable students to carry and administer their own medications if the parent or guardian, healthcare provider, and school nurse so advise.

Modify Physical Activities to Match Current Asthma Status

Students who follow their asthma management plans and keep their asthma under control can usually participate vigorously in the full range of sports and physical activities. Activities that are more intense and sustained—such as long periods of running, basketball, and soccer—are more likely to provoke asthma symptoms or an asthma episode. However, Olympic medalists with serious asthma have demonstrated that these activities are possible with good asthma management.

When a student experiences asthma symptoms, or is recovering from a recent asthma episode, exercise should be temporarily modified in type, length, and/or frequency to help reduce the risk of further symptoms. The student also needs convenient access to his or her medications.

Here are some actions to consider:

- Include adequate warm-up and cool-down periods. These help prevent or lessen episodes of exercise-induced asthma.

- Consult the student's asthma management plan, parent or guardian, or healthcare provider on the type and length of any limitations. Assess the student and school resources to determine how the student can participate most fully.

- Remember that a student who experiences symptoms or who has just recovered from an asthma episode is at even greater risk for additional asthma problems. Take extra care. Observe for asthma symptoms, and check the student's peak flow if he or she uses a peak flow meter. Review the student's asthma management plan if there are any questions.

- Monitor the environment for potential allergens and irritants, for example, a recently mowed field or refinished gym floor. If an allergen or irritant is present, consider a temporary change in location.

- Make exercise modifications as necessary to get appropriate levels of participation. For example, if running is scheduled, the student could walk the whole distance, run part of the distance, or alternate running and walking.

- Keep the student involved when any temporary but major modification is required. Ask the student to act, for example, as a scorekeeper, timer, or equipment handler until he or she can return to full participation. Dressing for a physical education class and participating at any level is better than being left out or left behind.

Recognizing Symptoms and Taking Appropriate Action

Recognizing asthma symptoms and taking appropriate action in response to the symptoms is crucial to asthma treatment and control.

Symptoms That Require Prompt Action

Acute symptoms require prompt action to help students resume their activities as soon as possible. Prompt action is also required to prevent an episode from becoming more serious or even life threatening. Following is a list of the symptoms that indicate an acute asthma episode and the need for immediate action. The student's asthma plan and the school's emergency plan should be easily accessible so that all staff, substitutes, volunteers, and aides know what to do.

Acute symptoms requiring prompt action include the following:

- Coughing or wheezing
- Difficulty in breathing
- Chest tightness or pressure—reported by the student
- Other signs, such as low peak flow readings as indicated on the asthma management plan

Symptoms of exercise-induced asthma (coughing, wheezing, pain, or chest tightness) may last several minutes to an hour or more. These symptoms are quite different from breathlessness (deep, rapid breathing) that quickly returns to normal after aerobic exercise.

Here are some actions to take:

- Stop the student's current activity.
- Follow the student's asthma management/action plan.
- Help the student use his or her inhaled medication.
- Observe for effect.

When to Get Emergency Help

Get emergency help if any of the following are true:

- If the student fails to improve.
- If any of the symptoms listed on the student's asthma plan as emergency indicators are present.
- If any of the following symptoms are present (consider calling 911):
  - The student is hunched over, with shoulders lifted, and straining to breathe.
  - The student has difficulty completing a sentence without pausing for breath.
  - The student's lips or fingernails turn blue.

Signs That May Indicate Poorly Controlled Asthma

Students may have symptoms that do not indicate an acute episode needing immediate treatment, but instead indicate that their asthma is not under complete control:

- A persistent cough
- Coughing, wheezing, chest tightness, or shortness of breath after vigorous physical activity, on a recurring basis
- A low level of stamina during physical activity, or reluctance to participate.

The teachers and coaches who supervise students' physical activities are in a unique position to notice signs that a child who struggles with physical activity might in fact have asthma. Because exercise provokes symptoms in most children with poorly controlled asthma, the student may need to be evaluated by his or her healthcare provider. It may also be that the student simply needs to follow his or her asthma management plan more carefully.

Here are some actions to consider:

- Share observations of the symptoms with the school nurse and the student's parents or guardians. Helping students get the medical attention they need is an important way to help children become active and take control of their condition.
- Provide students convenient access to their asthma medication.

491

Confusing Signs: Is It an Asthma Episode or a Need for More Support?

At times teachers and coaches may wonder if a student's reported symptoms indicate a desire for attention or a desire not to participate in an activity. At other times it may seem that students are overreacting to minimal symptoms.

It is always essential to respect the student's report of his or her own condition. If a student regularly asks to be excused from recess or avoids physical activity, a real physical problem may be present. It also may be that the student needs more assistance and support from his or her teacher and coach in order to become an active participant.

Here are some actions to consider:

- Talk with the student to learn his or her concerns about asthma and activity, offer reassurance that you understand the importance of appropriate modifications or activity limits, and develop a shared understanding about the conditions that require activity modifications or medications.

- Consult with the school nurse, the student's parent or guardian, or his or her healthcare provider to find ways to ensure that the student is safe, feels safe, and is encouraged to participate actively.

- If the student uses a peak flow meter, remind him or her to use it. This may help the student appreciate his or her asthma status and appropriate levels of activity.

Section 42.3

What Physical Educators and Coaches Need to Know about Asthma

As a coach or gym teacher, you may have helped, at some point along the way, to train or teach one of the multitude of Olympic medalists and professional athletes who have succeeded at the highest competitive levels—and have asthma.

It's important that you remember to support every young person's opportunity to reap the long-term physical and psychological health benefits of exercise to the best of your ability.

Each and every young person with asthma should be able to exercise and play sports with little, if any, limitation if the asthma is under good control and properly managed.

Be an integral part of the team that includes the youngster, parent, and pediatric pulmonologist. As a team member, encourage your athlete to adhere to his or her asthma treatment plan and communicate closely with parents and physicians.

Know the facts about asthma. Approximately one out of four elite, competitive athletes at the high school or college level have asthma or exercise-induced bronchospasm (the airway narrowing that occurs during or after physical exertion in susceptible young people). At least 10 percent of the youth population in general has asthma.

Be aware of the signs and symptoms suggestive of asthma.

Many young people are embarrassed or frightened to report symptoms. Some do not realize what is happening to them. Others may be afraid that they will no longer be able to exercise or play sports. Be cognizant of complaints about chest pain, chest tightness, difficulty "getting air in," dry cough, and redness in the face or extreme pallor during or immediately after aerobic exertion. These warning signs may warrant parent notification. Encourage your athlete or student to "get checked out" for possible asthma.

For gym teachers of younger individuals, the "one mile" or President's fitness run may provide the signal. For team coaches, the tip-off can be breathing difficulty with wind sprints or suicides (during practice and warm-up sessions). At the high school and college levels, underperformance for the level of conditioning may be a key indicator.

Your most important role as part of the asthma team is to help ensure that the young athlete trains hard, follows the individualized treatment plan, and consistently receives the encouragement that he or she can and will win even with the challenges and obstacles that asthma may present.

Be clear that there are certain times when a young person's asthma may present more of a challenge to outstanding athletic performance. These times may include seasonal allergies and upper respiratory infections or colds.

"Toughing it out" or "battling through" their symptoms is not the smart way to go. Instead, encourage and teach the youngster to adjust or increase their medicines as early as possible. This move decreases the chance of deterioration in asthma. Never discourage the use of asthma medications. Even at the professional and Olympic levels, many asthma medications are absolutely approved for use if deemed necessary, in advance, by the appropriate evaluation.

It's to a coach's or gym teacher's advantage to be in the know about asthma treatment.

Understand which medications should be used in advance and which should be introduced as rescue medications should symptoms occur. No two young people with asthma will likely be on the same asthma treatment plan—and each individual responds a little differently to various medications. Treatment trials and adjustments may be necessary, and, a combination of two or three medications may ultimately be necessary for optimal control.

If your athlete with asthma is not performing as well as expected, or, if more overt asthma symptoms arise, encourage them to take a break and incorporate their "rescue" strategies. They will most likely come back stronger in a short period of time.

Recognize an athlete or student in trouble and one who may be in need of emergency care.

When there is no symptom improvement within fifteen to twenty minutes of using a rescue inhaler (bronchodilator), it's a distress sign.

A youngster who is bent over with shoulders lifted, or is struggling to breathe, or has difficulty speaking, or has pulling in of the chest or neck muscles is definitely in trouble. A gray or bluish discoloration of the lips or nail beds is indicative of extreme distress.

Encourage your charge to remain calm by encouraging slow and steady deep breaths. Remain with your athlete or student and immediately ask someone to call 911.

Want to maximize physical exercise and athletic performance?

Encourage the consistent and proper use of a pre-medication inhaler(s) (if necessary), know the proper delivery techniques, and supervise your athlete whenever possible.

Actively encourage a moderate- to high-intensity warm-up for five to ten minutes. A focused warm-up goes a long way to decreasing the airway spasm that can occur. Cool-downs after workouts slow the changeover of air in the lungs from cold back to warm and lessen the chance of symptoms occurring after aerobic exercise.

If you coach or teach cold weather sports, encourage breathing through the nose as much as possible. Recommend your athlete cover his or her mouth with a scarf or ski gator. Cold air inhalation, accompanied by the usual airway dryness that occurs with increased ventilation generated with exercise, can easily trigger exercise-induced bronchospasm.

After serving as a source of encouragement and motivation all day long to athletes and students, coaches and gym teachers need an inspiring pep talk you can call your own. OK, here it is.

The better the athlete's state of physical condition, the better the asthma control. The better the asthma control, the better the athlete's performance. Now, get out there and help your youngster win over asthma.

Chapter 43

Asthma in Teens

Chapter Contents

Section 43.1

Dealing with Asthma: Tips for Teens

"How Can I Deal with My Asthma?" November 2009, reprinted with permission from www.kidshealth.org. Copyright © 2009 The Nemours Foundation. This information was provided by KidsHealth, one of the largest resources online for medically reviewed health information written for parents, kids, and teens. For more articles like this one, visit www.KidsHealth.org, or www.TeensHealth.org.

Asthma is more common these days than it used to be. The good news is it's also a lot easier to manage and control.

Since more teens have asthma, you're probably used to seeing people take a break from sports to use an inhaler or take a moment after school to test their airflow with a peak flow meter. But even though asthma is a part of so many people's daily lives, there are times when they can feel annoyed or frustrated at having asthma—just as they get annoyed or frustrated by anything else.

Different people have different reactions to the ways that asthma affects their lives. For example, some worry that they might have to avoid all physical activities—even those approved by their doctors—and miss out on fun. Others go to the opposite extreme, denying they have asthma at all and maybe forgetting or refusing to take the medications that can control it. Still others find that asthma is a convenient excuse to get out of chores or gym class.

Taking Action

If you have asthma and don't want it to have control over you, take control first.

The best tool for controlling asthma is something your doctor gives you called an asthma action plan. Following all the steps described in an action plan allows people with asthma to enjoy daily activities just like everyone else.

Your asthma action plan offers you the best protection against potentially dangerous (not to mention embarrassing) episodes—such as having an asthma attack at a party where people are smoking.

Unfortunately, people may not always stick with their plan, for lots of different reasons. Maybe they forget to take medications. Perhaps they don't completely understand why they're supposed to take certain steps or medications. A few might feel embarrassed about checking their airflow or using an inhaler in front of others. And some may mistakenly think they don't need medicine after they start feeling better—putting them at risk for potentially dangerous flare-ups.

More Tips

Here are some simple steps that can help you get around these common problems:

- **Understand your plan:** Ask your doctor to explain why each medication and step of the plan is important. You'll feel more in control if you understand exactly what's going on and what will happen if you follow (or don't follow) your plan. Check in with your doctor often and go over the plan, explaining where you may have had trouble with it and why.

- **Use asthma management tools:** Even if you're feeling absolutely fine, don't abandon tools like daily controller medicines and peak flow meters if they're a part of your treatment plan. Although it can be tempting to skip recommended daily meds and rely only on occasional rescue medicines, this usually doesn't work.

- **Set up a schedule:** It can be easy to slip up and forget to take a medication—but this is less likely to happen if you follow the steps on your action plan at the same time every day. Make your medicine part of your daily routine, like brushing your teeth.

- **Don't smoke:** Cigarette smoke is a common cause of asthma aggravation in teens. Talk to your parent or a doctor about how to quit if you smoke. If your friends smoke, don't stand nearby when they light up because secondhand smoke is a common trigger of asthma attacks. If someone in your family smokes, talk with him or her about quitting.

- **Control your environment:** Environmental triggers, such as dust mites and pet dander, can be hazardous if you have asthma. If you have pets, keep Fido or Fluffy out of your room. Also, try to keep your room dust free by cleaning it regularly, and talk to your doctor about using special mattress and pillow covers.

- **Get a flu shot every year:** Health officials now recommend that all kids and teens get a flu shot (for both seasonal flu and H1N1), and this is particularly important for people with asthma who have a greater chance of developing a more serious illness when they catch the flu.

- **Find a sport or activity that works for you:** Some sports, such as swimming and baseball, are less likely to trigger asthma flare-ups. Other sports may be more challenging for people with asthma, like endurance or cold-weather sports. Many athletes have found that with proper training and medication, they can participate in any sport they choose. Sports can boost your mood—a great help for those times when you may feel frustrated about having asthma.

Using a management plan to deal with asthma is good for more than your health. Getting used to following an asthma action plan can give you the discipline to stick with a plan and succeed in other areas of life as well.

Section 43.2

Parenting a Teen with Asthma

The teen years can be rough for kids, and they can be even rougher
for teens with asthma. The last thing they want their friends to know
is that they're "different." Here are some tips to make parenting an
adolescent with asthma a bit easier:

- Many teens don't want to take medication in front of their
  friends, so ask your doctor if your teen's daily controller medication can be taken at home in the morning and evening. This not
  only can make taking asthma medication part of a morning or
  nighttime routine, just like brushing teeth or showering, but also
  lets parents make sure their kids get all the medication they need.

- Many kids with asthma, especially teens, stop taking their daily
  controller medications and rely only upon their rescue medications. Controller medications work quietly in the background to
  control airway inflammation without the person actually feeling
  any immediate effects, so their benefits might go unnoticed. Not
  taking controller medications when needed can be dangerous
  and even fatal. If this becomes a concern, discuss it with your
  doctor immediately.

- It's very common for teens to be in denial about having asthma,
  and they may stop taking medications, which can lead to more
  symptoms and flare-ups. If this happens, you may need to monitor your teen's care until he or she is ready to do it alone. Many
  parents find it helpful to use a peak flow meter (a handheld tool
  that can be used at home to measure breathing ability) as the
  final word on whether (and how much) medication is needed to
  prevent a flare-up.

- When peak flow readings drop, it's a sign of increasing airway inflammation. The peak flow meter can detect subtle airway inflammation and obstruction, even when someone feels fine. In some cases, it can detect drops in peak flow readings two to three days before a flare-up occurs, providing plenty of time to treat and prevent it.

- Peak flow meters never lie, so kids can't deny they're having a problem—and parents are less likely to be seen as bad guys or overprotective, forcing their kids to take medication unnecessarily.

- Remember to maintain your teen's dignity and involvement when dealing with asthma. Older kids should be actively included in all discussions and treatment choices because they're the ones who ultimately have to take the medication regularly and deal with possible side effects.

- Uncontrolled asthma can lead to depression and low self-esteem. These feelings may manifest in emotional outbursts and poor school performance. However, early intervention by a school counselor, teacher, or physician can encourage compliance with doctors' orders and help keep your teen's asthma under control.

- Teens with asthma should be encouraged to live as normal a life as possible with the help of medications and thoughtful limitations. Some teens tend to shy away from normal activities such as sports and even school dances because they're afraid of having a flare-up. Others learn to use asthma as an excuse for getting out of activities and chores. Teens should understand how monitoring medication and breathing will let them do just about anything.

Part Six

Asthma in Other Special Populations

Chapter 44

Asthma and Pregnancy

Asthma Management

Early awareness of asthma symptoms and peak flow monitoring can help you and your doctor respond quickly to worsening of your asthma during pregnancy. It is important to identify and treat your asthma when the symptoms are still mild, so as to reduce the risk of a more serious episode. Common asthma symptoms may vary from person to person and include:

- cough;
- shortness of breath;
- tightness in the chest;
- wheeze;
- shortness of breath.

Many of these symptoms are common during pregnancy, and it sometimes may be difficult to tell if the cause is the increasing size of your baby or your asthma. A peak flow meter may enable you to tell the difference. A peak flow meter measures the airflow out of your lungs and can sometimes show a decrease hours or even a day before other asthma symptoms appear. Ask your doctor about using a peak flow meter to help monitor your asthma.

Asthma Action Plan for Your Pregnancy

An asthma action plan is a written plan based on changes in asthma symptoms and peak flow numbers, customized to your needs by your doctor to help you manage asthma worsening. It will give you information about when and how to use long-term control medicine and quick-relief medicine. It is a reminder of what to watch for and what steps to take so you will be able to make timely and appropriate decisions about managing your asthma during your pregnancy.

Severe Asthma Episodes During Pregnancy

When asthma symptoms and low peak flow numbers indicate your asthma is worsening, it is important to take action to ensure you and your baby receive enough oxygen. A severe asthma attack is a true medical emergency and you should seek medical assistance immediately. A small number of women with asthma may have an asthma episode severe enough to be hospitalized so that you and your baby can be closely monitored. A severe asthma attack is a true medical emergency and you should seek medical assistance immediately. Your treatment may include oxygen, frequent inhaled medications, and intravenous (IV) steroids, all of which can be given without risk to your baby.

Asthma Management During Labor and Delivery

It is important to continue long-term control medicines and have quick-relief medicines available throughout labor and delivery. Your breathing will be closely monitored, as will your baby's heart rate with a fetal monitor to make sure that he or she is not showing signs of distress. Plan ahead and discuss these decisions and potential problems with your healthcare providers. This will help decrease fears and problems that may arise once labor begins:

- Bring your own medications to the hospital, so everyone will understand what you have been taking. The hospital will then provide whatever medication is needed.

- Talk with your healthcare provider about pain control during delivery before your delivery date. If anesthesia is required, spinal anesthesia is preferred to general ("gas") anesthesia. If you receive anesthesia of this form, you may be able to use your inhaled medicine as directed by your doctor. If a Cesarean-section is required you may need IV steroids.

Breastfeeding When You Have Asthma

Research shows that breastfeeding for the first six to twelve months of life may help prevent or delay the development of certain allergies. The decision to breastfeed should be based on what you desire and your baby's needs. The medicines safe for use during pregnancy are generally used while breastfeeding without problems. Because your blood stream absorbs less medicine with inhaled medicine, less medicine passes into your breast milk. It is important to discuss your use of any medicines with your baby's doctor.

Asthma Medications

We would like to avoid all medicine during pregnancy. However, a pregnancy without medicine is not always possible or desirable. It is safer for pregnant women with asthma to be treated with asthma medications than for them to have asthma symptoms and exacerbations. Maintaining adequate control or asthma during pregnancy is important for the health and well-being of both the mother and her baby.

Medicine Safety Categories

The U.S. Food & Drug Administration has classified all medications into categories based on their safety for the mother and baby. Medicine is rated A, B, C, D, and X, where A is the safest and X is not safe. All medicines approved since 1980 are classified in one of these categories, and here are the categories relating to asthma medicines.

Category A: These are the medicines for which adequate, well-controlled studies in pregnant women have not shown an increased risk of fetal abnormalities. No medicines used to treat asthma fall into this category.

Category B: Category B indicates animal studies have revealed no evidence of harm to the fetus, however, there are no adequate and well-controlled studies in pregnant women. Some asthma medications fall in this category, and category B asthma drugs are generally considered safe for both mother and child.

Category C: Category C is one in which animal studies have shown an adverse effect and there are no adequate and well-controlled studies in pregnant women; or, no animal studies have been conducted and there are not adequate and well-controlled studies in pregnant women. Most of the medicine used to treat asthma fall into this category, and are generally considered safe for both mother and child.

Making Decisions about Medication During Pregnancy

It is important that your asthma be controlled to assure your baby's oxygen supply and decrease your health risk. By working closely with your doctor, you will be able to take the least medicine necessary for good asthma control:

- Review all the medicine you are taking with your doctor. This includes "over-the-counter medicine," vitamins, and any herbal supplement you may be taking. Even these seemingly harmless things can be harmful to your baby.

- Ask your healthcare provider about any medicine before you take it.

- Take only medicine your healthcare provider has approved or prescribed.

Long-Term Control Medicines and Pregnancy

Long-term control medicines are used daily to maintain control of asthma and prevent asthma symptoms, even when asthma is stable. They do not provide immediate relief of symptoms.

Inhaled steroids: Common inhaled steroids used during pregnancy include: Pulmicort (budesonide), category B; Vanceril, Beclovent, Qvar (beclomethasone), category C; and Flovent (fluticasone), category C.

All other inhaled steroids not listed here are in category C. Inhaled steroids prevent and reduce swelling in the airways and may decrease mucus production. They are the most effective long-term control medicine now available. They improve asthma symptoms and lung function, and they have been shown to decrease the need for oral steroids and hospitalization. Inhaled steroids are taken on a regular basis and cause few, if any, side effects in usual doses. Thrush, a possible side effect, is a yeast infection causing a white discoloration of the tongue. Using a spacer with inhaled steroids (metered-dose inhaler) and rinsing your mouth after inhaling the medicine reduces the risk of thrush.

Cromolyn sodium and nedocromil: Intal (cromolyn) and Tilade (nedocromil) are also long-term control medicines available in inhaled forms. They are in category B. They help to prevent asthma symptoms, especially symptoms caused by exercise, cold air, and allergies. When used routinely, each helps prevent swelling in the airways. They are often taken on a regular basis, but may also be used as a pre-treatment before exposure to things that make asthma worse. They are much less effective than inhaled steroids and leukotriene modifiers.

Leukotriene modifiers: Singulair and Accolate are category B long-term control medicine. They reduce swelling inside the airways and relax smooth muscles around the airways, and they are effective at improving asthma symptoms and lung function, but not as effectively as inhaled steroids. They are available as tablets. There have been fewer years of experience with this class of drugs than with other asthma medicine. For this reason, and because minimal data are currently available on the use of these drugs during pregnancy, they should be avoided.

Theophylline: Common theophyllines include Slo-Bid, Uniphyl, and T-Phyl. Theophylline relaxes the smooth muscles around the airways. Theophyllines are in category C. Studies and clinical experience confirm the safety of this drug at recommended doses that result in a serum theophylline level of 5–15 mcg/ml. But because of side effects (usually at higher serum levels) theophylline is not one of the first medicines used for long-term control of asthma. There are safer and more effective medicines available.

Quick-Relief Medicines and Pregnancy

Quick-relief medicines are used to treat asthma symptoms or asthma worsening.

Short-acting beta-agonists: Common inhaled beta-agonists include Proventil, Proventil HFA, Ventolin (albuterol); Xopenex (levalbuterol); Maxair (pirbuterol); and Combivent (albuterol and ipratropium).

These medicines are category C but have been used for decades and are deemed to be safe for both mother and fetus. Short-acting beta-agonists provide quick relief by relaxing the smooth muscles around the airways. If you use more than one of these metered-dose inhalers in a month talk with your doctor. This is a sign that your asthma is poorly controlled and your long-term control medicine may need to be adjusted. Remember, your asthma needs to be consistently under good control since you are "breathing for two."

Oral steroids: Common steroid pills and liquids include Deltasone (prednisone) and Medrol (methylprednisolone).

A short-term burst of oral steroids may be needed to decrease the severity of asthma symptoms and prevent an emergency room visit, but should be discontinued as soon as asthma control is achieved. Oral steroids are very effective at reducing swelling and mucus production in the airways. They also help other quick-relief medicine work better. Sustained use of oral steroids has been associated with preeclampsia, an undesirable condition associated only with pregnancy.

Inhaled medicine technique: It is crucial that you use your inhaled medicine correctly to get the full dosage and benefits from the medicine. If you are using a metered-dose inhaler you should use a spacer. This is especially important with inhaled corticosteroids. Ask your healthcare provider to watch your techniques with the inhaled medicine to make sure you are using it correctly.

Other Asthma-Related Medication Treatment

Annual influenza vaccine (flu shot): The annual flu shot is recommended for pregnant women with asthma during the second or third trimester.

Immunotherapy (allergy shots): Allergy shots should not be started during pregnancy. However, if you have been receiving allergy shots and have not shown any severe reactions, you may continue them at the same dose.

Chapter 45

Asthma in Older Adults

Chapter Contents

Section 45.1

Treating Asthma in Older Adults

Underdiagnosis of Asthma a Problem with Older People

Asthma is not just a childhood disease; it can occur at any age. The classic symptoms of asthma—coughing, wheezing, breathlessness, and tightness of chest—can easily be misinterpreted as part of normal aging or be misdiagnosed as other health problems in older adults. Older people may not report their symptoms; may attribute their symptoms to another illness or disease or normal aging; or may simply ignore their symptoms. Here are some of the most common reasons for unrecognized asthma in older people:

- Heart or lung diseases with similar symptoms to asthma, such as wheezing, can mask the presence of asthma.

- The actual symptoms of asthma might be dismissed as other conditions. For example, a chronic cough might be mistaken for bronchitis, or the inability to sleep during the night may be dismissed as insomnia.

Conditions which have symptoms in common with asthma in the elderly include:

- chronic obstructive pulmonary disease (COPD);

- chronic bronchitis, emphysema, or acute respiratory illness;

- rhinosinusitis with postnasal drip;

- tuberculosis;

- gastroesophageal reflux; and

- cardiac diseases such as congestive heart failure, acute myocardial infarction (heart attack), or cardiac arrhythmia (abnormal heart rhythm).

Different Triggers in Older Adults

Triggers for asthma attacks can differ in older adults with asthma from those most commonly affecting children with asthma. In older adults, viral respiratory illnesses (for example, colds and flu) and airborne allergens are the most common triggers. This is why it's important that older adults have an influenza vaccination every year. Pneumococcal vaccine is also recommended for all people who are over sixty-five.

Some medications used frequently in older adults are also known to trigger asthma or make symptoms worse. Examples include: aspirin and other anti-inflammatory medications used to treat arthritis and other pain; beta-blockers used to treat hypertension (high blood pressure) and heart disease; and beta-blocking eye drops used to treat glaucoma. For this reason, it is important to keep a list of all the medications you currently use and show it to your doctor at each visit.

Complications of Asthma in the Elderly

In addition to the issues above, changes in lung structure and function brought about by normal ageing may make the problems associated with asthma worse in the elderly.

Also, normal, age-related changes in the body mean that older people with asthma are more susceptible to adverse effects from the very medications they are taking to control their asthma. They may also be at risk of adverse interactions between different medications they are taking.

Remembering to take medications for chronic conditions, such as asthma, may be more of a challenge for older people than younger ones. Also, problems with coordination or arthritis of the hands may make using puffers and other asthma medication delivery devices difficult, and problems with eyesight may affect ability to read labels. If you have problems coordinating drug release and inhalation, you may find it easier using the puffer in conjunction with a spacer. Alternatively, you may be better off using a breath-activated device such as an Accuhaler, Autohaler, or Turbuhaler.

Questions for Older Adults Who Suspect They May Have Asthma

- Have you experienced an attack or recurrent attacks of wheezing?

513

- Have you had a troublesome cough or wheeze on waking up in the morning?

- Do you have a tendency to cough or wheeze after exercising?

- Do you experience a cough, wheeze, or chest tightness after exposure to airborne allergens or pollutants?

- Do colds go to your chest or take more than ten days to clear up?

What to Do

If asthma is suspected, see your doctor, who will make a diagnosis and prescribe the appropriate treatment. Making the diagnosis will probably involve doing some basic lung function tests, performed before and after using an asthma reliever medicine. Many doctors have such testing equipment in their offices and it can be done by them or their practice nurses. They may also order a chest x-ray to rule out other disorders or to diagnose coexisting conditions.

You should also follow the same recommended general rules for the control of asthma that all people with asthma are encouraged to follow—these will be incorporated in the written asthma action plan that you develop with your doctor.

Section 45.2

Asthma and Aged Care Facility Residents

Is Asthma Really an Issue in Aged Care?

- Ten percent of adults over sixty-five have currently diagnosed asthma.

- Thirty percent of elderly people may have undiagnosed asthma.

- The majority of deaths from asthma occur in people over the age of sixty-five.

- Many deaths from asthma are preventable.

What Can Aged Care Facility Staff Do to Help?

- Recognize asthma.

- Help residents take their medications effectively.

- Know what to do in an asthma emergency.

Recognize Asthma

Breathlessness and other respiratory symptoms are often considered by older people as a natural part of aging, but this is not true. Breathlessness can be a symptom of a number of different conditions, including asthma. Staff should particularly consider "Could it be asthma?" in residents who also show signs of wheezing or have a cough, especially at night or early in the morning.

Asthma is not just a childhood disease, and it can occur at any age or may return in someone who has not had symptoms for many years. Other health issues that can cause breathlessness should also be considered, such as chronic obstructive pulmonary disease (COPD), heart failure, and lung cancer, among others.

Seeking a medical review for diagnostic testing (such as spirometry, chest x-ray) as early as possible means you could help residents to better levels of health and activity quickly and effectively.

Help Residents Take Their Medications Effectively

Asthma medications can be complex and confusing with all the different medications and types of delivery devices. It is thought that up to 90 percent of people do not use their inhaler device correctly. This means they aren't getting the right amount of medication and so may not be receiving effective treatment.

You can support residents by learning how each of the medication devices is used and helping residents use them well. This may include contacting a doctor to tell them that a resident is not managing their current device, and suggesting it be changed to improve medication delivery.

Which device is right? The choice of device should always depend on the ability of the person using it. You should consider:

- breath intake;
- hand strength;
- coordination;
- understanding or confusion level of the resident;
- assisting devices, such as a spacer.

There are also special aids available to help people with poor grip strength to effectively use devices (e.g., Haleraid).

Some older people are particularly fond of using nebulizers, as they have experienced these in the past. Giving reliever medication via a puffer and spacer has been shown to be equally effective, and the dose can be delivered much faster. For this reason using a spacer device with a puffer is generally recommended over a nebulizer. It is also less costly over time to use a puffer with a spacer.

Note: It is also important to monitor any side effects from medications and to consider potential interactions with other drugs when a new medication is commenced.

Know What to Do in an Asthma Emergency: Know Asthma First Aid

An asthma attack can take minutes or days to develop. You should consider possible triggers for residents, and if you know what they are, try to minimize their exposure to them where possible.

Common triggers in aged care facilities are:

- cold or flu viruses;
- cleaning products;
- perfumes;
- changes in weather or temperature.

Recognize Worsening Asthma

Worsening asthma can be recognized by:

- shortness of breath;
- tightness in the chest; and/or
- wheezing and/or coughing, especially at night or early morning.

Note: These may also be symptoms of other illnesses, so should always be carefully monitored.

A written asthma action plan will also help you to recognize and respond to a change in a resident's asthma. The action plan is a written set of instructions from the resident's doctor that explains how to recognize changes in symptoms and what to do to treat them.

If a resident is having difficulty breathing, and you believe the cause to be asthma, follow asthma first aid immediately.

Chapter 46

Asthma in Athletes

Chapter Contents

Section 46.1

Asthma Management in Athletes

"Exercise-Induced Asthma Management in Athletes," © 2006 Colorado
Allergy and Asthma Centers (www.coloradoallergy.com). Reprinted with
permission. Revised by David A. Cooke, MD, FACP, May 2011.

Introduction

Most patients with asthma will experience asthma symptoms with
strenuous exercise. Usually, it is relatively easy to prevent exercise-
induced asthma (EIA) by using an inhaled bronchodilator (for example,
Proventil HFA, Ventolin HFA, or ProAir HFA) prior to exercise. However, in many athletes who exercise for sustained periods of time, simple
treatments are not effective. This is frustrating for many athletes who
see their asthma as causing a limitation of their ability to perform to
their maximal level. Additionally, there is a concern that many of the
asthma medications will not be allowed in competitive events, which
could lead to disqualification.

Fortunately, treatment plans for athletes with asthma have been
developed and successfully used in college-, Olympic-, and professional-
level sports. There are many medications which have been approved
(and some which have been banned!) in various arenas of athletic
competition, including international competition.

How Athletes Can Help Themselves Prevent EIA

It is important for you to develop a plan with your doctor to help
you prevent EIA. Every individual is different. Here is what we recommend to our patients with difficult-to-control EIA:

- Make sure your asthma is as well controlled as possible on a
  day-to-day basis.

- If possible, choose a sport that is the least likely to trigger asthma. Swimming is less "asthmagenic" than biking, and biking is
  less "asthmagenic" than running.

- Pay attention to environmental factors and their impact on your
  asthma during exercise. For example, elevated pollution levels

may affect your asthma during exercise, as may cold, dry air and pollen-filled air. Thus, exercising indoors at certain times may be preferable to outdoor exercise.

- Try to breathe through your nose during exercise as much as possible, since the nasal tissue's function is to clean, warm, and humidify air before it reaches your lungs.

- Physical training and conditioning is important, since it can increase how efficiently the heart and lungs work, thus allowing you to do a greater amount of work with less effort.

- A warm-up period, when used together with inhaled (and occasionally oral) medications before exercise, can help athletes avoid or control episodes of EIA during competition:

  - Begin by pre-medicating.

  - Warm-up with three to five minutes of very light aerobic activity. Proceed with a variety of stretching exercises.

  - Begin aerobic exercise (for example, jogging or running). Raise heart rate to 50 to 60 percent of your maximum and sustain it for five to ten minutes. This may cause the airways to "open up" to a slight extent, therefore getting more air into the lungs and more oxygen into the bloodstream. Proceed until your training session is complete. Follow with a cool-down period.

If EIA symptoms continue to interfere with exercise, contact your doctor for further evaluation.

Recommendations for Medication Use for Asthma and Upper Respiratory Symptoms in Competitive Athletes

It is important for every athlete who is or will be participating in college and/or Olympic sports to ensure that all of his or her medications are in compliance with the rules and regulations of sports governing bodies.

Different governing bodies have their own set of regulations regarding medications that are prohibited or restricted. Further, the particular form of a medication may make a difference in terms of its acceptability for use. In addition, certain medications require prior notification to the athletic governing body and/or other groups. Thus, it is essential that every competitive athlete contact the appropriate source(s) for information on all prescription and over-the-counter medications that he or she is using or is considering using. This includes all topical preparations.

It must be noted that if an athlete in the United States is using or considering using a medication obtained outside of the United States, its status must be determined through an appropriate source. It should also be noted that the United States Olympic Committee (USOC) and the National Collegiate Athletic Association (NCAA) have different lists for medications.

Here is a list of information sources for medication use for athletes:

- Sources for Olympic athletes:

  - Consult a USOC head team physician.

  - Consult a knowledgeable USOC medical staff member.

  - www.usantidoping.org has the most current Guide Book on Prohibited Substances.

  - USOC Olympic Drug Reference Line at 800-233-0393. This line is staffed on weekdays from 8:00 a.m. to 5:00 p.m. (Mountain Time), is confidential, and can assist athletes, coaches, parents, physicians, and others. For emergencies during weekends or after-hours, coverage is provided through an answering service.

  - Written information is available from the USOC.

  - It should be noted that the USOC has incorporated the principles and guidelines set forth by the International Olympic Committee (IOC). However, some medications may be prohibited by international federations.

- Sources for collegiate athletes:

  - Consult a trainer, coach, and/or team physician.

  - www2.ncaa.org This website provides general information that includes a "Banned Drug List." Click on "Legislation & Governance" at top of home page, click "Eligibility & Conduct," then click "Drug Testing."

  - NCAA, 700 W. Washington St., P.O. Box 6222, Indianapolis, IN 46206-6222, phone: 317-917-6222.

  - Written information is also available from the NCAA.

References

Huftel MA et al.: Finding and managing asthma in competitive athletes. *J Resp Dis* 1991; 12:1110.

Reiff DB et al.: The effect of prolonged submaximal warm-up exercise on exercise-induced asthma. *Am Rev Respir Dis* 1989; 139:479.

United States Olympic Committee Drug Education Program, Colorado Springs, Colorado, 80909, May 1999.

Athletic Drug Reference '99. Editors: Robert J. Fuentes, MS, Pharm D, Jack M. Rosenberg, Pharm D, PhD.

Section 46.2

Winning Strategies for Athletes with Asthma and Allergies

Competitive sports are as American as apple pie, and the late summer and early fall months see athletes of all ages gathering on fields. In much of the country, that means intense exercise in high heat and humidity—conditions that stress even the healthiest bodies.

Athletes with asthma or allergies face extra challenges. For many, exercise itself sets off asthma symptoms—although the warm, humid air of summertime may actually be easier on the lungs than cold, dry air. In addition, players practicing on outdoor fields in late summer and fall may have to deal with high levels of ragweed pollen and mold—two potent respiratory allergens—and air pollution.

Even so, there's no reason people with asthma can't play competitive sports, says Jack Becker, M.D., an allergist at St. Christopher's Hospital for Children, Philadelphia, and author of several studies on asthma and sports. "The way to avoid problems is to aggressively manage your asthma and take steps to reduce allergic reactions."

Create a Good Offense

Athletes with asthma should work with medical care providers to develop a management plan that minimizes symptoms.

Begin by understanding your individual asthma thumbprint. What sets off your asthma symptoms? Do you only experience breathing problems during exercise? Or is your asthma affected by other factors, such as allergies to dust mites, pets, mold, or pollen?

Asthma is a disease that involves inflammation in the airways. Exposure to an allergen, irritant, or activity that irritates those inflamed airways causes muscles around the airways to tighten up and twitch (bronchospasm), making you cough, wheeze, and have trouble breathing. The way to reduce symptoms and help your lungs deal with the stress of exercise, then, is to control inflammation and minimize exposure to allergens and irritants.

The most effective medications available to reduce airway inflammation are inhaled corticosteroids. These medications take time to reach full effect, so it's important to begin taking them before your athletic season begins. Many people with asthma take them year-round. Other medications that may be part of an aggressive asthma management plan include leukotriene modifiers and long-acting bronchodilators.

The best treatment for allergies is avoidance—but that is often impossible for athletes sensitive to airborne allergens such as pollen or mold. Since allergy medications also take time to build up effect, people with seasonal allergies should begin taking medications such as antihistamines or nasal corticosteroids two to three weeks before allergy season begins. Athletes with year-round allergies (such as mold) should talk with a physician about extra protection prior to the sports season. If you're allergic to airborne allergens such as pollen or mold you may want to consider allergy shots (immunotherapy).

Athletes with pollen or mold allergies who must exercise outdoors during pollen/mold seasons should also shower after outdoor exercise to wash allergens off their skin, hair, and eyes (particularly before bedtime) and consider using a nasal wash to help reduce allergy symptoms.

Air pollution is difficult to avoid when you practice outdoors, but many teams restrict practice on days with the worst air quality. Talk with your medical care team about what else you can do to control asthma symptoms on poor air quality days.

The Exercise Opponent

Experts think one reason exercise sets off asthma symptoms is that breathing through the mouth bypasses the built-in filtering and heating system of the nose and exposes lungs to allergens, pollutants, dry air, or cold air, any of which could cause airways to constrict, increase inflammation, or produce mucus. However, allergist Timothy Craig, DO, chair of the Sports Medicine Committee for both the American Academy of Allergy, Asthma & Immunology and the American College of Allergy, Asthma & Immunology says, "In the majority of cases, if your asthma is well controlled and you pretreat, you should be able to exercise with no problems."

To "pretreat," a recent report in the *Journal of Allergy & Clinical Immunology* (June 2007) recommends using a short-acting bronchodilator inhaler within fifteen minutes before exercise. This medication usually prevents asthma symptoms for about four hours. If you find your symptom relief doesn't last that long, make an appointment to talk with your medical care team about other ways to reduce exercise-induced symptoms.

You can also condition your airways with warm-up and cool-down exercises. Ten to fifteen minutes of stretching and calisthenics both before and after exercise will help your lungs handle the increased demand for oxygen during exertion and decreased demand afterward. Gradual temperature shifts lessen your chances of airway constriction and asthma symptoms.

Beat the Heat

Keeping your body well hydrated is also critical for safe sports—especially in heat and humidity. This is especially important to prevent dry airways for athletes with asthma.

Jon Almquist, a certified athletic trainer for the school system in Fairfax County, Virginia—an area well known for sticky summer days—says keeping the body hydrated should be a round-the-clock program for athletes, drinking plenty of fluids throughout the day, not just during exercise.

Beyond that, Almquist says building up slowly is the best way to prepare your body for the stress of heavy exercise in the summer heat. He recommends athletes not wait for the team tryouts—or even the team's preseason conditioning—to begin working out. Spend time before the season begins running or doing other high-intensity exercise in the heat of the day to get your body acclimated. That way, if you have to push your body to perform at its highest during a tryout, you'll be ready.

Dr. Craig points out that heavy sweating can deplete the body's levels of free water, potassium, magnesium, calcium, and sodium, which can worsen asthma symptoms, so he advises athletes with asthma be extra vigilant about replacing fluids after exercise with sports drinks that replace these essential salts. Check labels carefully, since not all sports drinks contain a full array of electrolytes.

On the Field

The single most important thing an athlete with asthma should remember is to always keep a bronchodilator inhaler handy.

Many school guidelines require athletes with asthma to have up-to-date management plans on file with the team that show specific steps the student should take to prevent or treat asthma symptoms. If players are prescribed a bronchodilator inhaler, they must have the medication with them at the field before they can practice or play.

The National Athletic Trainers Association (NATA) recommends using peak flow meters to help monitor players' lung function. These handheld devices can help coaches determine when a player is ready to get back into the practice or game.

Treatment guidelines based on peak flow meter readings will be different for each athlete. For instance, elite athletes may possess large lung capacities far beyond that of most people—and even beyond the range of some peak flow meters! What matters is not how a player's peak flow meter reading compares to the national average, but how it compares to his individual target: the number he should be able to reach when his lungs are working efficiently.

Dr. Craig explains that an athlete who needs to come off the field to use his inhaler might have unstable asthma, which should be monitored. "If the peak flow meter reading returns to the athlete's normal [target] within fifteen to twenty minutes after using his inhaler, he should be able to continue playing," says Dr. Craig. However, if the peak flow reading does not improve, the athlete should not return to the field.

Dr. Becker uses a 1-2-3 rule. "It's okay for an athlete to use his or her inhaler once before practice or before a game to prevent exercise-induced asthma symptoms. And it's okay if an athlete needs to use the inhaler a second time during the session. But if a player needs the inhaler a third time, they should not go back on the field that day. It may be a sign that the athlete's asthma is not well controlled and a visit to the physician may be necessary to help the athlete perform at his best on the field."

Coaches' Corner

Both athletes and coaches have a role to play in balancing performance with safety.

The National Athletic Trainers Association (NATA) warns, "Asthma can be difficult to diagnose and classify. Some individuals, especially elite athletes, do not display consistent signs or symptoms of asthma. Asthma symptoms may be present only during certain times (or seasons) of the year or only after exercise and may be highly variable."

With that in mind, NATA developed guidelines for trainers and coaches that include the following recommendations:

- Be aware of the major signs and symptoms of asthma, such as coughing, wheezing, tightness in the chest, shortness of breath, and breathing difficulty at night, upon awakening in the morning, or when exposed to certain allergens or irritants.

- Devise an asthma action plan for managing and referring athletes who may experience significant or life-threatening attacks or breathing difficulties.

- Have pulmonary function measuring devices, such as peak flow meters, at all athletic venues and be familiar with how to use them.

- Refer athletes with atypical symptoms, symptoms that occur despite proper therapy, or other complications that can exacerbate asthma (such as sinusitis, nasal polyps, severe rhinitis, gastroesophageal reflux disease, or vocal cord dysfunction) to a physician with expertise in sports medicine.

- Consider providing alternative practice sites for athletes with asthma. Indoor practice facilities that offer good ventilation and air conditioning should be taken into account for at least part of the practice.

- Schedule practices during times at which pollen counts are lowest.

- Encourage players with asthma to have follow-up examinations with their primary physician or specialist every six to twelve months.

- Identify athletes with past allergic reactions or intolerance to aspirin or nonsteroidal anti-inflammatory drugs (NSAIDs) and provide them with alternative medicines, such as acetaminophen.

Four steps to minimize asthma symptoms during sports or exercise:

1. Prevent or reduce airway inflammation (talk with your doctor).

2. Prevent or reduce allergic reactions through allergen avoidance, medication, or immunotherapy.

3. Pretreat airways before exercise to prevent bronchospasm.

4. Take time to condition your lungs by warming up before each exercise session and cooling down afterward.

Section 46.3

Swimming and Asthma

Having asthma doesn't mean you should avoid exercise. A healthy lifestyle and keeping fit arc important factors in managing your asthma effectively. If you are fit, you could have fewer asthma attacks.

Why Is Swimming a Good Exercise for People with Asthma?

Swimming can be a great exercise for people with asthma as you breathe in warm, moist air rather than the cold, dry air that can lead to asthma symptoms. Swimming can also help you develop good breathing practices.

Exercising in water suits many older people, as no stress is placed on weight-bearing joints such as the knees.

Will Exercise Trigger an Asthma Attack?

Exercise is a trigger for many people with asthma: at least 50 percent of people with asthma who use inhaled corticosteroid medicines find that exercise can bring on asthma symptoms. However, being fit can reduce the frequency of exercise-induced asthma, and a good warm-up can also help to prevent symptoms during exercise.

If you experience asthma symptoms while swimming or during another type of exercise, you should:

- stop the exercise and rest;

- take four separate puffs of your reliever medication; and

- not continue with the exercise until you can breathe comfortably and have no asthma symptoms.

If symptoms do not settle, or return again when you resume swimming (or another exercise), you may need emergency first aid treatment for your asthma symptoms, so you should follow the 4 x 4 x 4 Plan:

- Take four puffs of your reliever, one puff at a time, with four breaths after each puff;

- wait four minutes, and if no improvement, take four puffs again;

- if still no or little improvement, call an ambulance immediately, and continue with the four puffs every four minutes until help arrives.

For adults, up to eight puffs of reliever every five minutes can be given for a severe asthma attack, while waiting for the ambulance.

How Your Doctor Can Help

Always talk to your doctor before undertaking a new exercise program. Your doctor can help you with a written asthma management plan and evaluate your medicines and symptoms in the long-term.

To help assess your lung function and determine which medicines are best for you, your doctor may suggest you have lung function tests (spirometry).

Your doctor may prescribe medicines to prevent asthma symptoms from appearing while you're exercising.

Inhaled corticosteroids (preventers) can reduce the severity of exercise-induced asthma; however, they take two to three months to have their full effect. You will therefore probably need other medicines during this period, and possibly on an ongoing basis—your doctor may prescribe various medicines including long-acting beta-2 agonists (symptom controllers) or short-acting beta-2 agonists (relievers; taken just before exercising).

Symptom controllers and corticosteroid preventers are often given together in a combination inhaler.

In some mild cases of exercise-induced asthma, symptom controllers and/or relievers are given without preventers.

If you exercise often during the day you may be prescribed a preventer medicine such as montelukast (Singulair), zafirlukast (Accolate), nedocromil (Tilade), or sodium cromoglycate (Intal, Intal Forte).

Will Chlorine in Pools Affect My Asthma?

Chlorine in swimming pools can trigger and aggravate asthma symptoms. If you experience irritation in the pool, talk to your doctor about prevention and more effective management of your asthma.

Swimming is a great way to relax, and to have fun. Remember, SCUBA diving is not recommended for people with asthma, but snorkeling is a good alternative.

Chapter 47

Asthma and Minority Populations

Chapter Contents

Section 47.1

Asthma and African Americans

U.S. Department of Health and Human Services,
September 29, 2010.

- In 2009, about 2,380,000 African Americans reported that they currently have asthma.

- African American women were 30 percent more likely to have asthma than non-Hispanic white women, from 2001 to 2003.

- In 2006, African Americans were three times more likely to die from asthma-related causes than the white population.

- From 2003 to 2005, African American children had a death rate seven times that of non-Hispanic white children.

- African Americans had asthma-related emergency room visits 4.5 times more often than whites in 2004.

- Black children have a 260 percent higher emergency department visit rate, a 250 percent higher hospitalization rate, and a 500 percent higher death rate from asthma, as compared with white children.

- Children in poor families are more likely to ever have been diagnosed with asthma.

- While all of the causes of asthma remain unclear, children exposed to secondhand tobacco smoke exposure are at increased risk for acute lower respiratory tract infections, such as asthma, and children living below or near the poverty level are more likely to have high blood cotinine levels, a breakdown product of nicotine, than children living in higher income families.

Table 47.1. Estimated Average Annual Prevalence Percentages for Self-Reported Current Asthma, National Health Interview Survey, United States, 2001–2003

	African American	White	African American/ White Ratio
Men	8.2	5.8	1.4
Women	10.0	8.0	1.3
Both Sexes	9.2	6.9	1.3

Source: CDC 2007, National Surveillance for Asthma–United States, 1980–2004, Table 2, http://www.cdc.gov/mmwr/PDF/ss/ss5608.pdf

Table 47.2. Estimated Average Annual Prevalence Percentages for Self-Reported Asthma Attacks, National Health Interview Survey, United States, 2001–2003

	African American	White	African American/ White Ratio
Men	4.8	3.2	1.5
Women	5.9	4.7	1.3
Both Sexes	5.4	3.9	1.4

Source: CDC 2007, National Surveillance for Asthma–United States, 1980–2004, Table 6, http://www.cdc.gov/mmwr/PDF/ss/ss5608.pdf

Table 47.3. Percentage of Asthma Among Persons Eighteen Years of Age and Over, Ever Being Told They Had Asthma, 2009

Non-Hispanic Black	Non-Hispanic White	Non-Hispanic Black/ Non-Hispanic White Ratio
13.8	13.9	1.0

Source: CDC 2010, Summary Health Statistics for U.S. Adults: 2009, Table 4, http://www.cdc.gov/nchs/data/series/sr_10/sr10_249.pdf

Table 47.4. Percentage of Current Asthma Prevalence, 2009

Non-Hispanic Black	Non-Hispanic White	Non-Hispanic Black/ Non-Hispanic White Ratio
8.6	8.1	1.1

Source: CDC 2010, Summary Health Statistics for U.S. Adults: 2009, Table 4, http://www.cdc.gov/nchs/data/series/sr_10/sr10_249.pdf

Table 47.5. Deaths per 100,000, with Asthma as the Underlying Cause, National Vital Statistics System, 2006

Non-Hispanic Black	Non-Hispanic White	Non-Hispanic Black/ Non-Hispanic White Ratio
2.8	0.9	3.1

Source: CDC 2009, Deaths: Final Data for 2006, Table 17, http:// www.cdc.gov/nchs/data/nvsr/nvsr57/nvsr57_14.pdf

Table 47.6. Rate of Death with Asthma as the Underlying Cause per Million Population, National Vital Statistics System, United States, 2004

African American	White	African American/ White Ratio
30.6	10.4	2.9

Source: CDC 2007, National Surveillance for Asthma–United States, 1980-2004, Table 34, http://www.cdc.gov/mmwr/PDF/ss/ss5608.pdf

Table 47.7. Estimated Rate of Physician Office Visits with Asthma as the First Listed Diagnosis per 100 Persons with Asthma, National Ambulatory Medical Care Survey, 2004

African American	White	African American/ White Ratio
51.8	70.6	0.7

Source: CDC 2007, National Surveillance for Asthma–United States, 1980–2004, Table 15, http://www.cdc.gov/mmwr/PDF/ss/ss5608.pdf

Table 47.8. Estimated Rate of Outpatient Department Visits with Asthma as the First Listed Diagnosis per 10,000 Population, National Hospital Ambulatory Medical Care Survey, 2004

African American	White	African American/ White Ratio
116.4	24.0	4.9

Source: CDC 2007, National Surveillance for Asthma–United States, 1980–2004, Table 19, http://www.cdc.gov/mmwr/PDF/ss/ss5608.pdf

Table 47.9. Estimated Rate of Emergency Department Visits with Asthma as the First Listed Diagnosis per 10,000 Population, National Hospital Ambulatory Medical Care Survey, 2004

African American	White	African American/ White Ratio
195.0	43.6	4.5

Source: CDC 2007, National Surveillance for Asthma–United States, 1980–2004, Table 24, http://www.cdc.gov/mmwr/PDF/ss/ss5608.pdf

Table 47.10. Age-Adjusted Percentages for Children under 18 Years of Age, Ever Being Told They Had Asthma, 2009

Non-Hispanic Black	Non-Hispanic White	Non-Hispanic Black/ Non-Hispanic White Ratio
22.1	12.3	1.8

Source: CDC 2010, Summary Health Statistics for U.S. Children: National Health Interview Survey, 2009, Table 1, http://www.cdc.gov/nchs/data/series/sr_10/sr10_247.pdf

Table 47.11. Age-Adjusted Percentages for Children under 18 Years of Age Who Currently Have Asthma, 2009

Non-Hispanic Black	Non-Hispanic White	Non-Hispanic Black/ Non-Hispanic White Ratio
17.3	8.4	2.1

Source: CDC 2010, Summary Health Statistics for U.S. Children: National Health Interview Survey, 2009, Table 1, http://www.cdc.gov/nchs/data/series/sr_10/sr10_247.pdf

Table 47.12. Asthma Prevalence among Children 0–17 Years of Age, 2003–2005

Non-Hispanic Black	Non-Hispanic White	Non-Hispanic Black/ Non-Hispanic White Ratio
12.7	8.0	1.6

Source: CDC 2006, The State of Childhood Asthma, United States, 1980–2005, Table B, http://www.cdc.gov/nchs/data/ad/ad381.pdf

Table 47.13. Death Rates for Children 0–17 Years of Age, 2003–2005 (deaths per 1,000,000)

Non-Hispanic Black	Non-Hispanic White	Non-Hispanic Black/ Non-Hispanic White Ratio
9.2	1.3	7.1

Source: CDC 2006, The State of Childhood Asthma, United States, 1980–2005, Table B, http://www.cdc.gov/nchs/data/ad/ad381.pdf

Table 47.14. The Proportional Impact of Asthma Prevalence, Healthcare Use, and Mortality among Children 0–17 Years of Age, by Race and Ethnicity, United States, 2003–2004

	Non-Hispanic Black	Non-Hispanic White	Non-Hispanic Black/ Non-Hispanic White Ratio
Current prevalence (2004–2005)	146%	92%	1.6
Emergency department visit rate	254%	66%	3.8
Death rate	354%	50%	7.1

Source: CDC 2006, The State of Childhood Asthma, United States, 1980–2005, Table VIII, http://www.cdc.gov/nchs/data/ad/ad381.pdf

Section 47.2

Asthma and Asian Americans

U.S. Department of Health and Human Services, September 30, 2010.

- Asian Americans generally have lower rates of asthma than the white population, but they had a 40 percent greater death rate in 2006.

- Native Hawaiians/Pacific Islanders have a higher percentage of asthma than non-Hispanic whites.

- Chinese Americans also show a higher asthma rate than the white population.

- Native Hawaiian/Pacific Islander children were three times more likely to have asthma in 2008.

- Data on asthma conditions for Asian Americans is limited.

Table 47.15. Percentage of Asthma among Persons 18 Years of Age and Over, Currently Have Asthma, 2009

Asian	Non-Hispanic White	Asian/Non-Hispanic White Ratio
4.7	8.1	0.6

Source: CDC 2010, Summary Health Statistics for U.S. Adults: 2009, Table 4, http://www.cdc.gov/nchs/data/series/sr_10/sr10_249.pdf

Table 47.16. Percentage of Asthma among Persons 18 Years of Age and Over, Ever Being Told They Had Asthma, 2009

Asian	Non-Hispanic White	Asian/Non-Hispanic White Ratio
9.2	13.9	0.7

Source: CDC 2010, Summary Health Statistics for U.S. Adults: 2009, Table 4, http://www.cdc.gov/nchs/data/series/sr_10/sr10_249.pdf

Table 47.17. Percentage of Adults 18 Years of Age and Over with Asthma, 2004–2006

	Population	White	Population/ White Ratio
Total Asian	7.6	9.1	0.8
Native Hawaiian/ Pacific Islander & other	10.4	9.1	1.1
Chinese	11.2	9.1	1.2
Filipino	5.3	9.1	0.6
Asian Indian	6.0	9.1	0.7
Japanese	6.8	9.1	0.7
Vietnamese	8.0	9.1	0.9
Korean	5.8	9.1	0.6

Source: CDC 2008, Health Characteristics of the Asian Adult Population: United States, 2004–2006, Table 4, http://www.cdc.gov/nchs/data/ad/ad394.pdf

Table 47.18. Deaths per 100,000, with Asthma as the Underlying Cause, National Vital Statistics System, 2006

Asian	Non-Hispanic White	Asian/ Non-Hispanic White Ratio
1.3	0.9	1.4

Source: CDC 2009, Deaths: Final Data for 2006, Table 16 and Table 17, http://www.cdc.gov/nchs/data/nvsr/nvsr57/nvsr57_14.pdf

At a Glance: Treatment

The most recent National Surveillance for Asthma does not include data for Asian Americans.

Table 47.19. Age-Adjusted Percentages for Children under 18 Years of Age, Ever Being Told They Had Asthma, 2009

Asian	Non-Hispanic White	Asian/ Non-Hispanic White Ratio
11.3	12.3	0.9

Source: CDC 2010, Summary Health Statistics for U.S. Children: National Health Interview Survey, 2009, Table 1, http://www.cdc.gov/nchs/data/series/sr_10/sr10_247.pdf

Table 47.20. Asthma Prevalence among Children 0–17 Years of Age, 2003–2005

Asian	Non-Hispanic White	Asian/ Non-Hispanic White Ratio
4.9	8.0	0.6

Source: CDC 2006, The State of Childhood Asthma, United States, 1980–2005, Table B, http://www.cdc.gov/nchs/data/ad/ad381.pdf

Section 47.3

Asthma and Hispanic Americans

U.S. Department of Health and Human Services,
October 1, 2010

- In 2009, about 1,721,000 Hispanics reported that they currently have asthma.

- Puerto Rican Americans have over twice the asthma rate as compared to the overall Hispanic population.

- The rate of asthma attacks for Puerto Ricans was 2.5 times that of whites.

- Hispanics are twice as likely to use outpatient clinics for asthma visits, rather than physician offices.

- Hispanic children are 60 percent more likely to have asthma, as compared to non-Hispanic whites.

Table 47.21. Estimated Average Annual Prevalence Percentages for Self-Reported Current Asthma, National Health Interview Survey, United States, 2001–2003

	Population	White	Population / White Ratio
All Hispanic	5.4	6.9	0.8
Puerto Rican	14.5	6.9	2.1
Mexican	3.9	6.9	0.6

Source: CDC 2007, National Surveillance for Asthma–United States, 1980–2004, Table 2, http://www.cdc.gov/mmwr/PDF/ss/ss5608.pdf

Table 47.22. Estimated Average Annual Prevalence Percentages for Self-Reported Asthma Attacks, National Health Interview Survey, United States, 2001–2003

	Population	White	Population / White Ratio
Total Hispanic	3.3	3.9	0.8
Puerto Rican	9.6	3.9	2.5
Mexican	2.1	3.9	0.5

Source: CDC 2007, National Surveillance for Asthma–United States, 1980–2004, Table 6, http://www.cdc.gov/mmwr/PDF/ss/ss5608.pdf

Table 47.23. Percentage of Asthma among Persons 18 Years of Age and Over Ever Being Told They Had Asthma, 2009

Hispanic	Non-Hispanic White	Hispanic/ Non-Hispanic White Ratio
10.6	13.9	0.8

Source: CDC 2010, Summary Health Statistics for U.S. Adults: 2009, Table 4, http://www.cdc.gov/nchs/data/series/sr_10/sr10_249.pdf

Table 47.24. Percentage of Current Asthma Prevalence, Adults Ages 18 and Over, 2006–2008

	Population	Non-Hispanic White	Population / Non-Hispanic White Ratio
Total Hispanic	5.6	7.7	0.7
Puerto Rican	12.8	7.7	1.7
Mexican	4.2	7.7	0.5

Source: CDC 2010, Health Data Interactive, http://www.cdc.gov/nchs/hdi.htm [Accessed 09/21/2010]

Table 47.25. Percentage of Lifetime Asthma Diagnosis, Adults Age 18 and Over, 2006–2008

	Population	Non-Hispanic White	Population / Non-Hispanic White Ratio
Total Hispanic	9.1	12.1	0.8
Puerto Rican	21.1	12.1	1.6
Mexican	7.0	12.1	0.6

Source: CDC 2010, Health Data Interactive, http://www.cdc.gov/nchs/hdi.htm [Accessed 09/21/2010]

Table 47.26. Deaths per 100,000, with Asthma as the Underlying Cause, National Vital Statistics System, 2006

Hispanic	Non-Hispanic White	Hispanic/ Non-Hispanic White Ratio
1.0	0.9	1.1

Source: CDC 2009, Deaths: Final Data for 2006, Table 17, http://www.cdc.gov/nchs/data/nvsr/nvsr57/nvsr57_14.pdf

Table 47.27. Rate of Death with Asthma as the Underlying Cause per Million Population, National Vital Statistics System, United States, 2004

Hispanic	White	Hispanic/White Ratio
11.4	10.4	1.1

Source: CDC 2007, National Surveillance for Asthma–United States, 1980–2004, Table 34, http://www.cdc.gov/mmwr/PDF/ss/ss5608.pdf

Table 47.28. Number of Asthma Deaths per 100,000 Population, 2003

	Population	Non-Hispanic White	Population / Non-Hispanic White Ratio
Total Hispanic	1.3	1.1	1.2
Puerto Rican	4.4	1.1	4.0
Mexican	0.8	1.1	0.7

Source: CDC 2006, Health E-Stats, Asthma Prevalence, Health Care Use and Mortality: United States, 2003–05, Figure 7, http://www.cdc.gov/nchs/data/hestat/asthma03-05/asthma03-05.htm

Table 47.29. Estimated Rate of Physician Office Visits with Asthma as the First Listed Diagnosis per 100 Persons with Asthma, National Ambulatory Medical Care Survey, 2004

Hispanic	White	Hispanic/White Ratio
93.8	70.6	1.3

Source: CDC 2007, National Surveillance for Asthma–United States, 1980–2004, Table 15, http://www.cdc.gov/mmwr/PDF/ss/ss5608.pdf

Table 47.30. Estimated Rate of Outpatient Department Visits with Asthma as the First Listed Diagnosis per 10,000 Population, National Hospital Ambulatory Medical Care Survey, 2004

Hispanic	White	Hispanic/White Ratio
59.6	24.0	2.5

Source: CDC 2007, National Surveillance for Asthma–United States, 1980–2004, Table 19, http://www.cdc.gov/mmwr/PDF/ss/ss5608.pdf

Table 47.31. Estimated Rate of Emergency Department Visits with Asthma as the First Listed Diagnosis per 10,000 Population, National Hospital Ambulatory Medical Care Survey, 2004

Hispanic	White	Hispanic/White Ratio
57.5	43.6	1.3

Source: CDC 2007, National Surveillance for Asthma–United States, 1980–2004, Table 24, http://www.cdc.gov/mmwr/PDF/ss/ss5608.pdf

Table 47.32. Age-Adjusted Percentages for Children under 18 Years of Age Ever Being Told They Had Asthma, 2009

	Population	Non-Hispanic White	Population/Non-Hispanic White Ratio
Hispanic	12.9	12.3	1.0
Mexican	10.4	12.3	0.8

Source: CDC 2010, Summary Health Statistics for U.S. Children: National Health Interview Survey, 2009, Table 1, http://www.cdc.gov/nchs/data/series/sr_10/sr10_247.pdf

Table 47.33. Asthma Prevalence among Children 0–17 Years of Age, 2003–2005

Hispanic	Non-Hispanic White	Hispanic/Non-Hispanic White Ratio
12.7	8.0	1.6

Source: CDC 2006, The State of Childhood Asthma, United States, 1980–2005, Table B, http://www.cdc.gov/nchs/data/ad/ad381.pdf

Table 47.34. Death Rates for Children 0–17 Years of Age, 2003–2005 (deaths per 1,000,000)

Hispanic	Non-Hispanic White	Hispanic/Non-Hispanic White Ratio
1.8	1.3	1.4

Source: CDC 2006, The State of Childhood Asthma, United States, 1980–2005, Table B, http://www.cdc.gov/nchs/data/ad/ad381.pdf

Table 47.35. The Proportional Impact of Asthma Prevalence, Healthcare Use, and Mortality among Children 0–17 Years of Age, by Race and Ethnicity, United States, 2003–2004

	Hispanic	Non-Hispanic White	Hispanic/Non-Hispanic White Ratio
Current prevalence (2004–2005)	90%	92%	1.0
Emergency department visit rate	109%	66%	1.7
Death rate	69%	50%	1.4

Source: CDC 2006, The State of Childhood Asthma, United States, 1980–2005, Table VIII, http://www.cdc.gov/nchs/data/ad/ad381.pdf

Section 47.4

Asthma and American Indians and Alaska Natives

"Asthma and American Indians/Alaska Natives," U.S. Department of Health and Human Services, September 30, 2010.

- American Indian/Alaska Native adults are 20 percent more likely to have asthma than non-Hispanic whites.

- Data on asthma conditions for American Indian/Alaska Natives is limited.

Table 47.36. Percentage of Asthma among Persons 18 Years of Age and Over Ever Being Told They Had Asthma, 2009

American Indian/ Alaska Native	Non-Hispanic White	American Indian/Alaska Native Non-Hispanic White Ratio
14.2	13.9	1.0

Source: CDC 2010, Summary Health Statistics for U.S. Adults: 2009, Table 4, http://www.cdc.gov/nchs/data/series/sr_10/sr10_249.pdf

Table 47.37. Percentage of Adults 18 Years of Age and Over with Asthma, 2004–2008

American Indian/ Alaska Native	Non-Hispanic White	American Indian/Alaska Native Non-Hispanic White Ratio
14.2	11.6	1.2

Source: CDC 2010, Health Characteristics of the American Indian or Alaska Native Adult Population: United States, 2004–2008, Table 4, http://www.cdc.gov/nchs/data/nhsr/nhsr020.pdf

Table 47.38. Deaths per 100,000, with Asthma as the Underlying Cause, National Vital Statistics System, 2006

American Indian/ Alaska Native	Non-Hispanic White	American Indian/Alaska Native Non-Hispanic White Ratio
0.8	0.9	0.9

Source: CDC 2009, Deaths: Final Data for 2006, Table 16 and Table 17e, http://www.cdc.gov/nchs/data/nvsr/nvsr57/nvsr57_14.pdf

At a Glance: Treatment

The most recent National Surveillance for Asthma does not include data for American Indians and Alaska Natives.

Table 47.39. Age-Adjusted Percentages for Children under 18 Years of Age Ever Being Told They Had Asthma, 2009

American Indian/ Alaska Native	Non-Hispanic White	American Indian/Alaska Native Non-Hispanic White Ratio
10.1*	12.3	0.8

Source: CDC 2010, Summary Health Statistics for U.S. Children: National Health Interview Survey, 2009. Table 1, http://www.cdc.gov/nchs/data/series/sr_10/sr10_247.pdf

Note: Estimates are considered unreliable. Data shown have a relative standard error of greater than 30 percent.

Table 47.40. Age-Adjusted Percentages for Children under 18 Years of Age Who Currently Have Asthma, 2009

American Indian/ Alaska Native	Non-Hispanic White	American Indian/Alaska Native Non-Hispanic White Ratio
7.5*	8.4	0.9

Source: CDC 2010, Summary Health Statistics for U.S. Children: National Health Interview Survey, 2009, Table 1, http://www.cdc.gov/nchs/data/series/sr_10/sr10_247.pdf [PDF I1MB]

Note: Estimates are considered unreliable. Data shown have a relative standard error of greater than 30 percent.

Table 47.41. Asthma Prevalence among Children 0–17 Years of Age, 2003–2005

American Indian/ Alaska Native	Non-Hispanic White	American Indian/Alaska Native Non-Hispanic White Ratio
9.9	8.0	1.2

Source: CDC 2006, The State of Childhood Asthma, United States, 1980–2005, Table B, http://www.cdc.gov/nchs/data/ad/ad381.pdf

Chapter 48

Asthma Disproportionately Affects Low-Income Populations

Almost five million Californians have been diagnosed with asthma, and those living in poverty suffer more severe consequences from the condition than those in higher income brackets, according to a new report from the UCLA Center for Health Policy Research.

Low-income Californians with asthma experience more frequent symptoms, end up in the emergency room or hospital more often, and miss more days of work and school, researchers found.

Of the more than six hundred thousand Californians who experience frequent—daily or weekly—symptoms that can signal uncontrolled asthma, a significant proportion (39.1 percent) earn less than 200 percent of the federal government's poverty standard (FPL). In 2007, 200 percent of the FPL for a family of four was $41,300. By contrast, 19.3 percent of those with incomes of 400 percent of the FPL or higher suffer frequent symptoms from their asthma.

Analyzing data from the California Health Interview Survey from 2001 to 2007, the report's authors also found a relationship between poverty and a lack of access to quality healthcare and repeated exposure to environmental triggers for asthma symptoms, such as smoking and second-hand smoke.

The study calculates the prevalence of asthma among adults and children in California's counties. Those counties with a high percentage of families living in poverty had some of the highest proportions of people currently suffering from asthma. In all counties, however, poverty was associated with asthma.

"The poorest among us suffer most because they lack quality health-care and live in high-risk environments," said Ying-Ying Meng, a senior research scientist with the center and co-author of the report. "That disparity also burdens our health system with costly emergency care and hospitalizations and extracts the additional high cost of millions of lost days of work and school."

"Asthma has the potential to be debilitating," Meng added, "but it can be effectively controlled through appropriate medical care and avoidance of triggers."

Health insurance can provide access to the kind of continuous care needed to manage a complex chronic condition like asthma. Yet low-income Californians suffering from the disease were five times as likely to be uninsured (22.1 percent) as their counterparts with asthma earning twice as much (4.4 percent). They were also twice as likely to not have a usual source of care (19.0 percent vs. 8.6 percent)—a factor that also affects continuity and quality of asthma care.

Healthcare reforms should provide some relief by extending needed insurance to many low-income asthma sufferers, the report's authors say. But they also encourage policymakers to support asthma educa-tion and quality healthcare that includes access to a patient-centered medical home, case-management programs, specialty referrals, and access to around-the-clock advice from a health professional, as well as multilingual and culturally appropriate programs and educa-tion.

"These findings are illustrative of how where you live impacts your health. Low-income communities carry the highest disease burden, largely due to inequities that result in unhealthy environments," said Dr. Robert K. Ross, M.D., president and chief executive officer (CEO) of the California Endowment, which funded the study. "For example, you won't see diesel trucks driving through high-income communities, but you will see many driving through poor communities, spewing exhaust full of particulates that serve as asthma triggers."

The report's authors also call for improvements in substandard housing, restrictions on second-hand smoke and other policies that address the environmental factors that contribute to asthma.

Among the findings:

- **Asthma increasing in California:** The prevalence of asthma in California has increased from 11.3 percent in 2001 to 13.0 percent in 2007.

- **Higher rates in northern, central valley counties:** Many northern and central California counties—Lake, Tehama/Glenn, Sutter, Yuba, Contra Costa, Solano, Sacramento, Fresno, Kern, Merced, Madera and San Bernardino—have asthma rates significantly higher than the state average.

- **Lost productivity:** Californians missed an estimated 1.2 million days of work and 1.6 million days of school because of asthma in 2007. Income was a significant factor: Low-income sufferers missed an average of 2.2 days of work, compared with an average of 0.6 days of work missed by those with higher incomes. Low-income children missed twice as many days of school due to asthma as children from higher-income families.

- **Preventable urgent care:** Rates of emergency department visits for asthma were twice as high among lower-income adults as their higher-income counterparts (18.8 percent vs. 8.8 percent). Low-income children also sought emergency treatment more frequently (23.9 percent vs. 12.5 percent). Hospitalization rates were six times higher for low-income adults.

Part Seven

Additional Help
and Information

Chapter 49

Glossary of Asthma-Related Terms

action plan: A list of specific instructions drawn up by a healthcare professional for a person with asthma to follow at home. An asthma action plan includes a normal schedule for asthma medicines, as well as what to do if peak flow readings or asthma symptoms become worse than usual. Asthma action plans are usually split into zones: green zone, yellow zone, and red zone.

acute: Brief, not ongoing. Usually also implies relatively high intensity. For example, acute asthma symptoms may be ones that last a short time but are worse than a person's usual (see chronic) symptoms.

airways: Hollow tubes to and within the lungs through which air passes during breathing. Airways include the trachea, bronchi, and bronchioles.

allergen: Something that causes an allergic reaction.

allergy: A type of excessive immune system reaction to a substance in a person's environment. (Can also be called "hypersensitivity reaction.") Allergies can be triggered by eating, touching, or breathing in an allergen. Allergies are often associated with asthma, especially in children.

"All About Asthma: Glossary," © 2011 University of Chicago Asthma and COPD Center. Reprinted with permission. For additional information, visit http://asthma .bsd.uchicago.edu.

alveoli: The millions of tiny compartments within the lungs at the ends of the airways. (To imagine the shape, picture bunches of hollow grapes at the ends of hollow stems.) Also called "air sacs." Alveoli are where gas exchange takes place: that is, where the blood picks up oxygen (from the air a person has breathed in) and releases carbon dioxide (to be breathed out). (singular: alveolus)

aspirin-sensitive asthma: A type of asthma in which taking aspirin or nonsteroidal anti-inflammatory drugs (NSAIDs) triggers asthma symptoms. This particular kind of asthma usually starts in adulthood and is often accompanied by polyps (benign growths) in the nose and/or a chronically runny/stuffy nose (rhinitis). Aspirin-sensitive asthma may respond particularly well to leukotriene-modifying drugs.

atopy: The genetically determined tendency to be allergic to things.

attack: See episode.

beta-agonist: Also called beta-2-agonist or beta-adrenergic agonist. The most common type of bronchodilator medication. Albuterol is a beta-agonist. The name beta-agonist comes from the way the medicine works, which is to enhance the stimulation of a certain kind of autonomic nerve (the beta-2 type), which is responsible for relaxing the airway smooth muscle (thereby opening the airways).

bronchi: The airways that lead from the trachea to each lung, and then subdivide into smaller and smaller branches. They connect to the bronchioles. The walls of the bronchi are made of smooth lining tissue (called endothelium) over fibrous connective tissue, cartilage, and smooth muscle. They also have many glands to produce mucus. (singular: bronchus)

bronchial provocation testing: See challenge test.

bronchiole: The tiny (less than 1 millimeter in diameter), branching airways that lead from the bronchi to the alveoli. Bronchioles have elastic fibers and smooth muscle but (unlike bronchi) no cartilage. Most bronchioles also produce mucus.

bronchoconstriction: The reduction in the diameter of the bronchi, usually due to squeezing of the smooth muscle in the walls. This reduces the space for air to go through and can make breathing difficult.

bronchodilator: A medicine that relaxes the smooth muscles of the airways. This allows the airway to open up (to dilate) since the muscles are not squeezing it shut. Bronchodilator medicines do not help inflammation, however.

challenge test: A test done to determine whether or not a person's bronchi are hyperresponsive. The subject breathes in air containing carefully controlled amounts of a substance known to cause broncho-constriction. (Common substances used include methacholine, hista-mine, and vaporized salt water.) The bronchi of people with asthma respond to much smaller amounts of the substance than the bronchi of people who do not have asthma. This test is often used to confirm a diagnosis of asthma if there is uncertainty.

chronic: Lasting a long time. Asthma is a chronic illness because it is ongoing and does not just go away in a few days or weeks.

control: In the context of asthma, the degree to which a person has been able to reduce daily symptoms and acute episodes of the disease while participating fully in normal activities (such as exercising and sleeping through the night). This is usually achieved through taking medications and avoiding triggers.

corticosteroids: A type of medicine used to reduce inflammation. Corticosteroid drugs mimic a substance produced naturally by the body. In asthma, corticosteroids are often taken through an inhaler for long-term control. They may also be taken orally or given intravenously for a short time if asthma symptoms get out of control.

DPI: Stands for "dry powder inhaler." This variety of device provides a new way of taking inhaled medicine. The propellants used in regular metered dose inhalers can be bad for the environment. For this reason, drug companies are in the process of switching over to DPIs, which do not use a propellant at all. The medicine is in the form of a very fine powder, which is easily inhaled without the use of an aerosol spray device. There are advantages for patients, too. DPIs can be easier to use because the patient doesn't have to coordinate the timing of ac-tivating the inhaler and breathing in, and the problems of bad taste and unpleasant "feel" are also greatly reduced.

dust mites: Very tiny creatures (microscopic, or just barely visible) that live in the dust in people's homes. They are present both in vis-ible dust (under the bed or behind the couch, for example) and in soft places like pillows, mattresses, blankets, and stuffed animals. They thrive especially when the air is humid. Many people are allergic to dust mites, and trying to reduce the number of them in the home is part of many asthma control plans.

edema: Swelling due to collection of fluid within cells or tissues of the body.

eosinophil: A type of white blood cell whose major useful role seems to be in protecting against parasitic infections. It is also associated, however, with the inflammation that is at the root of asthma. People with asthma tend to have more eosinophils in their blood and, in addition, have an unusual number of eosinophils "migrate" into their lungs. It is still not entirely clear whether eosinophils cause some of the problems that asthmatics experience, or whether they are just associated with the process without doing damage themselves.

episode: In asthma, a period of markedly worsened symptoms. This may be brought on by exposure to a known trigger or by an upper respiratory infection (a cold), or it may not have a known explanation. An episode may come on suddenly or may develop gradually over days. Asthma episodes, at their worst, can be life threatening, and should always be taken seriously.

episodic: Intermittent, with periods of apparent normal function in between periods of symptoms.

exacerbation: See episode.

extrinsic: A classification of asthma that means about the same thing as "allergy-related." Extrinsic asthma has symptoms triggered by exposure to an allergen. (This term is not used much any more.)

FEV-1: The "forced expiratory volume in one second." In other words, this is the amount of air you are able to blow out in one second of blowing as hard as you can. This measurement, obtained through spirometry, gives your doctor an idea of the level of blockage you have in your airways due to inflammation, mucus, or bronchoconstriction.

FVC: "Forced vital capacity." This is the total amount of air you can blow out after you've taken a deep breath. It is one of the measurements doctors obtain through pulmonary function tests.

GERD: Gastroesophageal reflux disease. GERD is a chronic disorder in which some of the acid and enzymes that belong in the stomach are allowed to get up into the esophagus. This leads to the sensation of "heartburn" and sometimes also an unpleasant sour taste in the mouth. GERD and asthma can make a vicious circle: GERD is more common among people with asthma, and it also seems to make asthma worse in people who have it. Treatment of GERD can lead to an improvement in asthma symptoms.

histamine: A chemical made naturally in the body that is involved in inflammation, particularly inflammation related to an allergic reaction.

Antihistamines, as the name suggests, are medicines that block the effect of histamine. (Histamine made in a laboratory is sometimes also used in challenge testing.)

holding chamber: A device much like a spacer, which is also intended to help medicine from an MDI get into the lungs. The difference between a spacer and a holding chamber is that a holding chamber has a special valve on it that allows a person more time to breathe in the medicine (the breath does not need to be coordinated with the puff). In the real world, holding chambers are often called "spacers" also, even though they are slightly different things.

hyperreactivity: Same as hyperresponsiveness, below.

hyperresponsiveness: The "twitchiness" of the airways of people with asthma, resulting in excessive reaction to substances, smells, and activity. Even little things that would have no effect on the airways of nonasthmatic people cause the smooth muscle of the asthmatic's airway to squeeze and squeeze.

inflammation: A complex process in the body involving many types of cells (especially white blood cells) and chemicals (such as cytokines and leukotrienes). Inflammation may be protective or may be harmful. The typical signs of inflammation are redness, swelling, warmth, and pain. Loss of function (partial or complete) is often seen, and some kind of exudate is common. Inflammation of the airways is the main underlying problem in asthma.

inhaled corticosteroid: Anti-inflammatory medicine breathed directly into the lungs. The advantage to this is that the medicine goes directly to where the inflammation is, and has minimal effects on the rest of the body (and therefore fewer side effects than corticosteroids taken orally).

inhaler: See metered dose inhaler.

intrinsic: A classification of asthma that means the asthma symptoms are not caused by exposure to allergens. Aspirin-sensitive asthma is one kind of intrinsic asthma. (The term "intrinsic asthma" is not used much any more.)

intubation: The process of putting a tube down someone's throat into the trachea; the tube is connected to a machine (a respirator, or ventilator) that pushes measured amounts of air into the lungs (and then lets it out again) to help the person breathe. This can save the life of a person having a severe asthma episode but also has many risks and possible complications.

irritant: A substance that triggers asthma symptoms by irritating the airway when breathed in. Examples include cigarette smoke, fumes from a harsh cleaning fluid, or strong perfume. (Allergens are a different type of asthma trigger, which cause symptoms through an allergic reaction rather than by irritation.)

labile: Easily changing, unstable. If your asthma is labile, it means that you can go quickly and unpredictably from being perfectly fine to barely getting enough air.

leukotriene: A type of chemical involved in inflammation. Leukotrienes seem to play a particularly important role in the inflammation associated with asthma. Recently some asthma medicines have been developed that work to reduce leukotrienes or their effects (these are called "leukotriene modifiers" or "leukotriene inhibitors").

LRI: Lower respiratory infection. Some examples include pneumonia, bronchitis, and bronchiolitis.

metered dose inhaler: Often called "MDI." A device that allows delivery of medicine directly into the lungs. The medicine is in the form of a very, very fine powder, and a propellant is used to get the powder out in a cloud to be inhaled. Unfortunately, the propellant used in the standard MDI's is composed of CFC's (chlorofluorocarbons), which are involved in the destruction of the ozone layer. Different types of devices to deliver medicine to the lungs are now being designed, and some are already available to consumers (see DPI).

methacholine: A type of chemical used in challenge testing. Everybody's airways respond to it, but the airways of a person with asthma respond much more and at lower doses.

morbidity and mortality: Sickness and death. These words are usually used when looking at the effects of a disease in a population. For example, "asthma causes significant morbidity in this group" means "asthma makes a lot of people in this group sick." "Asthma mortality in this country is unacceptable," means "It is unacceptable if anyone in this country dies of asthma."

mucus: A substance secreted by various tissues in the body (the mucous membranes) made up of water, mucin (a glycoprotein), salts, and some cells. In the lungs, mucus serves to lubricate the insides of the airways and to trap inhaled foreign particles so that they can be coughed out. In asthma, however, an excess of mucus is produced and can actually block airways. Mucus also tends to be thicker and more viscous in asthmatics.

NSAID: Nonsteroidal anti-inflammatory drug, generally used to treat mild to moderate pain, especially pain that has a component of inflammation (such as arthritis pain). Some people (about 10 to 20 percent of all asthmatics) have their asthma symptoms triggered by these drugs (along with aspirin). Episodes triggered in this way can be quite severe and even life threatening. NSAID's include such medicines as ibuprofen (Motrin, Advil), naproxen (Naprosyn, Aleve, Anaprox), and a few related prescription medicines (such as Relafen, Daypro, Feldene, and Indocin).

nebulizer: A machine for getting medicine into the lungs. A nebulizer makes a mixture of liquid medicine and water into a mist that a person then inhales (through a mask or a mouthpiece). Nebulizers are often used for babies and children too small to be able to coordinate using a metered dose inhaler. They are also sometimes used for people having severe asthma symptoms, as many people find it easier to take in the medicine this way when they are having a lot of trouble breathing.

peak flow: The very fastest you can move air by blowing out as hard as you can. This measurement correlates pretty well with FEV-1 (a measurement obtained through spirometry in a doctor's office) but doesn't require expensive equipment and can be obtained easily at home with a peak flow meter.

peak flow meter: A device to measure how hard and fast a person can blow air out. This is an indication of how well the lungs and airways are doing. A peak flow meter is an important part of an asthma home-monitoring plan.

pulmonary function tests: Often called "PFT's." A series of tests done (usually in a lab in a hospital) to determine whether a person has breathing problems, and precisely what those problems are. These are used to differentiate among different diseases and disorders. It is sometimes hard for a doctor to tell just by a regular exam whether a person has asthma or another condition, and pulmonary function tests can help clarify the diagnosis. PFT's do not hurt. They involve things like holding your breath, blowing into a tube as hard as you can, and exercising while wearing a special mask.

reflux: See gastroesophageal reflux disease.

residual volume: The amount of air left in your lungs when you have exhaled as far as you can. (Your body doesn't let you exhale all the air in your lungs, because then your lungs would collapse.) This is one of the measurements obtained in pulmonary function testing.

respirator: See intubation.

severity: How bad or serious a disease is. In asthma, severity is generally broken up into four categories: mild intermittent, mild persistent, moderate persistent, and severe persistent. (Some experts also include a category for "severe intermittent" for those unusual people who most of the time have no asthma symptoms at all but occasionally have very serious or life-threatening asthma episodes.) Just as we do not know what causes asthma, we do not understand why individuals differ so much one from another in asthma severity.

sinusitis: An inflammation of the sinuses (hollow spaces in the bone of the cheeks and forehead) due to infection. Common symptoms of sinusitis include pain in the face, colored (not white or clear) secretions from the nose, and headache. A lot of people who have asthma also have problems with recurrent sinusitis. There is some evidence that a flare-up of sinusitis can trigger a worsening of asthma symptoms, but this is still not certain.

smooth muscle: Sometimes called involuntary muscle. A type of muscle found many places in the body, including the walls of the airways. (It is called smooth muscle simply because of how it looks under a microscope, to distinguish it from striated muscle, which is what makes up the heart as well as voluntary (skeletal) muscle.)

spacer: A device usually consisting of a plastic chamber that attaches to a metered dose inhaler on one end, with a mouthpiece on the other end. A spacer is intended to help medicine from a metered dose inhaler get into the lungs. Without a spacer, much of the medicine in an inhaler "puff" gets deposited on the tongue or in the back of the throat.

spirometry: The most commonly used pulmonary function test, done in a doctor's office or pulmonary function laboratory. The machine used measures how fast a person can blow out air, and how much air is blown. The results of this test include the FEV-1, the peak flow, and the FVC.

status asthmaticus: A severe episode of asthma that is not helped (or only partially helped) by inhaled bronchodilators, and that threatens a person's ability to breathe altogether. May require intensive bronchodilator therapy, systemic corticosteroids (oral or intravenous [IV]), or even intubation.

steroids: A general term for a wide variety of chemicals, natural and synthetic. In the context of asthma, "steroids" is usually a shorthand way of referring to corticosteroid medicines (taken to reduce asthma inflammation). Other steroids, including natural and synthetic sex hormones (such as the testosterone-like compounds sometimes used by athletes to build their muscles), are generally unrelated to asthma.

support group: A group of people all sharing a certain problem or concern (such as having asthma, or having a child with asthma) who meet to discuss how they are dealing with it. Support groups provide emotional support by decreasing a person's sense of isolation and can also provide practical advice, since other members of the group have experience confronting similar challenges. Social workers associated with local hospitals or clinics should have information on what support groups are available in your area.

systemic: Relating to or affecting the body as a whole (rather than one specific organ or part).

total lung capacity: The total amount of air in the lungs when a person has breathed in as far as possible. This is one of the measurements obtained in pulmonary function testing.

trachea: The largest breathing tube in the body, passing from the throat down to the chest (where it connects to the two bronchi leading to the lungs).

trigger: Anything that causes asthma symptoms to worsen in a given person. Different things are triggers for different people. Common triggers include exercise, cigarette smoke, pollen, dust, cold air, and aspirin/NSAIDs. Upper respiratory infections are perhaps the most common trigger for asthma symptoms.

URI: Upper respiratory infection. Medical term for a "cold."

ventilator: See intubation.

wheeze: A breathing sound that may be squeaky, whistling, or musical. Wheezes are often (but not always) a symptom of asthma. (Some people have asthma but never wheeze, and some people wheeze for reasons other than asthma.) Wheezes are due to air passing through a narrowed opening and are therefore usually accompanied by difficulty breathing.

zones: The way that asthma signs and symptoms are classified in an asthma action plan. Usually, the zones are the green zone (all is well, continue with regular medicines and activities); the yellow zone (trouble starting; follow doctor's instructions for yellow zone); and red zone (DANGER! Get to the emergency room as quickly as possible). These are determined by symptoms and peak flow readings.

Chapter 50

Directory of Asthma-Related Resources

Allergy & Asthma Network Mothers of Asthmatics
8201 Greensboro Drive, Suite 300
McLean, VA 22102
Phone: 800-878-4403
Fax: 703-288-5271
Website: http://www.aanma.org

American Academy of Allergy, Asthma & Immunology
611 East Wells Street
Milwaukee, WI 53202
Toll-Free: 800-822-2762
Website: http://www.aaaai.org

American Association for Respiratory Care
9425 North MacArthur Boulevard, Suite 100
Irving, TX 75063-4706
Phone: 972-243-2272
Fax: 972-484-2720
Website: http://www.aarc.org
E-mail: info@aarc.org

Resources in this chapter were compiled from several sources deemed reliable.
All contact information was verified and updated in May 2011.

American College of Allergy, Asthma & Immunology
85 West Algonquin Road, Suite 550
Arlington Heights, IL 60005
Toll-Free: 800-842-7777
Phone: 847-427-1200
Fax:847-427-1294
Website: http://www.acaai.org

American Lung Association
1301 Pennsylvania Avenue NW, Suite 800
Washington, DC 20004
Toll-Free: 800-548-8252
Phone: 202-785-3355
Fax: 202-452-1805
Website: http://www.lungusa.org
E-mail: info@lungusa.org

Asthma and Allergy Foundation of America
8201 Corporate Drive, Suite 1000
Landover, MD 20785
Toll-Free: 800-7-ASTHMA (800-727-8462)
Website: http://www.aafa.org
E-mail: info@aafa.org

Asthma Center Education and Research Fund
205 North Broad Street, Suite 300
Philadelphia, PA 19107
Phone: 215-569-1111
Website: http://www.theasthmacenter.org

Asthma Foundation NSW
Level 3, 486 Pacific Highway
Saint Leonards, NSW 2065
Phone: 02-9906-3233
Fax: 02-9906-4493
Website: http://www.asthmafoundation.org.au

Asthma Initiative of Michigan
Website: http://www.getasthmahelp.org
E-mail: info@getasthmahelp.org

Asthma Society of Canada
4950 Yonge Street, Suite 2306
Toronto, Ontario M2N 6K1
Canada
Toll-Free: 866-787-4050
Phone: 416-787-4050
Fax: 416-787-5807
Website: http://www.asthma.ca
E-mail: info@asthma.ca

Centers for Disease Control and Prevention
1600 Clifton Road
Atlanta, GA 30333
Toll-Free: 800-CDC-INFO (800-232-4636)
TTY: 888-232-6348
Website: http://www.cdc.gov
E-mail: cdcinfo@cdc.gov

Children's Asthma Education Centre
FE125 -685 William Avenue
Winnipeg, Manitoba
R3E 0Z2
Canada
Phone: 204-787-2551
Fax: 204-787-5040
Website: http://www.asthma-education.com
E-mail: caec@hsc.mb.ca

Cleveland Clinic
Toll-Free: 800-223-2273
Website: http://www.myclevelandclinic.org

Environmental Protection Agency
Ariel Rios Building
1200 Pennsylvania Avenue NW
Washington, DC 20460
Phone: 202-272-0167
TTY: 202-272-0165
Website: http://www.epa.gov

National Heart Lung and Blood Institute
NHLBI Health Information Center
Attention: Website
P.O. Box 30105
Bethesda, MD 20824-0105
Phone: 301-592-8573
Fax: 240-629-3246
TTY: 240-629-3255
Website: http://www.nhlbi.nih.gov
E-mail: nhlbiinfo@nhlbi.nih.gov

Ontario Lung Association
573 King Street East
Toronto, Ontario M5A 4L3
Canada
Toll-Free: 888-344-LUNG (888-344-5864)
Fax: 416-864-9916
Website: http://www.on.lung.ca
E-mail: info@on.lung.ca

Partners Asthma Center
15 Francis Street,
Boston, MA 02115
Toll-Free: 800-9PARTNERS (800-972-7863)
Phone: 617-732-7419
Website: http://www.asthma.partners.org
E-mail : asthma@partners.org.

University of Chicago Asthma and COPD Center
5841 South Maryland Avenue, MC 6076
Chicago, Illinois 60637
Phone: 773-702-0880
Fax: 774-834-0242
Website: http://asthma.bsd.uchicago.edu
E-mail: asthma@medicine.bsd.uchicago.edu

Index

Index

Page numbers followed by 'n' indicate a footnote. Page numbers in *italics* indicate a table or illustration.

Health Reference Series